Computational Intelligence and Soft Computing Applications in Healthcare Management Science

Muhammet Gul
Munzur University, Turkey

Erkan Celik
Munzur University, Turkey

Suleyman Mete
Gaziantep University, Turkey

Faruk Serin
Munzur University, Turkey

A volume in the Advances in Healthcare Information Systems and Administration (AHISA) Book Series

IGI Global
DISSEMINATOR OF KNOWLEDGE

Published in the United States of America by
IGI Global
Medical Information Science Reference (an imprint of IGI Global)
701 E. Chocolate Avenue
Hershey PA, USA 17033
Tel: 717-533-8845
Fax: 717-533-8661
E-mail: cust@igi-global.com
Web site: http://www.igi-global.com

Library of Congress Cataloging-in-Publication Data

Names: Gul, Muhammet, 1985- editor. | Celik, Erkan, 1984- editor. | Mete, Suleyman, 1985- editor. | Serin, Faruk, 1987- editor.
Title: Computational intelligence and soft computing applications in healthcare management science / Muhammet Gul, Erkan Celik, Suleyman Mete, and Faruk Serin, editors.
Description: Hershey, PA : Medical Information Science Reference, [2020] | Includes bibliographical references and index. | Summary: "This book explores the use of computational intelligence and soft computing in health services"-- Provided by publisher.
Identifiers: LCCN 2019041701 (print) | LCCN 2019041702 (ebook) | ISBN 9781799825814 (hardcover) | ISBN 9781799825821 (ebook)
Subjects: MESH: Medical Informatics Computing | Medical Informatics Applications
Classification: LCC R855.3 (print) | LCC R855.3 (ebook) | NLM W 26.5 | DDC 610.285--dc23
LC record available at https://lccn.loc.gov/2019041701
LC ebook record available at https://lccn.loc.gov/2019041702

This book is published in the IGI Global book series Advances in Healthcare Information Systems and Administration (AHISA) (ISSN: 2328-1243; eISSN: 2328-126X)

British Cataloguing in Publication Data
A Cataloguing in Publication record for this book is available from the British Library.

All work contributed to this book is new, previously-unpublished material.
The views expressed in this book are those of the authors, but not necessarily of the publisher.

For electronic access to this publication, please contact: eresources@igi-global.com.

Advances in Healthcare Information Systems and Administration (AHISA) Book Series

ISSN:2328-1243
EISSN:2328-126X

Editor-in-Chief: Anastasius Moumtzoglou, Hellenic Society for Quality & Safety in Healthcare and P. & A. Kyriakou Children's Hospital, Greece

MISSION

The **Advances in Healthcare Information Systems and Administration (AHISA) Book Series** aims to provide a channel for international researchers to progress the field of study on technology and its implications on healthcare and health information systems. With the growing focus on healthcare and the importance of enhancing this industry to tend to the expanding population, the book series seeks to accelerate the awareness of technological advancements of health information systems and expand awareness and implementation.

Driven by advancing technologies and their clinical applications, the emerging field of health information systems and informatics is still searching for coherent directing frameworks to advance health care and clinical practices and research. Conducting research in these areas is both promising and challenging due to a host of factors, including rapidly evolving technologies and their application complexity. At the same time, organizational issues, including technology adoption, diffusion and acceptance as well as cost benefits and cost effectiveness of advancing health information systems and informatics applications as innovative forms of investment in healthcare are gaining attention as well. **AHISA** addresses these concepts and critical issues.

COVERAGE

- IT Applications in Physical Therapeutic Treatments
- E-Health and M-Health
- Management of Emerging Health Care Technologies
- IS in Healthcare
- Clinical Decision Support Design, Development and Implementation
- Virtual health technologies
- Role of informatics specialists
- IT Applications in Health Organizations and Practices
- Medical Informatics
- Nursing Expert Systems

IGI Global is currently accepting manuscripts for publication within this series. To submit a proposal for a volume in this series, please contact our Acquisition Editors at Acquisitions@igi-global.com or visit: http://www.igi-global.com/publish/.

Titles in this Series

For a list of additional titles in this series, please visit:
http://www.igi-global.com/book-series/advances-healthcare-information-systems-administration/37156

Evaluating Challenges and Opportunities for Healthcare Reform
Raj Selladurai (Indiana University Northwest, USA) Charlie Hobson (Indiana University Northwest, USA) Roshini Isabell Selladurai (In His Image Family Medicine Residency, Ascension St. John Medical Center, USA) and Adam Greer (Ascension St. John Medical Cener, USA)
Medical Information Science Reference • © 2020 • 286pp • H/C (ISBN: 9781799829492) • US $275.00

Managing Patients' Organizations to Improve Healthcare Emerging Research and Opportunities
Francesca Costanza (University LUMSA, Palermo, Italy)
Medical Information Science Reference • © 2020 • 173pp • H/C (ISBN: 9781799826538) • US $195.00

Handbook of Research on Optimizing Healthcare Management Techniques
Nilmini Wickramasinghe (Swinburne University of Technology, Australia & Epworth HealthCare, Australia)
Medical Information Science Reference • © 2020 • 431pp • H/C (ISBN: 9781799813712) • US $365.00

Theory and Practice of Business Intelligence in Healthcare
Jiban Khuntia (University of Colorado, Denver, USA) Xue Ning (University of Colorado, Denver, USA) and Mohan Tanniru (Oakland University, USA)
Medical Information Science Reference • © 2020 • 322pp • H/C (ISBN: 9781799823100) • US $245.00

Smart Medical Data Sensing and IoT Systems Design in Healthcare
Chinmay Chakraborty (Birla Institute of Technology, India)
Medical Information Science Reference • © 2020 • 288pp • H/C (ISBN: 9781799802617) • US $275.00

IGI Global
DISSEMINATOR OF KNOWLEDGE

701 East Chocolate Avenue, Hershey, PA 17033, USA
Tel: 717-533-8845 x100 • Fax: 717-533-8661
E-Mail: cust@igi-global.com • www.igi-global.com

Table of Contents

Detailed Table of Contents

In this study, linear regression and neural network-based hybrid models are developed for modelling the daily ED visits. Month and week of the year, day of the week, and period of the day, are used as input variables of the linear regression model. Generated forecasts and the residuals are further processed through a multilayer perceptron model to improve the performance of forecasting. To obtain forecasts for daily number of patient visits, aggregation is used where the obtained periodical forecasts are summed up. By comparing the performances of models in generating periodical and daily forecasts, this chapter not only shows that hybrid model improves the forecasting performance significantly, but also aggregation fits well in practice.

One of the major concerns of the healthcare industry throughout the world is to provide better hospital service quality. Management and delivery of hospital healthcare services are achieved in a competitive environment in Turkey. For this reason, to make better decisions, the services provided by the public and private hospitals should be monitored and evaluated according to the viewpoint of medical stakeholders. This chapter presents a cause-and-effect, decision-making model in evaluating hospital service quality criteria. Since the decision-making process involves the vagueness of human judgments, a combination of fuzzy sets and decision-making trial and evaluation laboratory (DEMATEL) is used. Results of the study demonstrate that medical equipment level of the hospital, the attitude of nurses and medical staff to patients, pharmacists' advice on medicine preservation, medical staff with professional abilities, outpatient waiting time for medical treatment, and number and quality of the bathrooms available have more impact on the entire hospital service quality. In conclusion, the proposed approach will contribute to better providing of healthcare services at a higher quality level.

Transplantation of the organs is one of the principal treatment techniques for the people who have critical organ issues. One of the main steps of this treatment is getting the organ as quickly as possible to its recipient from a potential donor. To provide the aforementioned treatment, the spatial distributions of the organ transplant centers which maximize the donors/patients coverage become essential. In this chapter, the organ transplant process of Turkey which has 99 transplant centers (hospitals) in 81 cities is considered. The main goal of this study is to maximize the donor/patient coverage within the system constraints. As a potential demand source, 923 districts are determined using geographic information system (GIS). With the application of maximal covering location model, the number of covered donors/patients is maximized considering the cold ischemia time of organs. Optimal results are obtained for different scenarios based on heart, liver, and kidney.

Diabetes mellitus (DM) is a group of metabolic disorders with one common manifestation: elevated blood sugar or hyperglycemia. The diagnosis of diabetes is the most crucial point due to chronic hyperglycemia. This chapter improves the performance of the Classification and Regression Trees (CART) algorithm because the accurate classification of diabetes depends on the algorithm efficiency. Authors use the accuracy rate for the objective function in the prediction process by Genetic Algorithm (GA). The proposed GA-CART algorithm provides the best performance at 96.05%.

Emergency departments of hospitals are busy. In recent years, patient arrivals have significantly risen at emergency departments in Turkey like other countries in the world. The main important features of emergency services are uninterrupted service, providing services in a short time, and priority to emergency patients. However, patients who do not need immediate treatment can sometimes apply to this department due to several reasons like working time and short waiting time. This situation can reduce efficiency and effectiveness at emergency departments. On the other hand, computers solve complex classification problems by using machine learning methods. The methods have a wide range of applications, such as computational biology and computer vision. Therefore, classification of emergency and non-emergency patients is vital to increase productivity of the department. This chapter tries to find the best classifier for detection of emergency patients by utilizing a data set.

Healthcare inventory management is a complex task which contains critical decision phases. One of the efficient ways of healthcare inventory management is to classify inventory items into predefined categories in terms of their significant features. This chapter proposes a guideline to healthcare decision makers to implement appropriate inventory control methods. The proposed method combines Fuzzy AHP (Analytical Hierarchy Process), TOPSIS (Technique for Order of Preference by Similarity to Ideal Solution) and ABC (Always Better Control) analysis methods to determine the priority of inventory items. The corresponding method, which takes into account multiple criteria in the classification of inventory items, cope with the limits of the classical ABC method. It also helps to reduce the uncertainty in the inventory classification problem as the proposed method is based on the fuzzy logic approach. A real-life case study is conducted in a hospital laboratory to test the proposed method.

There are several ways to summarize the data set by using measures of locations, dispersions, charts, and so on. But how can the data set be represented or shown when uncertainty exists in the environment process? Usage of the fuzzy number can be a way to handle the uncertainty in the representation of the data set. This chapter focuses on the membership function construction from the data set and introduces the formulas for the interval Type-2 generalized bell-shaped fuzzy number generation based on the data set. The bispectral index scores (BIS) are processed to see the ability of the offered methods in the construction of the interval Type -2 generalized bell-shaped membership function in the real data set. The obtained membership functions are used for a classification problem of sedation stages according to BIS data sets. Classification accuracies are calculated.

Preface

Computational Intelligence provides a broad collection of nature inspired computational methodologies and approaches, and tools and techniques used to model and solve complex real-world problems in various areas of science and technology.

At the same time, soft computing presents techniques for coping with imperfect data in a mathematical manner. These two concepts have been recently become popular in the field of health care.

Healthcare area has various components such as hospitals and their crucial sub units (such as emergency room, inpatient unit, intensive care unit, outpatient clinic, laboratories, operating room and so on), home health care, public health, telemedicine.

Healthcare stakeholders around the world are facing new challenges in responding to trends from effective usage of resources in health delivery to combating chronic and epidemic diseases. However, at the same time, there is an increasing trend on developing new methodologies and applications to improve healthcare service quality, to reduce costs and to make people more prosperous. The Computational Intelligence and Soft Computing approaches are frequently studied and improved by researchers.

The book *Computational Intelligence and Soft Computing Applications in Healthcare Management Science* will aim to bring together researchers and practitioners in computational intelligence and soft computing technology especially those related to the areas of neural networks, fuzzy logic, analytical modeling, soft computing and simulation of health services.

The target audience of this book will be composed of professionals and researchers working in the field of computational intelligence and soft computing for health services. The engineers (computer, industrial, software and others), health care scholars and information scientists are those interested in these topics.

To satisfy the target audience and to meet the challenges, we have worked over a year on this book, and we had the honor of determining the best 13 chapters, presented below:

In the first chapter, **Gul et al.** proposed a NARX neural networks model for forecasting daily patient arrivals in the emergency department. Regarding measuring of service quality at the emergency departments (ED), essential parameters are length of stay (LOS) and waiting times. Patient arrivals, which is related to LOS and waiting times, is hard to forecast and is affected by many parameters. Therefore, it is employed a Nonlinear Autoregressive Exogenous (NARX) model for forecasting of ED arrivals. NARX models are used extensively in many applications that show non-linear and dynamic behavior, but as far as we know, the NARX method has not yet been used in the forecast of ED arrivals before. In this study, calendar and climatic variables are defined as input parameters. Patience arrivals is defined as output parameter. A commercial software, MATLAB, was used to train and test the data set. To find the best network architecture Levenberg-Marquardt (LM) and Bayesian Regularization (BR) algorithms, different lags and number of neurons are tested. R-squared and mean square error (MSE) are used to evaluate the accuracy of the tested networks.

In the second chapter, **Sarıyer and Taşar** studied modeling and forecasting daily number of emergency department visits using hybrid models. In this study, linear regression and neural network based hybrid models are developed for modelling the daily ED visits. Month and week of the year, day of the week, and period of the day, are used as input variables of the linear regression model. Generated forecasts and the residuals are further processed through a multilayer perceptron model to improve the performance of forecasting. In order to obtain forecasts for daily number of patient visits, aggregation is used where the obtained periodical forecasts are summed up. By comparing the performances of models in generating periodical and daily forecasts, this paper not only shows that hybrid model improves the forecasting performance significantly, but also aggregation fits well in practice.

In the third chapter, **Yucesan et al.** developed a fuzzy decision-making model for the key performance indicators of hospital service quality evaluation. One of the major concerns of healthcare industry over the world is to provide better hospital service quality. Management and delivery of hospital healthcare services in Turkey is achieved in a competitive environment. For that reason, to make better decisions, the services provided by the public and private hospitals should be monitored and evaluated according to the viewpoint of medical stakeholders. From this point on, this study aims to present a causal and effect decision making model in evaluating hospital service quality criteria. Since the decision-making process involves vagueness of human judgments, a combination of fuzzy sets and decision-making trial and evaluation laboratory (DEMATEL) is used. Through a case study, six main hospital service quality criteria and 32 sub-criteria are evaluated by questionnaires filled by 22 health experts from medical, administrative and auxiliary services. In conclusion, results of the proposed approach will contribute in better providing healthcare services at a higher quality level.

In the fourth chapter, **Özkan and Özceylan** proposed a maximal covering location model for the organ transplant organization. Transplantation of the organs is one of the principal treatment techniques for the people who have critical organ issues. One of the main steps of this treatment is getting the organ as quickly as possible to its recipient from a potential donor. To provide the aforementioned treatment, the spatial distributions of the organ transplant centers which maximize the donors/ patients coverage become essential. In this paper, the organ transplant process of Turkey which has 99 transplant centers (hospitals) in 81 cities is considered. The main goal of this study is to maximize the donor/patient coverage within the system constraints. As a potential demand source, 923 districts are determined using geographic information system (GIS). With the application of maximal covering location model, the number of covered donors/patients is maximized considering the cold ischemia time of organs. Optimal results are obtained for different scenarios based on heart, liver and kidney.

In the fifth chapter, **Pekel and Özmen** developed a computational intelligence approach for classification of diabetes mellitus using decision trees. Diabetes mellitus (DM) is a group of metabolic disorders with one common manifestation: elevated blood sugar or hyperglycemia. The diagnosis of diabetes is the most crucial point due to chronic hyperglycemia. This research paper aims to improve the performance of the Classification and Regression Trees (CART) algorithm because the accurate classification of diabetes depends on the algorithm efficiency. The chapter uses the accuracy rate for the objective function in the prediction process by Genetic Algorithm (GA). The proposed GA-CART algorithm provides the best performance at 96.05%.

In the sixth chapter, **Çil and Caliskan** presented machine learning applications for classification emergency and non-emergency patients. Emergency departments of hospitals are the busiest places. In recent years, the numbers of the patient arrivals have significantly risen at emergency departments in Turkey like other countries in the world. The main important features of emergency services are uninterrupted service, providing services in a short time and priority to emergency patients. However, patients who do not need immediate treatment can sometimes apply to this department in terms of several reasons which are working time, short waiting time and so on. This situation can cause to reduce efficiency and effectiveness emergency departments. On the other hand, computers are utilized to solve complex classification problems by using machine learning methods. The methods have wide range of applications, computational biology, computer vision, and so on. Therefore, classification of emergency and non-emergency patient is vital to increase productivity of the department in hospital. In this chapter, it is tried to find best classifier for detection of emergency patients by utilizing a data set.

In the seventh chapter, **Kabadayı and Dağ** proposed an integrated fuzzy method for multi-criteria inventory classification in healthcare supply chain. Healthcare inventory management is a complex task, which contains critical decision phases. One of the efficient ways of healthcare inventory management is to classify inventory items into predefined categories in terms of their significant features. This chapter aims to propose a guideline to healthcare decision makers to implement appropriate inventory control methods. The proposed method combines Fuzzy Analytic Hierarchy Process (AHP), Technique for Order of Preference by Similarity to Ideal Solution (TOPSIS), and Always Better Control (ABC) analysis methods to determine the priority of inventory items. The corresponding method, which takes into account multiple criteria in the classification of inventory items, copes with the limits of the classical ABC method. Additionally, it also helps reduce the uncertainty in the inventory classification problem as the proposed method is based on the fuzzy logic approach. Moreover, a real-life case study is conducted in a hospital laboratory to test the proposed method.

In the eighth chapter, **Nasibov and Peker** studied an interval type-2 fuzzy number generation from data set applied to sedation stage classification. There are several ways to summarize the data set by using measures of locations, dispersions, charts and so on. But how can be represent or show the data set when uncertainty exist in the environment, process. In that point, the usage of the fuzzy number can be a way to handle the uncertainty in the representation of the data set. In this chapter, the membership function construction from the data set is focused on and the formulas for the interval type-2 generalized bell shaped fuzzy number generation based on the data set are introduced. The bi-spectral index scores (BIS) are processed to see the ability of the offered methods in the construction of the interval type -2 generalized bell shaped membership function in the real data set. The obtained membership functions are used for a classification problem of sedation stages according to BIS data sets and classification accuracies are calculated.

In the ninth chapter, **Gulmez** dealt with detection of chronic disease in primary care with using artificial intelligence techniques. Chronic diseases are the leading causes of death and disability worldwide. By 2020, it is expected to increase to 73% of all deaths and 60% of global burden of disease associated with chronic diseases. For all these reasons, early diagnosis and treatment of chronic diseases is very important. Machine learning is an application of artificial intelligence that provides systems the ability to automatically learn and improve from experience without being explicitly programmed. Machine learning is the development of computer programs that can access data and use it learn for themselves. The learning process starts by searching for patterns in the examples, experiences, or observations. It will make faster and better decisions in the future based on all these. The primary purpose in machine learning is to allow computers to learn automatically without human help and affect. Considering all the reasons above, the aim of this chapter is to find the most appropriate artificial intelligence technique for the early detection of chronic diseases.

In the tenth chapter, **Shirazi et al.** investigated deep learning in the healthcare industry. Artificial Neural network (ANN) is a network composing of nodes that are joint to each other through weighted connections. Using an activation, an input is provided to some (or all) of the nodes and then by the weighted connections, the activation is spread throughout the network. Deep learning, as an extension of ANN, is a neural network model, but composed of different categories of layers: input layer, hidden layers and output layers. Input data are first fed into the first (input) layer. Then, the main process of the neural network is done within the hidden layers, ranging from a single hidden layer, to multiple ones. According to the type of model, the structure of the hidden layers is different, and according to the type of input data, different models can be applied. For example, for image data, convolutional neural networks are the most appropriate. On the other hand, for text or sequential and time series data, recurrent neural networks or long short-term memory models are better choices. In this chapter, the state-of-the-art deep learning methods applied to the healthcare industry is summarized.

In the eleventh chapter, **Manikandakumar** investigated smart cataract detector via an image processing based mobile application for cataract detection. Eye is an important part of the body. It reacts towards light. A common eye disease named as cataract that affects our lens badly and can cause blindness. Cataract is the clouding of the lens which leads to the decrease in vision. It can be in single or both eyes. Most major reason for cataract is ageing. Cataract is also found to occur in children is and can also occur due to eye injuries and inflammation. As mobile technology emerges in a greater extent, designing an application would help the normal people for self-check-up without meeting the doctors in person thus saving time and cost. The pre-diagnosis of cataracts is costly for poor people. Time taken by the machine to detect cataract is more and so the doctor could not attend more number of patients. So a cheap and reliable mobile application that helps in the diagnosis of cataract would cut down the cost and simplify the process of cataract diagnosis. This chapter proposes the development of smart phone application to detect the presence of cataract using image processing techniques.

In the twelfth chapter, **Satapathya** made survey and analysis to find dental implant issue in India. At present days, dental implantation are the ideal solution and best substitute option for missing teeth. Dental implants determined the replacements of root and non-working teeth after the loss of natural teeth. strengthening dental materials helps to fix the loss teeth. The teeth which is concerned by root disease, fault in bone density, dental implantation is very essential. While bridge work and dentures decline to reclaim the suitable chewing condition and turn the problem of missing teeth. Dental implant traces the solution of missing teeth. For more progress in dental concerned technology, an extensive growth in dental implants has been noticed during the last several years. So there is a large need of excellent quality dental materials. The selection of the implant materials, their generation system, manufacturing method, age-long durability, bio compatibility with medical principle and professional dental field of study are therefore essential.

We would like to congratulate and thank the authors for publishing their original work to this book. We also present our special gratitude to the reviewers who devoted their time selflessly and helped improve the overall quality of the chapters. We hope that this book will provide new insights to the readers and stimulate further work in Computational Intelligence and Soft Computing in Healthcare area.

Muhammet Gul
Munzur University, Turkey

Erkan Celik
Munzur University, Turkey

Suleyman Mete
Gaziantep University, Turkey

Faruk Serin
Munzur University, Turkey

Chapter 1
NARX Neural Networks Model for Forecasting Daily Patient Arrivals in the Emergency Department

Melih Yucesan
https://orcid.org/0000-0001-6148-4959
Munzur University, Turkey

Suleyman Mete
https://orcid.org/0000-0001-7631-5584
Gaziantep University, Turkey

Faruk Serin
https://orcid.org/0000-0002-1458-4508
Munzur University, Turkey

Erkan Celik
https://orcid.org/0000-0003-4465-0913
Munzur University, Turkey

Muhammet Gul
https://orcid.org/0000-0002-5319-4289
Munzur University, Turkey

ABSTRACT

Regarding measuring of service quality at the emergency departments (ED), essential parameters are length of stay (LOS) and waiting times. Patient arrivals, which is related to LOS and waiting times, is hard to forecast and is affected by many parameters. Therefore, authors employed a Nonlinear Autoregressive Exogenous

DOI: 10.4018/978-1-7998-2581-4.ch001

(NARX) model for forecasting of ED arrivals. NARX models are used extensively in many applications that show non-linear and dynamic behavior, but as far as authors know, the NARX method has not yet been used in the forecast of ED arrivals before. In this study, calendar and climatic variables are defined as input parameters. Patient Arrivals is defined as output parameter. A commercial software, MATLAB, was used to train and test the data set. To find the best network architecture Levenberg-Marquardt (LM) and Bayesian Regularization (BR) algorithms, different lags, and number of neurons were tested. R-squared and mean square error (MSE) are used to evaluate the accuracy of the tested networks.

INTRODUCTION

Emergency departments are the most crucial departments within hospitals, which meet emergency patient demand by delivering urgent care in normal and crisis times (Gul and Celik, 2018). These departments are the access points of a majority of patients looking for immediate treatment without appointment (Khaldi *et al.* 2019; Yeh and Lin, 2007). One of the most crucial processes in ED operations is patient arrivals. It is a measure of how many patients are visiting a healthcare provider at a specific point in time (Berglind, 2019). This process is usually predicted based on the ED patient arrival volume over a time period such as hourly, daily, weekly, monthly and annually (Gul and Celik, 2018; Hertzum, 2017; Gul and Guneri, 2016; Aladeemy *et al.* 2016). Accurate forecasting of ED arrivals contributes to better allocation of human resources and medical equipment (Yucesan *et al.* 2019) and decreasing of overcrowding on patient flow (Yucesan *et al.* 2018; Aladeemy *et al.* 2016).

In the literature, several approaches are developed to analyze ED patient arrivals. These include regression analysis and machine learning-based approaches (Sariyer *et al.* 2019; Ordu *et al.* 2019). For a detailed reading, scholars can refer to Gul and Celik (2018) to see what the forecasting themes, methods used to forecast ED arrivals, data characteristics and type used for forecasting of ED arrivals, study objectives and performance measures and publication trends are. Some previous studies have modeled the approximation as a linear combination of independent variables using calendar data and in some cases climate data (Gul and Celik, 2018). Later studies attempted more sophisticated statistical models like the Autoregressive Integrated Moving Average (ARIMA) models and seasonal ARIMA models that model the approximation based on the historical time series within a short range (Berglind, 2019). Also, neural network models such as back-propagation neural network (BPNN) and radial basic function neural network (RBFNN) are widely used. But the available methods have a slow convergence and data overfitting problem can mislead decision makers. NARX neural networks perform well in the ANN-based algorithm pool in terms of learning ability, convergence rate, generalization performance and high accuracy (Lipu *et al.* 2018; He *et al.* 2004). Therefore, in this chapter, we have employed a NARX model to forecast ED patient arrivals. By the chapter, NARX model has been applied to such problem for the first time in the literature. As inputs for the study, calendar and climatic variables were used. Two different algorithms of LM and BR have been tested to find the best network architecture for the problem.

BACKGROUND

NARX neural networks models are recurrent dynamic networks which assume that the value of the prediction variable at time *t* is dependent on the historical values of this variable as well as on the local values of the exogenous variable. NARX models have been applied to many different areas from energy to water resource management. However, they have not yet been applied to prediction of patient arrivals at the EDs which is one of the most important problems of health care management. Forecasting of patient arrivals at the EDs have been previously studied using ANN by Gul and Guneri (2016), Menke et al. (2014) and Xu et al. (2013) and using ARIMAX method by Yucesan et al. (2018). The use of the NARX method, which incorporates the strengths of neural networks and time series, in the prediction of ED patient arrivals will bring novelty to the literature. In this section, forecasting studies by NARX models in various fields are reviewed. Table 1 shows a brief summary of the previous forecasting studies using NARX models.

Pisoni et al. (2009) present an NARX forecasting model to air pollution time series. Chang et al. (2013) estimated contaminated water quality by using NARX network. They used easily-measured water quality variables as input variables. Marcjasz et al. (2018), forecasted electricity price by using NARX. Pham et al. (2010) presents NARX model and autoregressive moving average (ARMA) model for long-term machine state forecasting. Ozcan, and Oguducu (2018) propose a link prediction in evolving heterogeneous networks using a NARX. Piazza et al. (2016) used NARX model to perform hourly solar irradiation and wind speed forecasting. Lipu et al. (2018) present NARX neural network-based estimation with particle swarm optimization (PSO) algorithm for finding the Network properties. Banihabib et al. (2018) proposed monthly Autoregressive Moving Average (MARMA) and NARX model to improve the accuracy of monthly flow forecasts. Guzman et al. (2017) simulate daily groundwater levels by using NARX. They used (LM) and (BR) training algorithms. Wunsch et al (2018), forecasted water level with NARX. Hubicka et al. (2019) proposed a novel concept in energy forecasting. Rahimi et al. (2018) performed rainfall prediction with using NARX. Sarkar et al. (2019) used NARX, ANN and NAR methods for wind speed forecasting and then they compared results.

Table 1. Summary of previous forecasting studies NARX

Author/s (Year)	Aims	Sectors	Independent Variables	Dependent Variable
Pisoni et al. (2009)	To forecast ozone concentrations	Environment	Ozone concentration delay, Temperature, Temperature delay	Ozone concentration
Chang et al. (2013)	Arsenic concentration determination	Hydrology	Power of hydrogen, Alkalinity, Cadmium ion, Chlorine ion, Total dissolved solid, Electrical conductivity, Sodium ion, Sulfate ion, Potassium ion, Dissolved oxygen, Magnesium ion, Temperature	Arsenic concentration
Marcjasz et al. (2018)	To estimate electricity price	Energy	Hourly resolution, Locational marginal price, Day-ahead predictions of zonal and system loads	Electricity price
Pham et al. (2010)	Long-term machine state forecasting based on vibration data	Manufacturing	Vibration data	Machine state
Ozcan, and Oguducu (2018)	Link prediction	Information science	Calculated similarity score, Link information, Link type	Future similarity scores
Piazza et al. (2016)	Solar irradiation and wind speed forecasting	Energy	Temperature	Solar irradiation and wind speed
Lipu et al. (2018)	State of charge prediction of a lithium-ion battery	Energy	Current, Voltage and temperature	State of charge
Banihabib et al. (2018)	To forecast reservoir inflow	Water Resources Management	Rainfall, Flow data of hydrometric stations	Reservoir inflow
Guzman et al. (2017)	To simulate daily groundwater	Water Resources Management	Precipitation	Groundwater level
Wunsch et al (2018)	To forecast ground water level	Water Resources Management	Temperature, Precipitation	Groundwater level
Hubicka et al. (2019)	Energy price forecast	Energy	Day-of-the-week, Day-ahead load	Electricity price
Rahimi et al. (2018)	Weather forecasting	Water Resources Management	Precipitable water vapor	Rainfall
Sarkar et al. (2019)	Wind speed forecast	Energy	Wind speed past value, Temperature	Wind speed

While many different versions of NARX models have been used to predict a wide variety of problems mentioned above, ED patient arrival prediction by NARX has not yet been studied. A case study to show the applicability of the NARX model is performed in a Turkish hospital. The results obtained from two different learning algorithms were compared. MAPE values of the prediction models were calculated and their validities were proved.

MATERIAL AND METHOD

Data Source and Analysis

In this study, ED patient arrivals were determined as independent variables. The selected hospital is in Marmara region of Turkey. Daily data were used between 1 January 2011 and 31 December 2012. Calendar, climate variables (maximum temperature of day) and holidays were used as dependent variables to estimate the ED patient arrival. A total of 21 independent variables are used. Binary dummy variables are used in data regarding month of the year, day of the week and holiday (weekend holiday). While "0" value means that the related date does not belong to that month or that day or weekend holiday, "1" means belonging. The dummy variables are utilized in the data set instead of the original categorical variable. The data for climatic variables is obtained from an association named as Infoclimat, France (http://www.infoclimat.fr). A detailed description for each variable is provided in Table 2.

Table 2. Descriptive statistics of variables

Variable	Unit	Type	Total Number of variables	Mean (Standard) deviation)
Month of the year	Binary dummy	Input	12	-
Day of the week	Binary dummy	Input	7	-
Holiday (weekend)	Binary dummy	Input	1	-
Maximum temperature (°C)	Numerical	Input	1	19 (9)
Number of daily ED patient arrival	Numerical	Output	1	692 (88)

Nonlinear Auto Regressive Models with Exogenous Inputs (NARX)

NARX model aims to create a nonlinear static function by using input and output functions and historical values of these functions. The problem is composed of finding the static mapping between these inputs and the current output (Pisoni et al. 2009; Lin et al. 1997).

NARX models are the nonlinear extension of the Autoregressive models with exogenous (ARX) models, which constitute a standard tool in linear black-box model identification (Ljung, 1999). These models can express nonlinear relationships and behaviors and are used extensively in various disciplines (Leontaritis and Billings, 1985). The general form of the polynomial NARX model is as follows: (Pisoni et al., 2009)

$$y(t) = a_0 + \sum_{r=1}^{l}\sum_{i_1=1}^{n}\sum_{i_2=1}^{i_1}\cdots\sum_{i_r=1}^{i_{r-1}} a_{i_1}, i_2, \cdots i_r x_{i_1} x_{i_2} \cdots x_{i_r} + \xi(t) \tag{1}$$

where

$$x = \left[y(t-1), \cdots, y(t-n_y), u(t-1), \cdots, n(t-n_u)\right]$$

is the $n = n_u + n_y$ dimensional vector of the base regressors. In other words, y(t) is obtained from a linear regression of terms past values of u and y. $n_u \; and \, n_y$ are the respective maximum lags. ξ is a noise term, generally assumed gaussian and white. The function y(t) in modeled by means of artificial neural networks.

Mean Squared Error (MSE) and R^2 are used to measure the accuracy of networks. They are defined as in Eq. (2-3)

$$\frac{1}{n}\sum_{i=1}^{n}(y_i - \tilde{y}_i) \tag{2}$$

Where n is the number of the data, y_i represent the actual values and $\tilde{y}_i$ forecasted values.

$$R^2 = 1 - \frac{SS_{residuals}}{SS_{total}} \tag{3}$$

Where SS_{total} refers to the total sum of squares (proportional to the variance of the data), and $SS_{residuals}$ indicate the sum of squares of residuals.

Levenberg – Marquardt (LM)

LM is one of the algorithms used for network prediction and training. This algorithm is similar to Gaussian Newton algorithm. The purpose of this algorithm is to find the minimum value of the function and to optimize the result. It uses an approximation of the Hessian matrix as given below (Guzman et al. 2017; Sahoo, and Jha 2013).

$$\Delta w = \left[J^T J + \mu I\right]^{-1} J^T\left(w\right)e\left(w\right) \tag{4}$$

Where w is the weights J^T represents the Hessian matrix J is the jacobian matrix μ is the learning constant I is the identity matrix and e represents the vector of errors.

Bayesian Regularization

BR training algorithm is one of the algorithms aiming to reduce the effect of large weights. Regularization reduces the possibility of overfitting by adjusting optimal performance function based on Bayesian techniques (Foresee and Hagan 1997; Yucesan et al. 2017).

In general, the training phase aims to minimize the error function between the model output and its objective. Bayesian regularization attach an extra term to this equation:

$$F = \beta E_D + \alpha E_w \tag{5}$$

where F is the objective function, E_D is the sum of squared errors, E_w is sum of square of the network weights, and α and β are objective function parameters (MacKay, 1992; Ticknor, 2013)

RESULTS AND DISCUSSION

In this study, MATLAB commercial software was used to analyze the data set. The model was tested with different delays and neurons. In ANN based modeling, randomized arrangement of the training validation and test data is strongly preferred versus ordered arrangement. Therefore, training, validation and test data were used randomly at a ratio of 70:15:15. This means that 70% of the data points were used as training the network, 15% for validation and 15% for test phases. The data was trained with Levenberg – Marquardt and Bayesian Regularization learning algorithms. The structured LM network was demonstrated in Figure 1. The 21 explanatory variables were represented by ED patient arrivals with 8 hidden neurons and 3 delay. The hidden layer consists of eight neurons with tangent sigmoid transfer functions. The output layer is one neuron with a linear transfer function, which returns *y(t)*.

Figure 1. The applied NARX network structure trained with LM

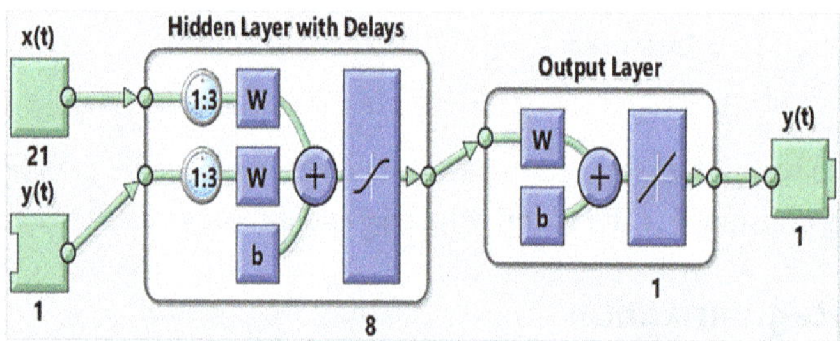

Input variables 731 x 21 and target matrix 731 x 1. It was aimed to determine the optimal network structure by changing the number of hidden neurons between 1-10 and delay number 1-3. The performance of the tested networks by applied NARX network structure trained with LM is presented in Table 3. The training, test, validation and the whole data performance of the best network were demonstrated using regression plots in Figure 2. The plot shows that they are almost close since coefficient of determination is close to 1.

Figure 3 shows the observed (actual) and forecasted values of daily ED visits for the NARX model. The plot shows that the lines representing each of actual and forecasted values by the NARX model follow a similar pattern. Also, there is an overlapping in the values of the curves. The upward and downward changes in actual values are consistent with the pattern in forecasted values.

Similarly, BR algorithm was tested under the same dataset. The network structured by BR algorithm is shown in Figure 4. The hidden layer consists of ten neurons with tangent sigmoid transfer functions. The output layer is one neuron with a linear transfer function, which returns y(t). Several models were run with various number of hidden neurons and delay. The obtained results are shown in Table 4.

The validation performance and regression plot of the best network are presented in Figure 5.

Table 3. Experiments with different number of hidden neurons and delay (with LM model)

Number of Hidden Neurons	Delay	Training	Validation	Test	All	Training (MSE)	Validation (MSE)	Testing (MSE)
1	1	0.719	0.771	0.537	0.705	0.012	0.015	0.018
1	2	0.702	0.585	0.749	0.697	0.013	0.012	0.011
1	3	0.737	0.570	0.671	0.700	0.011	0.015	0.015
2	1	0.813	0.785	0.740	0.797	0.008	0.008	0.013
2	2	0.831	0.799	0.768	0.816	0.007	0.009	0.014
2	3	0.741	0.715	0.699	0.731	0.011	0.014	0.011
3	1	0.804	0.681	0.791	0.787	0.009	0.010	0.010
3	2	0.825	0.732	0.607	0.777	0.007	0.014	0.014
3	3	0.859	0.756	0.767	0.830	0.006	0.008	0.011
4	1	0.812	0.797	0.712	0.786	0.008	0.011	0.013
4	2	0.825	0.718	0.800	0.804	0.008	0.011	0.009
4	3	0.811	0.731	0.702	0.784	0.009	0.010	0.011
5	1	0.817	0.651	0.747	0.784	0.008	0.012	0.013
5	2	0.829	0.713	0.746	0.795	0.008	0.012	0.011
5	3	0.896	0.849	0.701	0.861	0.005	0.007	0.011
6	1	0.832	0.708	0.776	0.807	0.007	0.011	0.009
6	2	0.871	0.813	0.692	0.836	0.006	0.009	0.015
6	3	0.895	0.715	0.682	0.838	0.005	0.014	0.011
7	1	0.835	0.745	0.781	0.814	0.007	0.010	0.010
7	2	0.765	0.702	0.764	0.755	0.010	0.012	0.010
7	3	0.872	0.788	0.712	0.838	0.006	0.009	0.011
8	1	0.779	0.795	0.629	0.764	0.010	0.009	0.010
8	2	0.813	0.692	0.768	0.787	0.009	0.010	0.014
8	**3**	0.892	0.809	0.792	0.861	0.005	0.008	0.010
9	1	0.826	0.779	0.831	0.818	0.007	0.011	0.009
9	2	0.852	0.692	0.778	0.817	0.007	0.012	0.010
9	3	0.854	0.806	0.705	0.823	0.006	0.009	0.013
10	1	0.868	0.717	0.738	0.822	0.006	0.013	0.019
10	2	0.884	0.805	0.639	0.835	0.005	0.010	0.014
10	3	0.902	0.705	0.707	0.844	0.005	0.012	0.017

Figure 2. Regression analysis of NARX model with LM algorithm

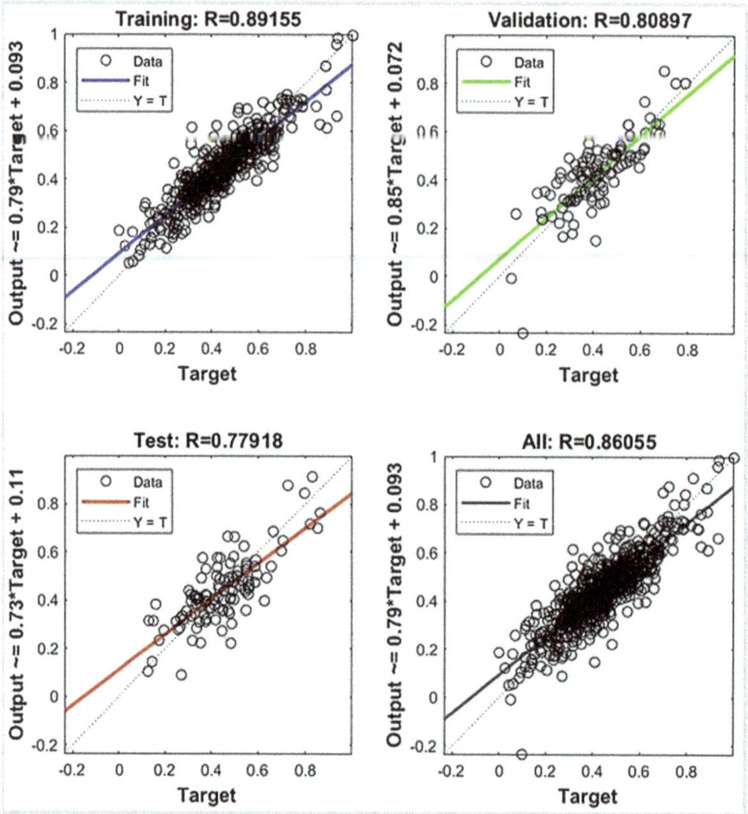

Figure 3. Comparison of actual values and forecasted output values

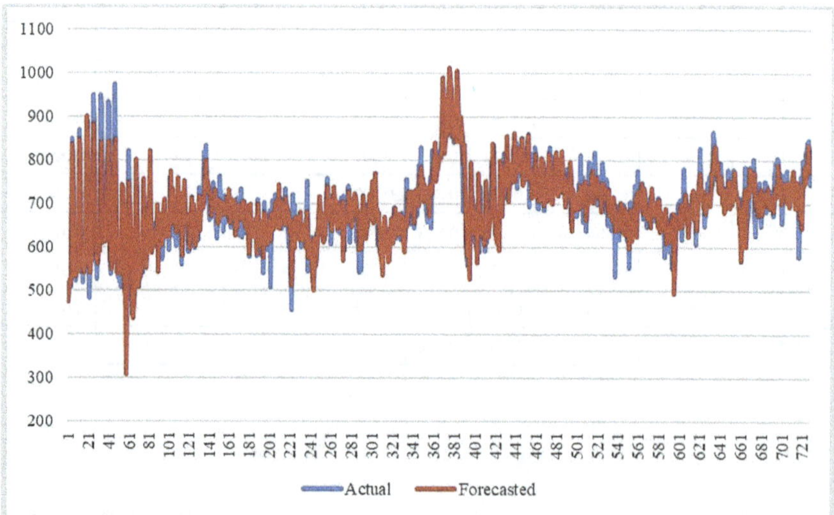

Figure 4. The applied NARX Network Structure trained with BR

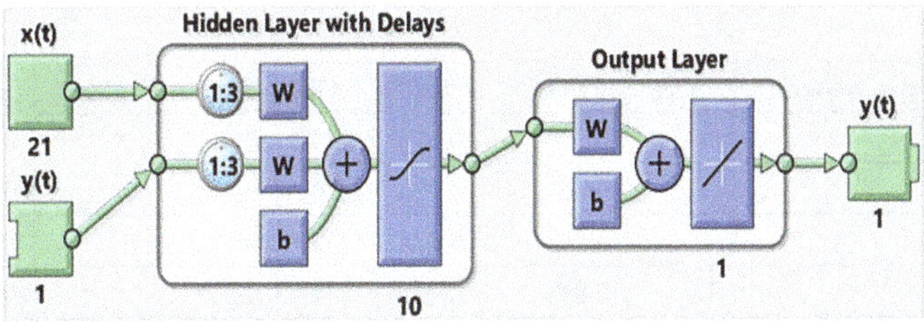

According to the regression plot, R (coefficient of determination) values of training, testing and all data are close to 1 (93%, 70% and 90%, respectively). When investigated the comparison of the actual and forecasted values of daily ED visits by NARX model structure trained with BR, it was seen a similar pattern (Figure 6). That verifies the BR model fits well to the problem.

In order to discuss the obtained results from both algorithms, we have made a full factorial design. We have considered three main factors with their levels as follows:

- **Factor A:** Type of model (Level 1: LM, Level 2: BR),
- **Factor B:** Number of hidden neurons (10 levels from 1 to 10), and
- **Factor C:** Delay (Level 1: 1, Level 2: 2, Level 3: 3)

Then, we have investigated effects of these three factors on MSE values of the test data. We have demonstrated the results with main effect plots as shown in Figure 7. These results suggest that it is possible to reduce MSE values. Especially, reducing the MSE values of test data is achieved by modification of factor A and C (Type of model and Delay). Changing type of model from LM to BR enables to reduce MSE values. Also, increasing delay from 1 to 3 decreases MSE values for the test data. Regarding factor B, it is observed that changing the number of hidden neurons causes both increases and decreases on mean MSE values. This is an expected result. The lowest MSE value is obtained under a hidden neuron number of 5. There is no exact and optimal point for this factor to be achieved.

CONCLUSION

Emergency departments are one of the most important units in hospitals, which meet essential needs in society by delivering emergency healthcare services. One of the vital processes in ED operations is patient arrivals. It means that how many patients are visiting an ED at a specific point in time. It is usually forecasted based on the

Table 4. Experiments with different number of hidden neurons and delay (with BR model)

Number of Hidden Neurons	Delay	Training	Test	All	Training (MSE)	Testing (MSE)
1	1	0.720	0.613	0.701	0.011	0.017
1	2	0.701	0.738	0.707	0.012	0.011
1	3	0.744	0.628	0.729	0.011	0.012
2	1	0.818	0.775	0.811	0.008	0.010
2	2	0.825	0.802	0.821	0.008	0.008
2	3	0.827	0.888	0.839	0.007	0.008
3	1	0.843	0.718	0.825	0.007	0.010
3	2	0.855	0.706	0.830	0.006	0.014
3	3	0.866	0.811	0.858	0.006	0.008
4	1	0.862	0.710	0.839	0.006	0.012
4	2	0.862	0.723	0.844	0.006	0.010
4	3	0.879	0.747	0.863	0.005	0.009
5	1	0.844	0.834	0.842	0.007	0.008
5	2	0.871	0.815	0.863	0.006	0.007
5	3	0.889	0.824	0.879	0.005	0.008
6	1	0.868	0.733	0.843	0.006	0.013
6	2	0.893	0.842	0.882	0.005	0.009
6	3	0.893	0.813	0.880	0.005	0.008
7	1	0.886	0.736	0.865	0.005	0.009
7	2	0.910	0.764	0.885	0.004	0.011
7	3	0.910	0.784	0.895	0.004	0.008
8	1	0.869	0.803	0.857	0.005	0.012
8	2	0.906	0.709	0.877	0.004	0.012
8	3	0.918	0.801	0.895	0.003	0.012
9	1	0.854	0.824	0.849	0.006	0.009
9	2	0.902	0.833	0.890	0.004	0.009
9	3	0.937	0.679	0.895	0.003	0.015
10	1	0.878	0.771	0.863	0.005	0.009
10	2	0.925	0.701	0.891	0.004	0.013
10	**3**	0.931	0.698	0.899	0.003	0.020

Figure 5. Regression analysis of NARX model with BR algorithm

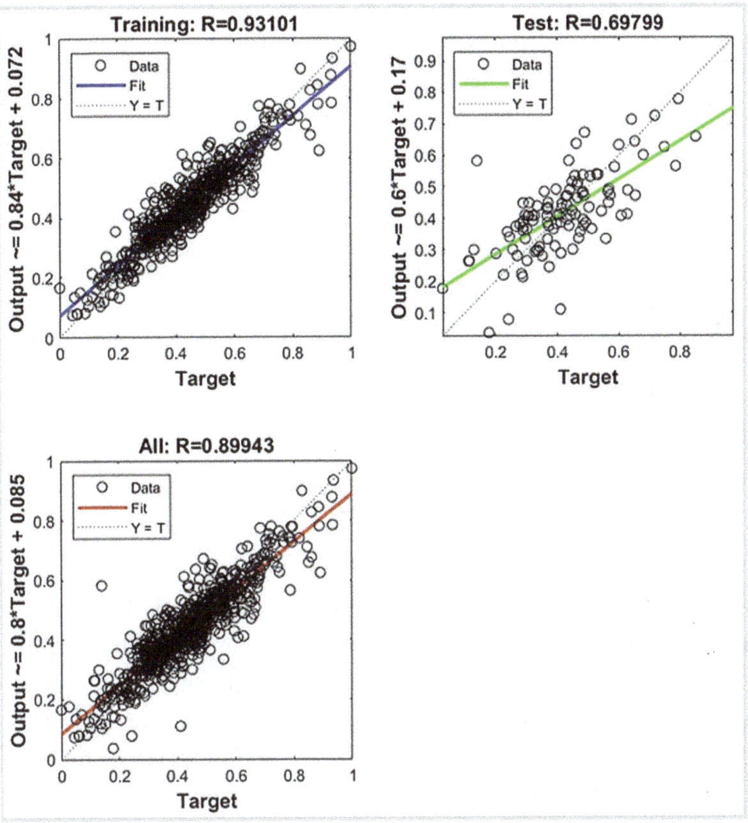

Figure 6. Comparison of actual values and forecasted output values

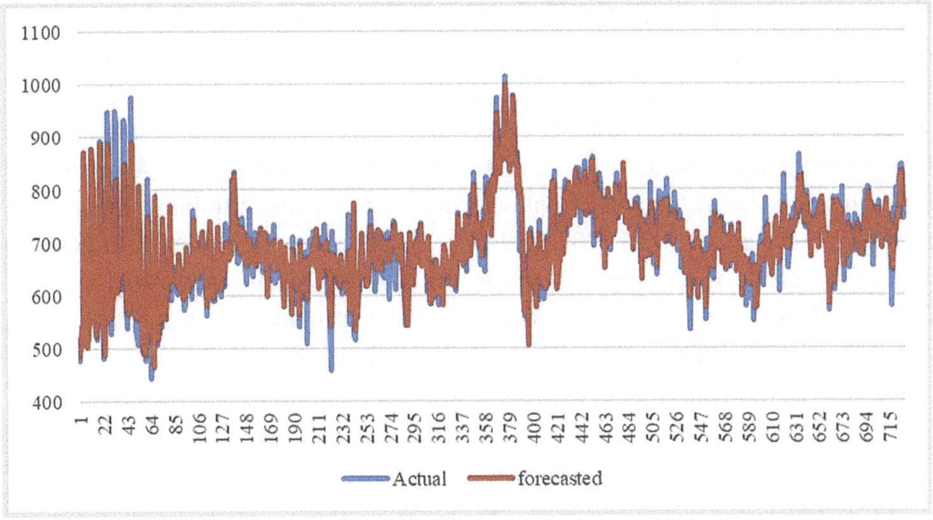

Figure 7. Main effects plot of three variables (A, B, and C) on MSE values of test data

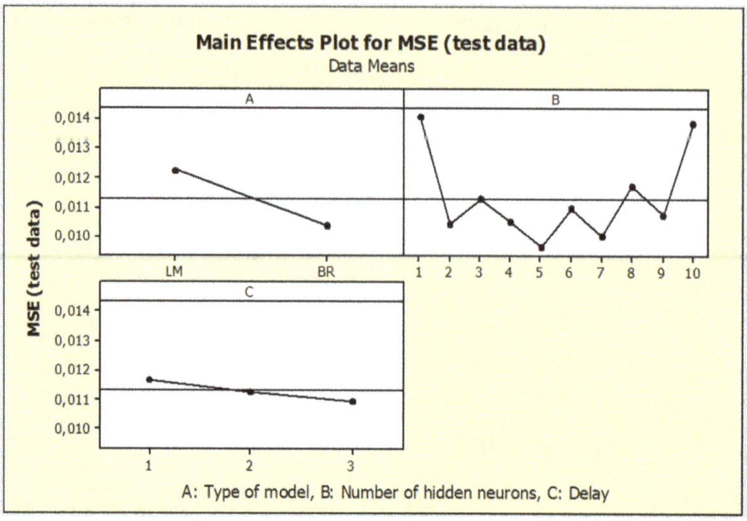

ED patient arrival volume over a time period using hourly, daily, weekly, monthly and annually demand. Predicting of ED arrivals in a higher accuracy contributes to decrease the overcrowding on patient flow and better allocation of resources (human and medical equipment). In this study, we predicted ED patient arrivals using NARX neural networks since they have a good performance in terms of learning ability, convergence rate, generalization performance and high accuracy. According to our knowledge, NARX model has been firstly applied to the demonstrated problem in the literature.

In this study, case of a selected hospital in Marmara region of Turkey is handled. Patient arrival data between 1 January 2011 and 31 December 2012 has been used. As inputs of the study, calendar and climatic variables have been used. Two different algorithms of LM and BR different delays and neurons have been tested to find the best network architecture for the problem. 70% of the data points are used for training of the network, 15% for validation and 15% for test phases. According to the regression plot, R (coefficient of determination) values of training, testing and all data are close to 1 (93%, 70% and 90%, respectively). For future studies, the authors are planning to extend the NARX model considering additional external factors such as Google trend data and air pollution to provide a more accurate result, although it is not considered in this particular case study.

REFERENCES

Abbas, F., Feng, D., Habib, S., Rahman, U., Rasool, A., & Yan, Z. (2018). Short term residential load forecasting: An Improved optimal nonlinear auto regressive (NARX) method with exponential weight decay function. *Electronics (Basel)*, *7*(12), 432. doi:10.3390/electronics7120432

Adeloye, A. J., & De Munari, A. (2006). Artificial neural network based generalized storage–yield–reliability models using the Levenberg–Marquardt algorithm. *Journal of Hydrology (Amsterdam)*, *326*(1-4), 215–230. doi:10.1016/j.jhydrol.2005.10.033

Banihabib, M. E., Ahmadian, A., & Valipour, M. (2018). Hybrid MARMA-NARX model for flow forecasting based on the large-scale climate signals, sea-surface temperatures, and rainfall. *Hydrology Research*, *49*(6), 1788–1803. doi:10.2166/nh.2018.145

Berglind, J. (2019). Temporal convolutional networks for forecasting of patient volumes in a digital healthcare setting. Degree project in computer science and engineering, Second cycle, Stockholm, Sweden.

Chang, F. J., Chen, P. A., Liu, C. W., Liao, V. H. C., & Liao, C. M. (2013). Regional estimation of groundwater arsenic concentrations through systematical dynamic-neural modeling. *Journal of Hydrology (Amsterdam)*, *499*, 265–274. doi:10.1016/j.jhydrol.2013.07.008

Di Piazza, A., Di Piazza, M. C., & Vitale, G. (2016). Solar and wind forecasting by NARX neural networks. *Renewable Energy and Environmental Sustainability*, *1*, 39. doi:10.1051/rees/2016047

Foresee, F. D., & Hagan, M. T. 1997: Gauss-Newton approximation to Bayesian learning. *Proceedings IEEE International Conference on Neural Networks, 3,* 1930-1935. 10.1109/ICNN.1997.614194

Foresee, F. D., & Hagan, M. T. (1997, June). Gauss-Newton approximation to Bayesian learning. *Proceedings of International Conference on Neural Networks (ICNN'97)* (Vol. 3, pp. 1930-1935). IEEE. 10.1109/ICNN.1997.614194

Gul, M., & Celik, E. (2018). An exhaustive review and analysis on applications of statistical forecasting in hospital emergency departments. *Health Systems (Basingstoke, England)*, 1–22. doi:10.1080/20476965.2018.1547348

Gul, M., & Guneri, A. F. (2016). Planning the future of emergency departments: Forecasting ED patient arrivals by using regression and neural network models. *International Journal of Industrial Engineering*, *23*(2), 137–154.

Guzman, S. M., Paz, J. O., & Tagert, M. L. M. (2017). The use of NARX neural networks to forecast daily groundwater levels. *Water Resources Management, 31*(5), 1591–1603. doi:10.100711269-017-1598-5

He, W., Williard, N., Chen, C., & Pecht, M. (2014). State of charge estimation for Li-ion batteries using neural network modeling and unscented Kalman filter-based error cancellation. *International Journal of Electrical Power & Energy Systems, 62*, 783–791. doi:10.1016/j.ijepes.2014.04.059

Hertzum. M. (2017). Forecasting Hourly Patient Visits in the Emergency Department to Counteract Crowding. *The Ergonomics Open Journal, 10*(1).

Hubicka, K., Marcjasz, G., & Weron, R. (2018). A note on averaging day-ahead electricity price forecasts across calibration windows. *IEEE Transactions on Sustainable Energy, 10*(1), 321–323. doi:10.1109/TSTE.2018.2869557

Infoclimat, France. Retrieved from (http://www.infoclimat.fr) [Access in 30.05.2019]

Khaldi, R., El Afia, A., & Chiheb, R. (2019). Forecasting of weekly patient visits to emergency department: Real case study. *Procedia Computer Science, 148*, 532–541. doi:10.1016/j.procs.2019.01.026

Leontaritis, I., & Billings, S. (1985a). Input–output parametric models for non-linear systems—Part I:deterministicnon-linearsystems. *International Journal of Control, 41*(2), 303–328. doi:10.1080/0020718508961129

Lin, T. N., Giles, C. L., Horne, B. G., & Kung, S. Y. (1997). A delay damage model selection algorithm for NARX neural networks. *IEEE Transactions on Signal Processing, 45*(11), 2719–2730. doi:10.1109/78.650098

Lipu, M. H., Hussain, A., Saad, M. H. M., Ayob, A., & Hannan, M. A. (2018, April). Improved recurrent NARX neural network model for state of charge estimation of lithium-ion battery using pso algorithm. *Proceedings 2018 IEEE Symposium on Computer Applications & Industrial Electronics (ISCAIE)* (pp. 354-359). IEEE. 10.1109/ISCAIE.2018.8405498

MacKay, D. J. (1992). A practical Bayesian framework for backpropagation networks. *Neural Computation, 4*(3), 448–472. doi:10.1162/neco.1992.4.3.448

Marcjasz, G., Uniejewski, B., & Weron, R. (2018). On the importance of the long-term seasonal component in day-ahead electricity price forecasting with NARX neural networks. *International Journal of Forecasting*.

Menke, N. B., Caputo, N., Fraser, R., Haber, J., Shields, C., & Menke, M. N. (2014). A retrospective analysis of the utility of an artificial neural network to predict ED volume. *The American Journal of Emergency Medicine*, *32*(6), 614–617. doi:10.1016/j.ajem.2014.03.011 PMID:24736127

Ordu, M., Demir, E., & Tofallis, C. (2019). A comprehensive modelling framework to forecast the demand for all hospital services. *The International Journal of Health Planning and Management*, *34*(2), 1257–1271. doi:10.1002/hpm.2771 PMID:30901132

Ozcan, A., & Oguducu, S. G. (2018). Link prediction in evolving heterogeneous networks using the NARX neural networks. *Knowledge and Information Systems*, *55*(2), 333–360. doi:10.100710115-017-1073-x

Pham, H. T., & Yang, B. S. (2010). A hybrid of nonlinear autoregressive model with exogenous input and autoregressive moving average model for long-term machine state forecasting. *Expert Systems with Applications*, *37*(4), 3310–3317. doi:10.1016/j.eswa.2009.10.020

Pisoni, E., Farina, M., Carnevale, C., & Piroddi, L. (2009). Forecasting peak air pollution levels using NARX models. *Engineering Applications of Artificial Intelligence*, *22*(4-5), 593–602. doi:10.1016/j.engappai.2009.04.002

Rahimi, Z., Shafri, H. Z. M., & Norman, M. (2018). A GNSS-based weather forecasting approach using Nonlinear Auto Regressive Approach with Exogenous Input (NARX). *Journal of Atmospheric and Solar-Terrestrial Physics*, *178*, 74–84. doi:10.1016/j.jastp.2018.06.011

Sahoo, S., & Jha, M. K. (2013). Groundwater-level prediction using multiple linear regression and artificial neural network techniques: A comparative assessment. *Hydrogeology Journal*, *21*(8), 1865–1887. doi:10.100710040-013-1029-5

Sariyer, G., Taşar, C. Ö., & Cepe, G. E. (2019). Use of data mining techniques to classify length of stay of emergency department patients. *Bio-Algorithms and Med-Systems*, *15*(1). doi:10.1515/bams-2018-0044

Sarkar, R., Julai, S., Hossain, S., Chong, W. T., & Rahman, M. (2019). A Comparative Study of Activation Functions of NAR and NARX Neural Network for Long-Term Wind Speed Forecasting in Malaysia. *Mathematical Problems in Engineering*.

Ticknor, J. L. (2013). A Bayesian regularized artificial neural network for stock market forecasting. *Expert Systems with Applications*, *40*(14), 5501–5506. doi:10.1016/j.eswa.2013.04.013

Wunsch, A., Liesch, T., & Broda, S. (2018). Forecasting groundwater levels using nonlinear autoregressive networks with exogenous input (NARX). *Journal of Hydrology (Amsterdam)*, *567*, 743–758. doi:10.1016/j.jhydrol.2018.01.045

Xu, M., Wong, T. C., & Chin, K. S. (2013). Modeling daily patient arrivals at Emergency Department and quantifying the relative importance of contributing variables using artificial neural network. *Decision Support Systems*, *54*(3), 1488–1498. doi:10.1016/j.dss.2012.12.019

Yeh, J. Y., & Lin, W. S. (2007). Using simulation technique and genetic algorithm to improve the quality care of a hospital emergency department. *Expert Systems with Applications*, *32*(4), 1073–1083. doi:10.1016/j.eswa.2006.02.017

Yucesan, M., Gul, M., & Celik, E. (2018). A multi-method patient arrival forecasting outline for hospital emergency departments. *International Journal of Healthcare Management*, 1–13. doi:10.1080/20479700.2018.1531608

Yucesan, M., Gul, M., & Erkan, E. (2017). Application of artificial neural networks using Bayesian training rule in sales forecasting for furniture industry. *Drvna industrija: Znanstveni časopis za pitanja drvne tehnologije, 68*(3), 219-228.

Yucesan, M., Gul, M., Mete, S., & Celik, E. (2019). A forecasting model for patient arrivals of an emergency department in healthcare management systems. In *Intelligent Systems for Healthcare Management and Delivery* (pp. 266–284). IGI Global. doi:10.4018/978-1-5225-7071-4.ch012

Chapter 2
Modeling and Forecasting the Daily Number of Emergency Department Visits Using Hybrid Models

Görkem Sarıyer
https://orcid.org/0000-0002-8290-2248
Yasar University, Turkey

Ceren Öcal Taşar
Yaşar University, Turkey

ABSTRACT

In this study, linear regression and neural network-based hybrid models are developed for modelling the daily ED visits. Month and week of the year, day of the week, and period of the day, are used as input variables of the linear regression model. Generated forecasts and the residuals are further processed through a multilayer perceptron model to improve the performance of forecasting. To obtain forecasts for daily number of patient visits, aggregation is used where the obtained periodical forecasts are summed up. By comparing the performances of models in generating periodical and daily forecasts, this chapter not only shows that hybrid model improves the forecasting performance significantly, but also aggregation fits well in practice.

DOI: 10.4018/978-1-7998-2581-4.ch002

INTRODUCTION

Health services have become one of the largest industries globally and emergency departments (EDs) constitute the main component of these services. EDs are very important for health services as they provide prompt and essential care for patients (Sariyer, Taşar and Cepe, 2019). EDs are also determined as critical bottlenecks, since they are often the entry point for patients through a hospital for an unscheduled care (Holm and Dahl, 2011). Since visits to EDs occur without an appointment, unknown or random demand of these departments creates a great concern for the hospital management. Besides, increases in expectations from health services, average ages, and population rates continuously accelerate the number of visits to EDs. This growing demand for emergency services has created circumstances such that overcrowding in EDs is becoming a threat for public health (Taşar and Sariyer, 2018; Sariyer, Ataman and Kızıloğlu, 2018). Since providing prompt care, especially for life-critical situations, is vital for EDs having an unknown demand and an overcrowded environment, improving timeliness of emergency care should be main goal of service providers. Although, increasing resources should be a possible approach to improve timeliness of care, it is generally not recommended since it is not feasible and economic (Hoot and Aronsky, 2008). Thus, with the given amount of resources, effective demand management is indispensable in EDs to generate better plans for operations and consequent improved outcomes. Many researchers and policy makers have argued that for an organization to be able to generate efficient plans, anticipating the future is vital (i.e., Milner, 1997). Thus, generating real-like forecasts for number of ED visits can be used as a main parameter for demand management and efficient planning.

In literature, variety of techniques are proposed in forecasting demand in health services over time, for an exhaustive review see Gul and Celik (2018). Time series methods are most widely used in this context. For non-seasonal and stationary data, researchers prefer to apply simple techniques such as moving average and exponential smoothing in forecasting based on their practicability and superiority (i.e. Bergs et al., 2014; Ozudogru and Gorener, 2016; Sariyer, 2018a; Taylor, 2008). When the variability of the demand data increases, such as data is no-longer stationary, researchers require to apply more complex methods such as multivariate time series modelling (Jones et al., 2009), auto regressive integrative moving average-ARIMA (Hertzum, 2017, Sariyer, 2018b), or neural network models (Gul and Guneri, 2016; Xu, Wong and Chin, 2013). More recent approach used by researchers in forecasting demand of services is to use of hybrid models (Hadavandi et al., 2012; Yucesan, Gul and Celik, 2018).

In this study, following the recent approach of literature, linear regression (LR) and neural network (ANN) based hybrid models are developed for modelling the daily ED visits. Different time-based parameters, month and week of the year, day of the week, and period of the day, are used as input variables of the linear regression model. With the linear regression model, forecasts for total number of patients arriving in each period (for the given month, week and day), are obtained. These periodical forecasts with the residuals (difference between actual patient volume and forecasted one for each period) of the linear regression model are then put through a neural network-based model by applying multilayer perceptron algorithm to improve the performance of forecasting. In order to obtain forecasts for daily number of patient visits, aggregation is used where the obtained periodical forecasts are summed up. By comparing the performances of models in generating periodical and daily forecasts, this paper not only shows that hybrid model improves the forecasting performance significantly, but also aggregation fits well in practice. Thus, while use of neural network based hybrid models and aggregation strategy can provide insights to researchers, the proposed models, which are applied in real life demand data, can also shed light to practitioners in managing demand efficiently and coping with the overcrowded environment. This chapter contributes to the literature by the following aspects: *(i)* To the best of the knowledge, no studies have combined hybrid model and aggregation approach in forecasting ED visits, *(ii)* The model includes and highlights the importance of within day variations in ED visits by defining periods as a time-based input variable, *(iii)* The model presented in this study shows LR-ANN hybridization and aggregating periodical forecasts obtained by this model to predict daily number of ED visits fits well in practice.

This study is structured as follows: Section 2 summarizes related literature for forecasting ED visits. Section 3 presents methodology of the study where details on data, LR and ANN methods are provided. Section 4 summarizes main descriptive results on data, and hybrid model results for forecasting periodical and daily number of ED visits. Section 5 represents conclusion, limitations and future research directions.

LITERATURE REVIEW

Since EDs are main component for health services, managing resources and quality of them is critical from practical viewpoint. In this context, predicting number of patient visits becomes a rapidly expanding topic due to the fact that operational plans are generally based on generated predictions. Variety of techniques are applied to predict patient volumes for ED visits. This section summarizes the current status of literature and cutting edge approaches that concentrates on solutions to forecast demand in EDs. General interpretation about literature studies is techniques applied for forecasting demand in ED processes are mostly time series, regression and data mining based models. More importantly, cutting edge studies go toward the way of hybrid models that integrate two or more techniques to generate more accurate predictions which is also the focus of this study.

Hadavandi et al. (2012) represents a hybrid artificial intelligence model to build a fuzzy rule-based system to generate forecasts of number of outpatient visits of the department of internal medicine in a hospital in Taiwan and four big hospitals in Iran. Hybrid model employs genetic algorithms to provide evolving knowledge base for the fuzzy system that is named as Genetic Fuzzy Systems (GFS). Descriptive rule induction approach is applied to discover meaningful patterns of data to produce forecasts. Their study is the first expert system that uses GFS approach to produce forecasts of outpatient visits. Clustering technique is used to create GFS so their study is named as Clustering-Based Genetic Fuzzy System (CGFS). Hybrid model is based on evolutionary computation that integrates fuzzy rules with genetic algorithms for more accurate forecasts.

Another hybrid study to predict ED visits is proposed by Xu et al. (2013) that models daily ED arrivals of non-critical patients and quantifying the related contributing features related by using regression and artificial neural network. Research questions of this study are "What are the variables directly associated with patient arrivals in the ED?", " What is the nature of association between these variables and patient arrivals?" and "Which variable is the most influential and why?". They describe the study in three main steps. Firstly, defining the directly correlated parameters by using a data-driven descriptive method and second step is designing ANN to describe association between contributing parameters and daily patient arrival to ED. By using the same attributes, another two models are generated with nonlinear least square regression (NLLSR) and multiple linear regression (MLR). MAPE is used to compare the performance of that models. In the third step, relative importance of input attributes based on ANN are tested by MLR based relative importance values. Their study emphasize the importance of data-driven selection of attributes for complex systems and predictions on patient volume on strategic decision-making process of EDs.

Gul and Guneri (2016) analyzed annual, monthly and daily ED arrivals data from a hospital in Istanbul, Turkey to generate predictions of patient volume to contribute planning of physical capacity requirements, staffing, budgeting and arranging staff schedules. Regression and neural network models are designed to be compared. Comparison results indicate that higher accuracy values in prediction are achieved by ANN model. Generally, the authors focus on the fact that generating more accurate predictions greatly contributes to short and long term planning of ED departments to better allocate the resources.

Xu et al. (2016) introduced hybrid models for forecasting patient visits in ED and compared the performances of the models to achieve best fit model with highest accuracy rate. A hybrid model that integrates autoregressive integrated moving average (ARIMA) and linear regression (LR) is designed to recognize the seasonal trend and effects of contributors. Another hybrid approach they define is to integrate ARIMA and ANN where the training data set consists of patient visit data from three different hospitals in China. Performances of all models are compared with generalized linear model (GLM), ARIMA (only) and ARIMA with explanatory attributes (ARIMAX). In conclusion, they achieve the result of hybrid model ARIMA-LR best fits with the shape and pattern of data and generates most accurate predictions.

Golmohammadi (2016) builds a prediction model for hospital admissions to support decision making and help reduction of ED boarding in a local hospital. Demographic and clinical contributing factors are focused while designing the prediction model. Logistic regression and ANN models are tested to perform comparison to draw conclusions. Based on their descriptive analysis, age, encounter reason and radiology exam type are determined as most contributing factors for hospital admission prediction. The study claims that it is proved that a model that uses both demographic and clinical factors can accurately predict patient admission that concludes in reduction of ED boarding and congestion.

Hu et al. (2017) represents a comparison study to predict return visits to ED for pediatric patients. Return visits are one of the reasons of medical resource consumption and quality bottlenecks. Supervised learning methods are applied to compare performance of the models. Naive Bayes, CART (classification and regression tree), random forest and logistic regression models are developed by using the independent predictors of return visits. Decision tree based models (random forest and CART) show better performances comparing the others.

Yucesan et al. (2018) represents a hybrid study for hospital EDs which they named as multi-method patient arrival forecasting outline. Different models that include single and multiple methods are compared in their study. Single methods are linear regression, ARIMA, ANN and exponential smoothing. Tested hybrid methods are ARIMA-ANN and ARIMA-LR. Hybrid methods are applied to draw the effects of integration in final prediction outcomes. Prediction performance is evaluated by mean absolute percentage error (MAPE). Results show that most accurate prediction outcomes are generated by ARIMA-ANN. Contribution to ED literature in strategic decision making and scheduling policy planning is addressed in their study.

Tasar and Sariyer (2018) addresses the problem of overcrowding in EDs. Recent enhancements in data mining and machine learning techniques are pointed out to provide improvement of operational planning and decision-making strategies for EDs. A study which applies data mining and neural network for forecasting patient volume in an emergency department is represented. Data is sourced from a large-scaled hospital ED that has average 800 patients in a day. Different point of the study is that train data set covers summer in 2016 whereas test data set is sourced from summer in 2017 as separate real life data. Instead of using train test split on training data set, accuracy results are evaluated by employing totally diverse data set. Random forest and ANN are compared and results show that multilayer perceptron model of ANN achieves better results.

Jilani et al. (2019) designed a tool for EDs in UK by focusing on the problems about reaching 95% National Health Service (NHS) access standards caused by unexpected changes in the number of the patients. Maximizing efficiency, minimizing risks, accessing NHS standards and optimal allocating physical and human resources are main objectives of the study. ARIMA and ANN models are built up to compare with heuristic based fuzzy time series model. Results indicate that fuzzy time series model outperform compared to ARIMA and ANN for both short- and long-term predictions.

Summarization of literature review is given in Table 1 by considering the dimensions such as applied methods, objective of the studies, data characteristics and coverage to better declare the contribution of this study and address the literature gap.

As seen in Table 1, this study combines hybrid model with aggregation approach which is one of the highlighted difference that aims to fulfill the literature gap. Additionally, impact of periodical data to predict number of patients is examined in the proposed model.

METHODS

Study Design

This is a retrospective study to model daily number of visits at a single ED. The local institutional review board approves this study and waives the requirement for informed consent.

Study Setting and Participants

The data of this research is obtained from a large-scaled urban training hospital having an average daily number of around 1,000 patients in İzmir, Turkey. Data set covers one year period from 1st January to 31st December 2017. All patients register to this ED during the study period are included in the study.

Data Sources and Variables

Data of this study are extracted from the hospital's electronic data warehouse. This database includes protocol numbers, time stamps and different demographics of

Table 1. Summarization of literature review

Author(s)-Year	Method(s)	Objective	Data Characteristics - Coverage	Performance Metric(s)
Hadavandi et al. (2012)	Fuzzy Rule Based System, Genetic Algorithms	Developing a hybrid model that named as clustering based genetic fuzzy system to predict outpatient visits in hospitals	Daily – Data from 1 June 2007 to 1 September 2010	MAPE
Xu et al. (2013)	Regression, ANN	Modeling daily ED visits to quantify the contributing parameters related	Daily - A whole year data of patient arrivals	MAPE
Gul and Guneri (2016)	Regression, ANN	Forecasting ED arrivals in short and long term to better allocate ED resources	Daily, Monthly, Yearly - 266,693 patient records from 1 January to 31 December in 2012	Standard error, R-squared
Xu et al. (2016)	ARIMA, LR	Building up a hybrid model (ARIMA+LR) to predict patient visits in ED	Daily – Data from 1 January 2012 to 31 December 2013	RMSE, MAPE
Golmohammadi (2016)	Logistic Regression, ANN	Building up a prediction model for hospital admission to support decision making and reduce ED boarding	Daily - 15,050 Data from January 2012 to August 2012	MSE, R, MAE
Hu et al. (2017)	Naive Bayes, CART, Random Forest, Logistic Regression	Determining contributing predictors for return visits to EDs in pediatric patients	Daily- 125,940 Data from 1 January 1998 to 31 December 2009	Sensitivity, Specifity, Accuracy, AUC
Yucesan et al. (2018)	ARIMA, LR, ANN	Representing a multi method/hybrid patient arrival forecasting outline (ARIMA+LR, ARIMA+ANN)	Daily - Data from 1 May 2015 to 30 April 2017	MAPE
Tasar and Sariyer (2018)	Random Forest, ANN (Multilayer Perceptron (MLP))	Building and comparing models for patient volume prediction in an ED.	Daily - Data from 1 June 2016 to 31 August 2016	MAPE, RMSE
Jilani et al. (2019)	Heuristic based fuzzy time series model, ARIMA, ANN	Short and long term prediction of number of patients to achieve standards of NHS and optimal allocation of resources in EDs	Daily, Monthly – Data from January 2011 to December 2015	MAPE
This Study	LR, ANN(MLP)	A hybrid approach (LR+ANN) for modelling and forecasting daily number of visits by considering periodical impact with aggregation	Daily, Periodically, Data from 1 January 2017 to 31 December 2017	MAE, RMSE, MAPE

registered patients. Only the protocol numbers and time stamps are considered in this study. Protocol numbers are used in data preprocessing to ensure each specific visit is used for once. Although different time stamps (registration time, departure time, time stamps for diagnostic tests etc.) are coded for patients, registration times which are stored in the system with the following form: "dd.mm.yyyy hh:mm:ss", are used in this study since periodical and daily visits to this ED is aimed to be modelled. The output variable of this study is defined as daily number of ED visits which are obtained by aggregating the periodical visits. Time based input variables are defined as month and week of the year, day of the week, period of the day.

Statistical Analysis

Proposed hybrid approach that focuses on improving daily and periodically prediction results by combining linear regression and artificial neural network is presented in Figure 1.

Figure 1. Architecture of a hybrid model

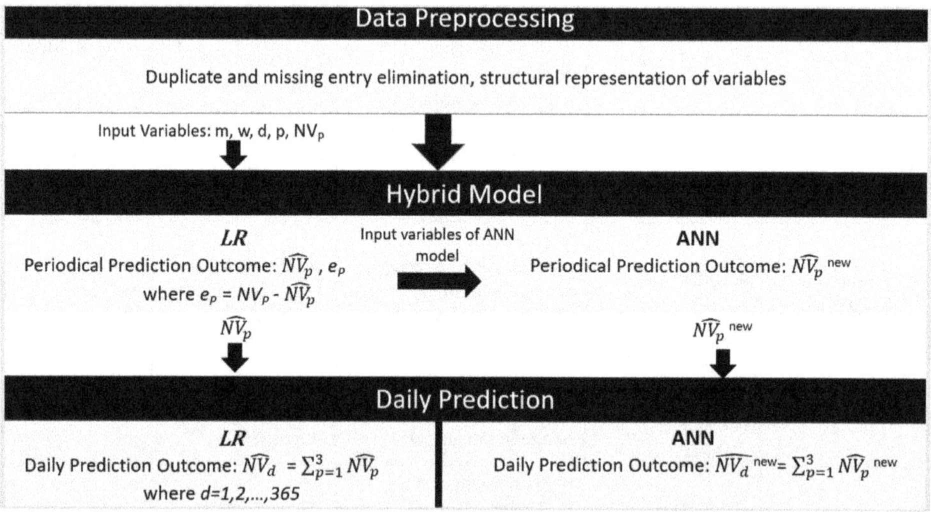

Data Preprocessing

In preprocessing step, data with missing entries and duplicate data are removed from the data set. Protocol number, which is a unique identifier of a patient for each of his/her visit (for the arrivals representing different times, different numbers are assigned), can be seen repetitively in the data set in case of patients having more than one diagnosis. Thus, in order not to count the same visit repetitively, the duplicate protocol numbers are removed from the data set. Similarly, since input variables of this study are defined based on the registration time stamp, the entries having missing values for registration time stamp is removed.

After this, structured data set is formed by defining the time stamps of the remaining data in accordance with study design. The month of arrival is considered as the first input variable of structured data set and it takes values between 1 to 12 (1: January, 2: February, 3: March, 4: April, 5: May, 6: June, 7: July, 8: August, 9: September, 10: October, 11: November, 12: December). Week of year is used as second input taking values between 1 and 53. Day of the arrival represents the third variable of the structured data set. For this variable, values 1 through 7 are assigned (1: Monday, 2: Tuesday, 3: Wednesday, 4: Thursday, 5: Friday, 6: Saturday, 7: Sunday). The last variable is related with the period of the arrival. The period is designated as series of binary variables; P1 and P2 (if both of them are entered as 0, period is identified as P3). If the registration time stamp of patient falls [00:00:00-08:00:00), then binary variable P1 takes the value of 1, if it falls between [08:00:00-16:00:00) then the binary variable P2 takes the value 1, and for the others, arriving during [16:00:00-00:00:00), both P1 and P2 take the 0 values. . The number of patients having the same values for each time based input variable, for example month=January, week=1, day=Monday, period=P1, is summed up to obtain number of patients arriving in periods for each month, week, and day of the year. A small instance of the structured data set is represented in Table 2.

Table 2. Instances from data set

Month	Week	Day	P1	P2	# of Periodical visits
1	1	7	1	0	246
1	1	7	0	1	528
1	1	7	0	0	620
⋮	⋮	⋮	⋮	⋮	⋮
12	53	4	1	0	144
12	53	4	0	1	486
12	53	4	0	0	593

Linear Regression

Linear regression (LR) is a method for statistical predictive analysis that focuses on finding the dependence for corresponding features. Dependence refers the statistical relationship between the prediction target and one or more predictor features. Simple linear regression model is used to find relation between two continuous variables whereas multiple linear regression serves to generate relation between target and more than one features. Detailed view to LR and definitions are found in the literature (Montgomery, Peck and Vining, 2012). LR model is designed based on the Equation (1):

$$E(Y|X = x_i) = \alpha_i + \beta_1 x_{i1} + \ldots + \beta_p x_{ip} + e^i \ (i = 1,\ldots,n) \tag{1}$$

Where $E(Y|X = x_i)$ is the expected value of the output, α_i is the model constant, x_{ij}'s are independent input features, β_i's are the model coefficients, e^i $(i = 1,\ldots,n)$ is the error term.

In this study, LR model is generated using structured data set to predict the number of patient visits in ED for the corresponding time based parameters for each day of the year. Results are evaluated by comparing the actual and predicted values to achieve residuals for further interpretation by artifical neural network model. Since time based input variables of this study are categorical where categories are ordered and number of categories are five and more, ordinal approximation of a continuous variable is used and independent variables are then assumed as continuous variables (Johnson and Creech, 1983; Norman, 2010; Sullivan and Artino, 2013; Zumbo and Zimmerman, 1993).

Artificial Neural Network (ANN)

Artificial neural networks are gaining popularity and attention from researchers in various disciplines. ANNs are applied for different problems such as prediction/forecasting, classification, pattern recognition, image classification/recognition and optimization. Massive parallelism, learning ability, adaptivity, fault tolerance and generalization ability are the most critical and underlined features of an ANN (Jain, Mao and Mohiuddin, 1996).

Multilayer perceptron (MLP) which is one of the artificial neural network-based algorithm is used for regression to generate hybrid model in this study. This model follows supervised learning procedure. Instead of the technique of learning with observation, learning by example is the focus of supervised learning. Learning model is builded with training data set by using backpropagation algorithm. Main principle behind MLP algorithm is providing a multilayer feed-forward neural network for learning and computation of connected weights of the network. Set of weights in the layers are iteratively learned by the model until finding the weights with the best score (Arora and Suman, 2012). 3 types of layers are the key components of MLP which are input layer, hidden layer and output layer. Input layer represents the features of train data set. For the given input features $x_1, x_2, x_3, \ldots, x_n$ and target output, MLP learn a non-linear function approximator for either classification or regression. General structure of a MLP network is illustrated in Figure 2 (Han, Kamber and Pei; 2011).

Figure 2. General structure of a MLP network
[Han, Kamber and Pei; 2011]

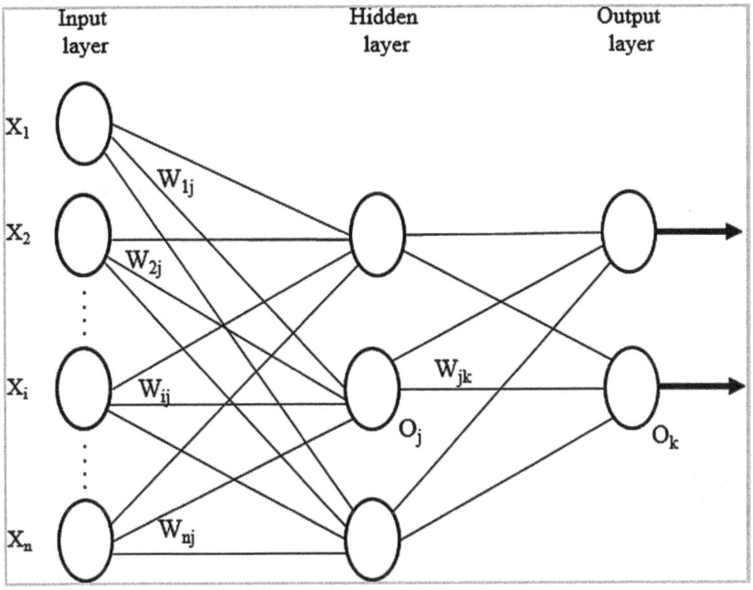

Machine learning library of Python which is named "sklearn" is employed for this study. To build up a MLP network in Python development environment, MLPRegressor class of the sklearn library that performs regression with supervised neural network is used. Parameters of MLP network is tuned for corresponding shape and nature of input data to find the best prediction results. Main parameters influencing the performance of MLPRegressor are learning rate, momentum, number of hidden layers, solver function and activation function of hidden layer. Learning rate defines the training speed of the network. Critical thing to consider for learning rate is as it increases, network trains faster with the cost of the probability of an unstable network generation. Momentum is a role player for this problem, it balances the network and is used to avoid the problem of instability caused by tuning of learning rate (Baba, 1989). As the number of hidden layers increases, more target functions and combinations of input features are tested (Minsky and Papert, 1969). Options for solver functions defined in sklearn are "lbfgs", "sgd" and "adam". "lbfgs" is an optimizer in the family of quasi-Newton method (Zhu, Byrd, Lu and Nocedal, 1997) "sgd" stands for stochastic gradient descent (Rumelhart, Hinton and Williams, 1986) "adam" refers to gradient-based optimizer solution (Kingma and Ba, 2014). Values for the activation function parameter are "identity", "logistic", "tanh" and "relu". "identity" is used to implement linear bottleneck (f(x) = x), "logistic" is the logistic sigmoid function (f(x) = 1/ (1+exp(-x))), "tanh" is the hyperbolic tan function (f(x) = tanh(x)) and "relu" refers to the rectified linear unit function (f(x) = max(0,x)).

Outcome Measure

In this study, mean absolute percentage error (MAPE) is used to evaluate the performance of the forecasting models. The mean absolute error (MAE) and root mean square error (RMSE) values are also presented for the models. For each model of this study, MAPE, MAE and RMSE values are computed as follows:

$$MAPE = \frac{1}{n}\sum_{i=1}^{n}\left|\frac{\widehat{Y_i} - Y_i}{Y_i}\right| * 100 \tag{2}$$

$$\text{MAE}=\frac{1}{n}\sum_{i=1}^{n}\widehat{Y_i} - Y_i \tag{3}$$

$$\text{RMSE}=\sqrt{\frac{1}{n}\sum_{i=1}^{n}\left(\widehat{Y_i} - Y_i\right)^2} \tag{4}$$

In equations 2 through 4, Y_i shows the observed value in period i and $\widehat{Y_i}$ is the generated forecast value of the model for the same period, *n* represents the length of forecasting period.

RESULTS

Descriptive Statistics

During the study period, 454,645 patients are arrived to this ED. After preprocessing, data of 434,734 patients left in the structured data set. Thus, around 4.57% of data are removed in this step. Main descriptive statistics of this data based on the input variables month, day and period are shown in Figures 3 through 5.

Figure 3. Box plot for periodical ED visits for each month of the year

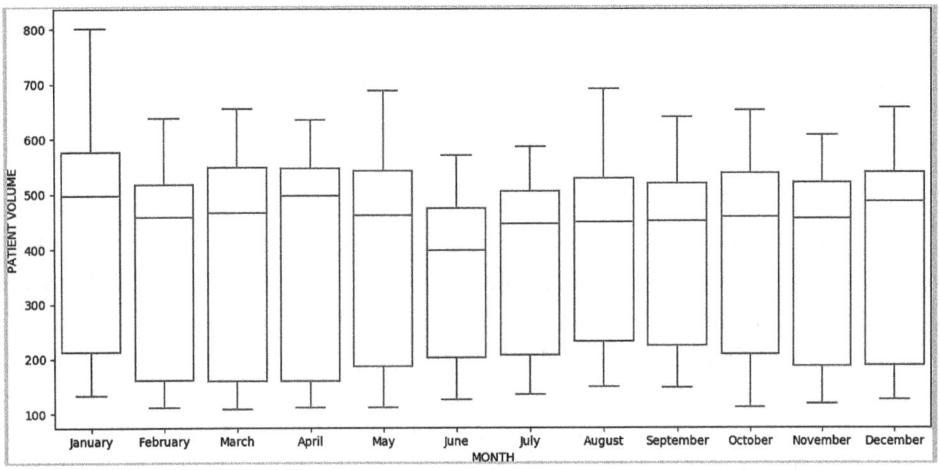

Figure 3 shows that data has similar statistics based on months of the year; distributions are observed to be left skewed, median values are close to be each other around 450, minimum and maximum values are also close to each other. Similar observation can also be made in Figure 4 for the distribution based on days. However, from this figure it is also seen that while the basic statistics for weekdays are closer to each other compared to weekends, statistics of weekends are closer. Figure 5 shows that number of visits to this ED is highest in P3, and lowest in P1. It is observed that number of visits during P2 and P3 are close to each other. For periods P1 and P3, number of visits are seen to have a symmetric distribution, whereas for P2 it is seen as right skewed.

Forecasting Results for Periodical Data

LR model outputs are shown in Table 3.

Table 3. Results of estimated LR model

Predictor	Coefficient	SE Coeff	t	p
Constant	529.145	4.942	107.07	0.000
Month	5.425	5.277	1.03	0.304
Week	-1.364	1.209	-1.13	0.259
Day	4.411	0.780	5.65	0.000
P1	-368.849	3.723	-99.07	0.000
P2	-74.573	3.723	-20.03	0.000
Model summary: S= 50.295 R-Sq=80.65% R-Sq (adj)=80.25% R-Sq(pred)=80.15%				
Analysis of Variance				
Source	**DF**	**SS**	**MS**	**F, p-value**
Regression	5	27865304	5573061	2203.14 (p=0.000)
Residual error	1089	2754729	2530	
Total	1094	30620033		

As seen in Table 3, the four time-based variables are the inputs of the LR model. Although, in general the dependent and independent variables of LR model are continuous, this model should also be applied when the dependent variable is continuous, and independent variables are ordinal (McCullagh, 1980). Since existing studies also show that ordinal approximation of a continuous variable can be used when number of categories of considered ordinal scaled input variables are five or more (Johnson and Creech, 1983; Norman, 2010; Sullivan and Artino, 2013;

Figure 4. Box plot for periodical ED visits for each day of the week

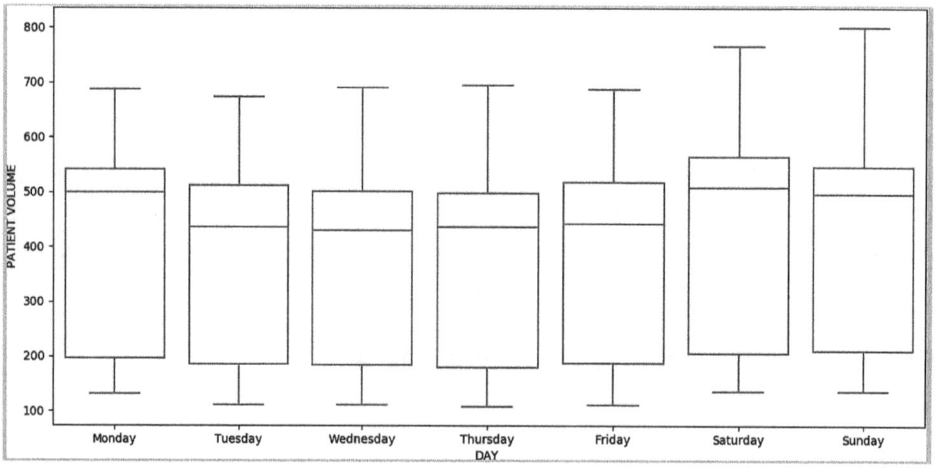

Figure 5. Box plot for periodical ED visits for each period of day

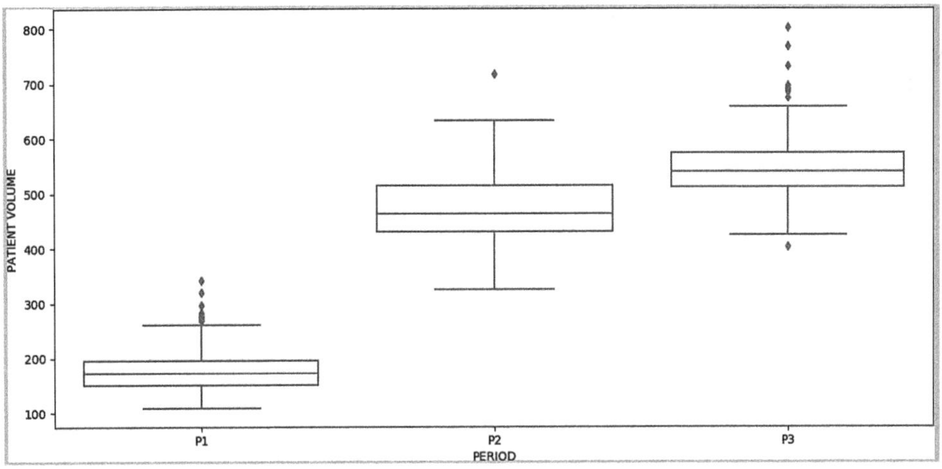

Zumbo and Zimmerman, 1993), the first three input variables (month and week of year, and day of week) are used as continuous variables in this study since number of categories of them are 12, 53, and 7 respectively. However, since the last input variable, period, has just three categories, it is defined as series of binary variables coded as 0 and 1. Negative model coefficients for periodical binary variables show an increase in number of ED visits on P3, since model does not contain a variable for P3. Additionally, model coefficients shown in this table highlights the importance of day of the week and periods of day in the regression model (related p values are <0.001). The value of coefficient of determination is 80.65%. This statistic implies that 80.65% of the variability in periodical number of ED visits can be explained by the estimated regression model and the considered time-based input variables. Remaining 19.35% of the variability can be explained by many of the other input variables; such as weather, environmental, air quality effects or others. The standard error of regression value, which is 50.30, shows to the difference between the actual number of ED visits and the forecasted ones per period. The predicted R-squared, which is 90.15%, regression model fits well in predicting future observations. The regression equation for modeling periodical number of patient visits is given as:

$$\widehat{y_p} = \begin{cases} 160.3 + 5.4 * month - 1.4 * week + 4.4 * day \; for \; p = 1 \\ 454.6 + 5.4 * month - 1.4 * week + 4.4 * day \; for \; p = 2 \\ 529.1 + 5.4 * month - 1.4 * week + 4.4 * day \; for \; p = 3 \end{cases} \quad (5)$$

The generated forecasts and residuals are further processed with ANN based MLP model for obtaining better outcomes. For MLP model, tuning of the parameters are performed with the listed values: learning rate = 0.01, momentum = 0.1, number of hidden layers = 10, solver = "adam" and activation = "relu".

The performance statistics of LR and hybrid models for the periodical data are given in Table 4.

Table 4. Performance statistics of LR and hybrid models for periodical data

Forecasting Model	MAE	RMSE	MAPE
LR	38.12	50.15	11.28%
Hybrid (LR-ANN)	1.04	1.06	0.35%

According to the MAPE statistic of LR model represented in Table 4, it can be interpreted that this model performs well in predicting number of ED visits, since it is smaller than 15% (Lewis, 1982). This result is also in line with summary results of regression model presented in Table 3. However, forecasting performance significantly increases in hybrid models, where prediction error gets close to zero, compared to LR.

Figures 6 and Figure 7 represent the actual and predicted values, for both LR and hybrid models, for each values of the time based inputs; month, day and period.

From Figure 6 and Figure 7, it is mainly concluded that actual values and hybrid model predictions are almost the same, where LR model predictions differ from them. Similar patterns are discovered in Figure 6 and 7. However, Figure 7 shows that while LR model generally overestimates for the periods P1 and P3, it underestimates for P2.

Forecasting Results for Daily Data

The daily forecasts are obtained based on the aggregation principle. Thus, the obtained periodical forecasts for each day are summed up for both of the models to form daily forecasts generated by the models. Then, the similarity between the actual daily visits and aggregated forecasts is measured. Table 5 summarizes the results.

When the results of Table 5 are compared with the results of Table 4, it is concluded that MAPE value for both models are improved when aggregation is used to predict daily number of visits in comparison with forecasting the periodical visits separately. It is also observed that improvement rate is higher for LR model; MAPE decreases from 18.12% to 6.92%.

Figure 6. Actual and predicted values for each month of the year

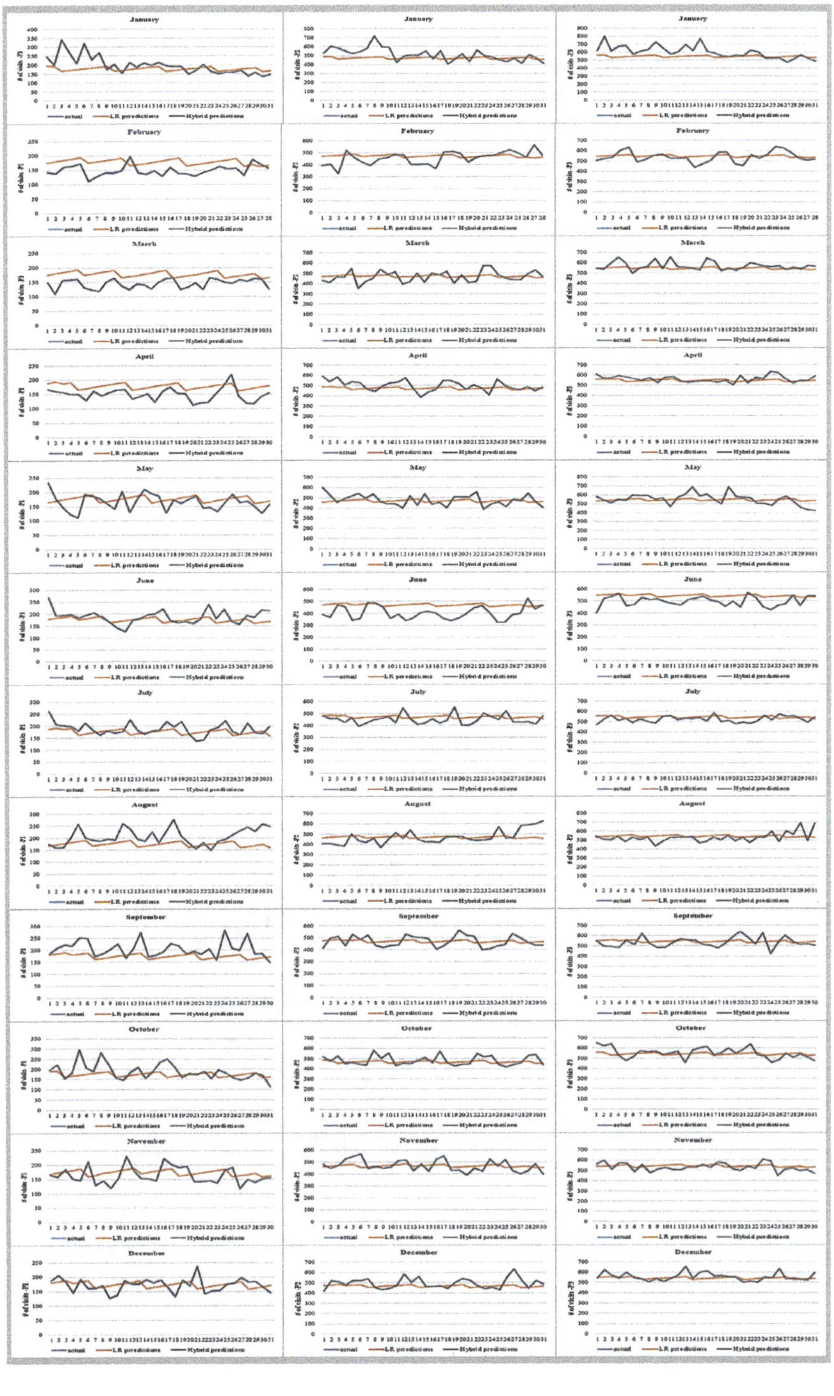

Figure 7. Actual and predicted values for each day of the week

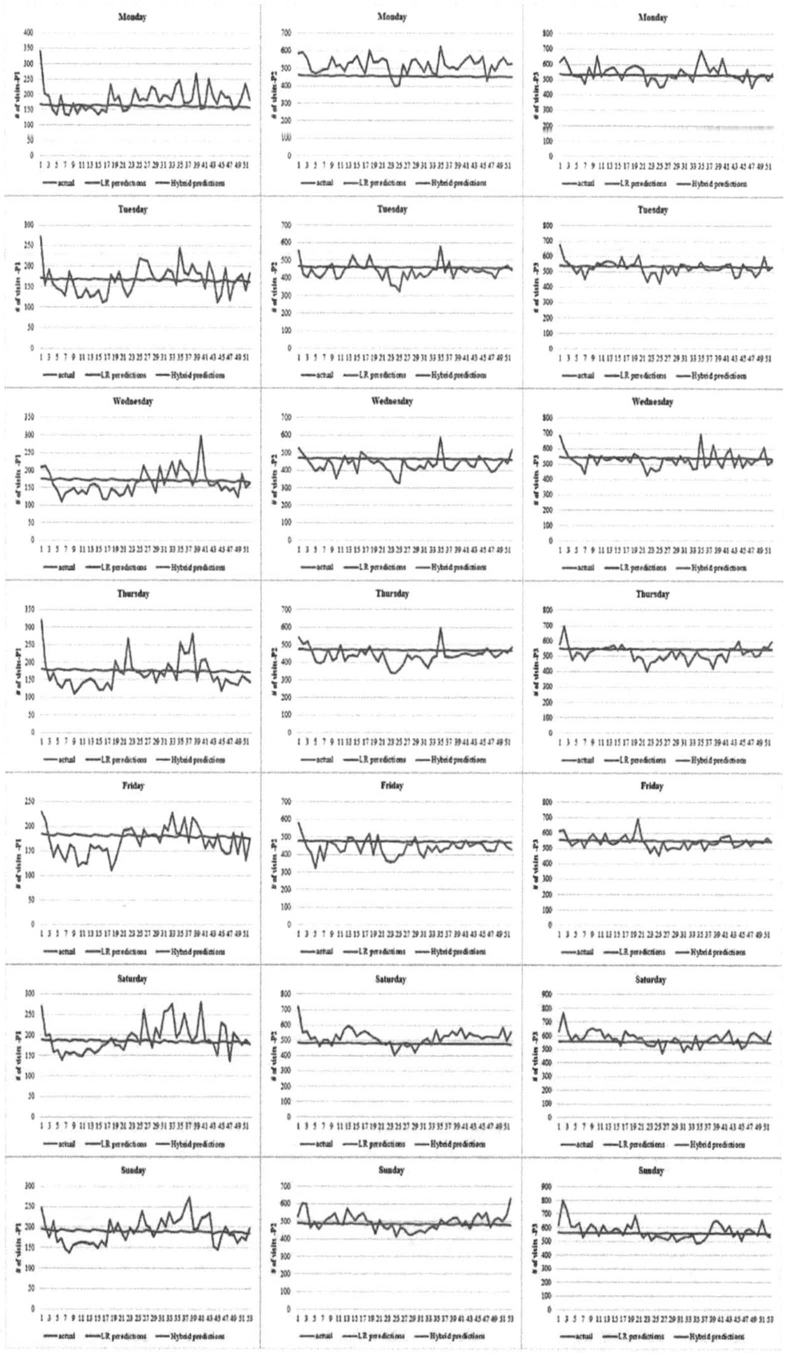

Table 5. Performance statistics of LR and hybrid models for aggregated data

Forecasting Model	MAE	RMSE	MAPE
LR	82.81	108.30	6.94%
Hybrid (LR-MP)	3.10	3.13	0.26%

Actual and predicted values of daily number of visits are also presented in Figure 8.

Figure 8. Actual and predicted values (daily)

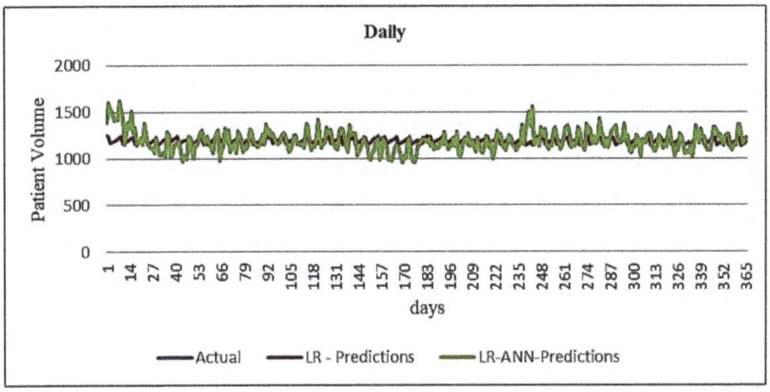

As in Figure 6 and Figure 7, it is also observed from Figure 8 that actual values of daily number of ED visits are almost the same with the aggregated periodical predictions generated by the hybrid model. It is also seen that, aggregated forecasts obtained by LR are more similar to actual values in Figure 8 when compared with Figure 6 and Figure 7.

CONCLUSION

In this study, different time-based input variables such as month and week of the year, day of the week, and period of the day are used in forecasting periodical/daily number of visits to ED of a large scaled urban hospital. Day of the week and period of the week are found as significant predictors of linear regression model having periodical number of ED visits as a dependent variable. Forecasts obtained from linear regression model and the model residuals are further processed with an ANN type MP algorithm. Obtained periodical forecasts via LR and LR-MP hybrid models are then aggregated to obtain forecasts of daily number of ED visits for the two corresponding models. When the performances of these models are evaluated, it is mainly concluded that hybrid model outperforms the LR model in forecasting both of the periodical and daily number of visits. It is also concluded that generating daily forecasts by aggregating the periodical forecasts fits well in practice. The proposed approaches, applying hybrid models and aggregation, can be applied in forecasting short term (periodical and daily) ED visits. Since a case study where the proposed models are applied and tested in a real-life data is presented in this study, it provides a basis for demand and capacity management decisions for EDs in practice (from practical viewpoint). It is believed that, the proposed model provides ED practitioners a useful tool for planning and managing operations which will result in improving the quality of ED services. The first step of future studies is planned as using different time series models such as autoregressive integrative moving average (ARIMA), seasonal ARIMA (SARIMA), and ARIMA with additional explanatory variables (ARIMAX), as a basis of hybrid model and comparing the results of existing LR-MP hybrid model with those models. When the best performing model with the highest accuracy is decided, developing a user-friendly decision support tool that can be used in this ED for managing periodical and daily number of patient visits is planned as the next future research direction.

REFERENCES

Arora, R., & Suman, S. (2012). Comparative analysis of classification algorithms on different datasets using WEKA. *International Journal of Computers and Applications*, *54*(13).

Baba, N. (1989). A new approach for finding the global minimum of error function for neural networks. *Neural Networks*, *2*(5), 367–373. doi:10.1016/0893-6080(89)90021-X

Bergs, J., Heerinckx, P., & Verelst, S. (2014). Knowing what to expect, forecasting monthly emergency department visits: A time-series analysis. *International Emergency Nursing*, *22*(2), 112–115. doi:10.1016/j.ienj.2013.08.001 PMID:24055373

Golmohammadi, D. (2016). Predicting hospital admissions to reduce emergency department boarding. *International Journal of Production Economics*, *182*, 535–544. doi:10.1016/j.ijpe.2016.09.020

Gul, M., & Celik, E. (2018). An exhaustive review and analysis on applications of statistical forecasting in hospital emergency departments. *Health Systems (Basingstoke, England)*, 1–22. doi:10.1080/20476965.2018.1547348

Gul, M., & Guneri, A. F. (2016). Planning the future of emergency departments: Forecasting ED patient arrivals by using regression and neural network models. *International Journal of Industrial Engineering*, *23*(2).

Hadavandi, E., Shavandi, H., Ghanbari, A., & Abbasian-Naghneh, S. (2012). Developing a hybrid artificial intelligence model for outpatient visits forecasting in hospitals. *Applied Soft Computing*, *12*(2), 700–711. doi:10.1016/j.asoc.2011.09.018

Han, J., Kamber, M., & Pei, J. (2011). *Data mining: concepts and techniques. The Morgan Kaufmann series of data management systems* (pp. 230–240). Elsevier.

Hertzum, M. (2017). Forecasting Hourly Patient Visits in the Emergency Department to Counteract Crowding. *The Ergonomics Open Journal, 10*(1).

Holm, L. B., & Dahl, F. A. (2011). Using soft systems methodology as a precursor for an emergency department simulation model. *OR insight, 24*(3), 168-189.

Hoot, N. R., & Aronsky, D. (2008). Systematic review of emergency department crowding: Causes, effects, and solutions. *Annals of Emergency Medicine*, *52*(2), 126–136. doi:10.1016/j.annemergmed.2008.03.014 PMID:18433933

Hu, Y. H., Tai, C. T., Chen, S. C. C., Lee, H. W., & Sung, S. F. (2017). Predicting return visits to the emergency department for pediatric patients: Applying supervised learning techniques to the Taiwan National Health Insurance Research Database. *Computer Methods and Programs in Biomedicine*, *144*, 105–112. doi:10.1016/j.cmpb.2017.03.022 PMID:28494994

Jain, A. K., Mao, J., & Mohiuddin, K. M. (1996). Artificial neural networks: A tutorial. *Computer*, *29*(3), 31–44. doi:10.1109/2.485891

Jilani, T., Housley, G., Figueredo, G., Tang, P. S., Hatton, J., & Shaw, D. (2019). Short- and Long-Term Predictions of Hospital Emergency Department Attendances. *International Journal of Medical Informatics*, *129*, 167–174. doi:10.1016/j.ijmedinf.2019.05.011 PMID:31445251

Johnson, D. R., & Creech, J. C. (1983). Ordinal measures in multiple indicator models: A simulation study of categorization error. *American Sociological Review*, *48*(3), 398–407. doi:10.2307/2095231

Jones, S. S., Evans, R. S., Allen, T. L., Thomas, A., Haug, P. J., Welch, S. J., & Snow, G. L. (2009). A multivariate time series approach to modeling and forecasting demand in the emergency department. *Journal of Biomedical Informatics*, *42*(1), 123–139. doi:10.1016/j.jbi.2008.05.003 PMID:18571990

Kingma, D. P., & Ba, J. (2014). Adam: A method for stochastic optimization. *Proceedings International Conference on Learning Representations* (pp. 1-15). Academic Press.

Lewis, C. D. (1982). *Industrial and business forecasting methods: A practical guide to exponential smoothing and curve fitting*. Butterworth-Heinemann.

McCullagh, P. (1980). Regression models for ordinal data. *Journal of the Royal Statistical Society. Series B. Methodological*, *42*(2), 109–127. doi:10.1111/j.2517-6161.1980.tb01109.x

Milner, P. C. (1997). Ten-year follow-up of ARIMA forecasts of attendances at accident and emergency departments in the Trent region. *Statistics in Medicine*, *16*(18), 2117–2125. doi:10.1002/(SICI)1097-0258(19970930)16:18<2117::AID-SIM649>3.0.CO;2-E PMID:9308136

Minsky, M. L., & Papert, S. (1969). *Perceptrons: an introduction to computational geometry*. USA: MIT Press.

Montgomery, D. C., Peck, E. A., & Vining, G. G. (2012). *Introduction to linear regression analysis* (Vol. 821). John Wiley & Sons.

Norman, G. (2010). Likert scales, levels of measurement and the "laws" of statistics. *Advances in Health Sciences Education: Theory and Practice*, *15*(5), 625–632. doi:10.100710459-010-9222-y PMID:20146096

Ozudogru, A. G., & Gorener, A. (2016). Method Selection for Demand Forecasting: Application in a Private Hospital. *International Journal of Decision Sciences & Applications-IJDSA*, *1*(1), 22–34.

Rumelhart, D. E., Hinton, G. E., & Williams, R. J. (1986): Learning internal representations by error propagation. In Parallel distributed processing: Explorations in the microstructure of cognition, 1, 318-362, Bradford Books.

Sariyer, G. (2018b). Acil Servislerde Talebin Zaman Serileri Modelleri ile Tahmin Edilmesi. *Uluslararası Mühendislik Araştırma ve Geliştirme Dergisi*, *10*(1), 66–77.

Sariyer, G. (2018a). Sizing capacity levels in emergency medical services dispatch centers: Using the newsvendor approach. *The American Journal of Emergency Medicine*, *36*(5), 804–815. doi:10.1016/j.ajem.2017.10.027 PMID:29055616

Sarıyer, G., Ataman, M. G., & Kızıloğlu, İ. (2018). Factors affecting length of stay in the emergency department: A research from an operational viewpoint. *International Journal of Healthcare Management*, ▪▪▪, 1–10.

Sariyer, G., Taşar, C. Ö., & Cepe, G. E. (n.d.). Use of data mining techniques to classify length of stay of emergency department patients. *Bio-Algorithms and Med-Systems*. doi:10.1515/bams-2018.0044

Sullivan, G., & Artino, A. R. Jr. (2013). Analyzing and Interpreting Data From Likert-Type Scales. *Journal of Graduate Medical Education*, *5*(4), 541–542. doi:10.4300/JGME-5-4-18 PMID:24454995

Taşar, C. Ö., & Sariyer, G. (April, 2018). The use of data mining and neural networks for forecasting patient volume in an emergency department (abstract). 4th International Researchers, Statisticians, and Young Statisticians Congress. Izmir, Turkey

Taylor, J. W. (2008). A comparison of univariate time series methods for forecasting intraday arrivals at a call center. *Management Science*, *54*(2), 253–265. doi:10.1287/mnsc.1070.0786

Xu, M., Wong, T. C., & Chin, K. S. (2013). Modeling daily patient arrivals at Emergency Department and quantifying the relative importance of contributing variables using artificial neural network. *Decision Support Systems*, *54*(3), 1488–1498. doi:10.1016/j.dss.2012.12.019

Xu, Q., Tsui, K. L., Jiang, W., & Guo, H. (2016). A hybrid approach for forecasting patient visits in emergency department. *Quality and Reliability Engineering International*, *32*(8), 2751–2759. doi:10.1002/qre.2095

Yucesan, M., Gul, M., & Celik, E. (2018). A multi-method patient arrival forecasting outline for hospital emergency departments. *International Journal of Healthcare Management*, 1–13. doi:10.1080/20479700.2018.1531608

Zhu, C., Byrd, R. H., Lu, P., & Nocedal, J. (1997). Algorithm 778: L-BFGS-B: Fortran subroutines for large-scale bound-constrained optimization. *ACM Transactions on Mathematical Software*, *23*(4), 550–560. doi:10.1145/279232.279236

Zumbo, B. D., & Zimmerman, D. W. (1993). Is the selection of statistical methods governed by level of measurement? *Canadian Psychology*, *34*(4), 390–400. doi:10.1037/h0078865

Chapter 3
A Fuzzy Decision-Making Model for the Key Performance Indicators of Hospital Service Quality Evaluation

Melih Yucesan
https://orcid.org/0000-0001-6148-4959
Munzur University, Turkey

Suleyman Mete
https://orcid.org/0000-0001-7631-5584
Gaziantep University, Turkey

Muhammet Gul
https://orcid.org/0000-0002-5319-4289
Munzur University, Turkey

Erkan Celik
https://orcid.org/0000-0003-4465-0913
Munzur University, Turkey

ABSTRACT

One of the major concerns of the healthcare industry throughout the world is to provide better hospital service quality. Management and delivery of hospital healthcare services are achieved in a competitive environment in Turkey. For this reason, to make better decisions, the services provided by the public and private hospitals should be monitored and evaluated according to the viewpoint of medical stakeholders. This chapter presents a cause-and-effect, decision-making model in evaluating hospital service quality criteria. Since the decision-making process

DOI: 10.4018/978-1-7998-2581-4.ch003

involves the vagueness of human judgments, a combination of fuzzy sets and decision-making trial and evaluation laboratory (DEMATEL) is used. Results of the study demonstrate that medical equipment level of the hospital, the attitude of nurses and medical staff to patients, pharmacists' advice on medicine preservation, medical staff with professional abilities, outpatient waiting time for medical treatment, and number and quality of the bathrooms available have more impact on the entire hospital service quality. In conclusion, the proposed approach will contribute to better providing of healthcare services at a higher quality level.

INTRODUCTION

One of the major concerns of the healthcare industry all over the world is to provide better hospital service quality (Yucesan and Gul, 2020 Chang, 2014; Akdag et al. 2014; Taşkin et al. 2015). Management and delivery of hospital services are achieved in a competitive environment in Turkey. For this reason, to make better decisions, the services provided by the public and private hospitals should be assessed in terms of key performance indicators. According to the recent official figures, a number of healthcare facilities and infrastructures has been improved by the end of 2017. In the year 2017, the number of hospitals under the auspices of the ministry of health has increased compared to the previous year. Similarly, the number qualified beds have an increase of 14% by the year 2017 compared to 2016. Moreover, statistics for the indicators such as total number of intensive care unit beds, number of neonatal intensive care unit beds, number of hemodialysis centers, number of MRI, CT and Ultrasound devices in inpatient health care facilities, number of primary health care facilities, number of family health center medical examination rooms and number of ambulances have been improved at the year 2017 compared to the previous years. On the other hand, the utilization of healthcare services in Turkey has been made better (Republic of Turkey Ministry of Health, 2018). Despite the continuous increase in the number of patients admitted and the number of hospitals in Turkey, it does not have enough attempts about service quality evaluation according to hospital types. On the other hand, many people continue to receive health services from public hospitals, although private hospitals are increasingly located in the Turkish health care system. Therefore, a causal and effect decision-making model is needed in order to evaluate both public and private hospital service quality key performance indicators.

In this study, therefore, a multi-criteria decision-making (MCDM) model in evaluating hospital service quality criteria is presented. MCDM is an important field of management science, which clearly reflects multiple criteria in decision-making environments. It includes several kinds of methodologies for decision-makers and practitioners. MCDM based methods heavily include human participation and judgments (Kubler et al. 2016). It deals with evaluating, prioritizing or selecting alternatives under conflicting criteria with respect to decision-maker(s) preferences (Gul et al. 2016). The main mechanisms of an MCDM method are itemized as alternatives, criteria against evaluated alternatives, scores of alternatives on the criteria, and criteria weights reflecting the relative importance of each criterion as compared with others (Gul et al. 2016). DEMATEL is one of the MCDM methods applied to various fields, from manufacturing to the service sector. In healthcare service quality evaluation literature, researchers apply DEMATEL mostly to determine the importance weights of service quality criteria (Behdioğlu et al. 2019; Roy et al. 2018; Gul et al. 2014; Shieh et al. 2010). Since the decision-making process involves the vagueness of human judgments, a combination of fuzzy sets theory and the DEMATEL method is used in this study.

Fuzzy set theory is used to take vagueness and uncertainty of subjective evaluations into consideration. The integrated fuzzy DEMATEL provides more autonomy to decision-makers in articulating their ideas about the vagueness and uncertainty of the considered MCDM problem. Considering the interdependence among criteria, proposed fuzzy DEMATEL reflects the causal relationships among criteria through a cause-effect relationship diagram. Through a case study, six main hospital service quality criteria and 32 sub-criteria are evaluated by two questionnaires (one for main criteria and the latter is for sub-criteria) filled by 22 health experts. The expert group includes employers from medical, administrative, and auxiliary services such as governmental medical department, hospital administration, quality deployment department, medical staff from emergency department, intensive care unit, audiometry, and other inpatient units (doctor, nurse, technician, etc.) and ward service provider. They are also well-experienced in the healthcare delivery and workflow of the hospitals. By the obtained results, an effective tool for evaluating hospital service quality will be gained.

The rest of the chapter is structured as follows: A literature review on the general view of healthcare service quality and MCDM based hospital service quality evaluation is given in Section 2. Preliminaries on fuzzy sets, DEMATEL, and proposed approach using fuzzy DEMATEL are examined in Section 3. The Application of the integrated approach with a case study is given Section 4. Results and discussions are presented in Section 5. Conclusions are emphasized in the last section.

LITERATURE REVIEW

In this section, we briefly review the literature from two aspects. For one thing, we analyze the researches on SERVQUAL-based healthcare service quality evaluation.

For another, we review the literature related to the methods that applied a single or hybrid MCDM-based healthcare service quality evaluation.

SERVQUAL is a commonly used tool to measure service quality in the literature and refers to the abbreviated form of *service quality* (Parasuraman et al. 1988). This method is a survey analysis based on the evaluation of perceived and expected service quality by the customer's point of view. With the results of the evaluation, the gap between service expectations (e.g, required quality as important-unimportant) and the performance level of the service (e.g. good-poor perceived quality) determines the quality of the service. In other words, evaluation of service quality in SERVQUAL analysis is based on calculating the difference between the scores in which the customers respond to the pairs of expressions "expectation-perception" (Demir et al. 2018). SERVQUAL is applied to many service industries such as healthcare, transportation, education, finance, and safety (Altuntas et al. 2012; Kayapınar and Erginel, 2018; Lupo, 2013; Ali and Raza, 2017; Demir et al. 2018). Regarding healthcare service quality, SERVQUAL is mentioned by many researchers. Singh and Praser (2019) present an integration of fuzzy set theory and SERVQUAL methodology to measure the service quality of four hospitals from the Punjab state of India. Behdioğlu et al. (2019) proposed a fuzzy SERVQUAL approach for evaluating service quality in a physiotherapy and rehabilitation hospital. Pekkaya et al. (2019) aim to measure/evaluate ongoing healthcare service quality and patient satisfaction via the SERVQUAL scale with respect to the outpatients' view. Al-Neyadi et al. (2018) evaluate the quality of healthcare services by investigating the factors affecting patient satisfaction in private and public hospitals in the UAE based on five service quality dimensions of the SERVQUAL, namely; tangibles, reliability, responsiveness, assurance, and empathy. Ali et al. (2018) applied a SERVQUAL framework for quality measurement of Indian commercial hospitals. Raziei et al. (2018) propose a hybrid approach incorporating group decision-making, SERVQUAL, and Quality function deployment (QFD) to improve service quality in hospitals. Lupo (2016) analyzed the public healthcare sector of the Sicily region by a SERVQUAL based framework. Handayani et al. (2015) used a different dimension to classical SERVQUAL called professionalism. Demirer and Bülbül (2014) comparatively explored the suitability of SERVQUAL and the relationship between perceived service quality, patient satisfaction, and patient preference for the public and private hospitals in Turkey. Altuntas et al. (2012) measured hospital service quality by using the analytic hierarchy process (AHP) and analytic network process (ANP) to acquire the relationship and the level of the importance among the SERVQUAL dimension. Afkham et al. (2012) proposed a fuzzy-based method using fuzzy AHP and technique for order preference by similarity to an ideal solution (TOPSIS). SERVQUAL model was used to evaluate the respondents' judgments of service quality. Chakravarty (2011) evaluated the service quality of hospital outpatient departments using SERVQUAL. Similarly, Teng et al. (2007) focused on surgical hospitalization using SERVQUAL. Lee et al. (2000) proposed three different methods for measuring health-care service quality as the constant-sum rating method, the single-item global rating method, and multi-item rating method. Shieh et al. (2010) and Gul et al. (2014) combined SERVQUAL and DEMATEL methods in identifying key success factors of hospital service quality.

Apart from SERVQUAL-based studies, the limited number of studies stand in the literature in conjunction with MCDM, fuzzy sets, and healthcare (in particular "hospital") service quality evaluation. Yucesan and Gul (2020) proposed an integrated model based on Pythagorean fuzzy AHP and fuzzy TOPSIS in hospital service quality evaluation. Liu et al. (2019) proposed a Grey relational analysis (GRA)-based method for evaluating medical service quality. Tuzkaya et al. (2019) applied interval-valued intuitionistic fuzzy PROMETHEE (IVIF-PROMETHEE) for service quality evaluation based on patients' views in a real-life case study of a public hospital in Istanbul, and the results were compared with the results from IVIF-TOPSIS method. Aktas et al. (2015) developed a service quality index in order to present a basis for the classification of hospitals by using MCDM tools with respect to the criteria in the literature. Lin et al. (2013) integrated hierarchical balanced scorecard with fuzzy linguistic for evaluating operating room performance in hospitals. Taskın et al. (2015) and Chang (2014) benefited from VIKOR method in hospital service quality evaluation. Both studies applied the fuzzy MCDM approach to determine the importance weights of evaluation criteria and the VIKOR method to prioritize feasible alternatives. For each of them, an empirical case involving 33 evaluation criteria, 2 public and 3 private medical centers in Turkey and Taiwan assessed by 18 evaluators from various fields of medical industry was presented. Akdag et al. (2014) applied the TOPSIS method separated from Taskın et al. (2015) and Chang (2014) to evaluate the service quality of some Turkish hospitals. In this study, the importance weights of criteria were found with AHP. Then, TOPSIS and Yager's min-max approach was applied to rank hospitals. As a follow-up study, an aggregation of performance criteria with Ordered Weighted Averaging (OWA) and Compensatory AND operators are looked at instead of the TOPSIS method and min-max approach, and the obtained results were compared.

This study focuses on the ranking of 6 main criteria and 32 sub-criteria of the hospital service quality using the fuzzy DEMATEL method based on the service quality perceptions of medical, administrative, and auxiliary services staff. In selecting these criteria, the related literature on the service quality criteria, which is summarized in the case study section, is taken into account.

METHODOLOGY

Fuzzy Sets and its Extensions

Fuzzy logic, introduced in 1965 by Lotfi A. Zadeh, is a robust tool to deal with the vagueness, ambiguity, and uncertainty of human judgments, and assessment in making decisions process. In real-world decision-making problems, many decisions involve imprecision since goals, constraints, and possible actions are not known precisely (Zadeh, 1965). Instead of combining various experiences, opinions, ideas, and motivations of an individual or group decision-maker, it is better to convert the linguistic terms into fuzzy numbers (Akyuz and Celik, 2015; Celik and Akyuz, 2016). Therefore, the problems of group decision-making have necessarily produced fuzzy numbers in practice. A triangular fuzzy number can be defined as a triplet $\tilde{A} = \left(l, m, u\right)$ where *l, m,* and *u* denotes lower, medium and upper numbers of the fuzzy which is crisp and real numbers ($x \leq y \leq z$). The membership function of a triangular fuzzy number can be defined as follows.

$$\mu_{\tilde{A}} = \begin{cases} 0, & x < l \\ \left(x - l\right) / \left(m - l\right), & l \leq x \leq m \\ \left(u - x\right) / \left(u - m\right), & m \leq x \leq u \\ 0, & x \geq u \end{cases} \tag{1}$$

Figure 1. Triangular fuzzy number

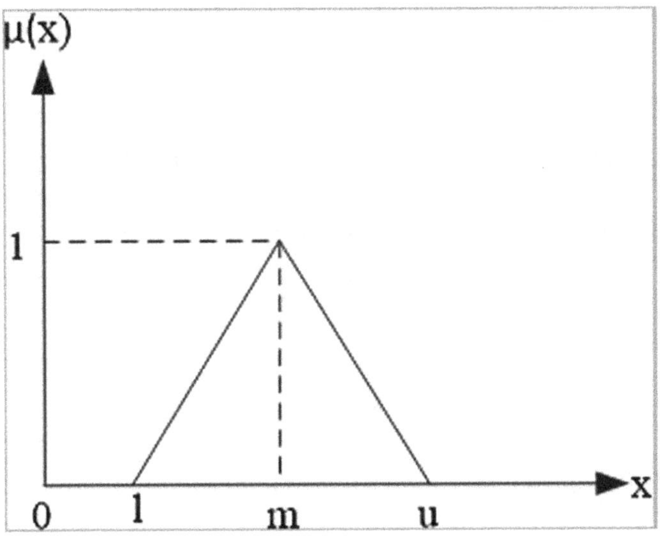

In this context, Figure 1 shows a triangular fuzzy number. The corresponding relationship between the linguistic terms and triangular fuzzy numbers is determined in accordance with Table 1. Accordingly, fuzzy ratings and their membership function are illustrated in Figure 2.

Table 1. Corresponding relationship between linguistic terms and fuzzy numbers

Linguistic Terms	Triangular Fuzzy Numbers
No influence (No)	(0, 0, 0.25)
Very low influence (VL)	(0, 0.25, 0.5)
Low influence (L)	(0.25, 0.5, 0.75)
High influence (H)	(0.5, 0.75, 1)
Very high influence (VH)	(0.75, 1, 1)

Figure 2. Fuzzy ratings and their membership function

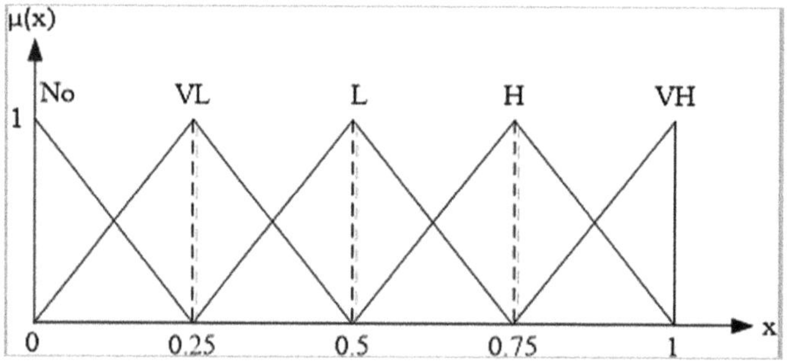

For any two triangular fuzzy numbers $\tilde{A}_1 = (l_1, m_1, u_1)$ and $\tilde{A}_2 = (l_2, m_2, u_2)$, the mathematical calculation of the two triangular fuzzy numbers can be defined as follows:

The addition operation between the triangular fuzzy numbers;

$$\tilde{A}_1 + \tilde{A}_2 = (l_1 + l_2, m_1 + m_2, u_1 + u_2) \tag{2}$$

The subtraction operation between the triangular fuzzy numbers;

$$\tilde{A}_1 - \tilde{A}_2 = (l_1 - u_2, m_1 - m_2, u_1 - l_2) \tag{3}$$

The multiplication operation between the triangular fuzzy numbers;

$$\tilde{A}_1 x \tilde{A}_2 = \left(l_1 x l_2, m_1 x m_2, u_1 x u_2\right) \tag{4}$$

The arithmetic operation for the triangular fuzzy numbers;

$$k x \tilde{A}_1 = \left(k x l_1, k x m_1, k x u_1\right), \left(k > 0\right) \tag{5}$$

$$\frac{\tilde{A}_1}{k} = \left(\frac{l_1}{k}, \frac{m_1}{k}, \frac{u_1}{k}\right), \left(k > 0\right) \tag{6}$$

Fuzzy DEMATEL

In this section, fuzzy sets and DEMATEL methods are combined to perform the sensitive evaluation. The main steps of the method are defined as follows (Chen-Yi et al., 2007; Wu and Lee, 2007; Liou et al., 2008; Balin et al.,2018; Başhan and Demirel, 2019).

Step 1 Select a Group of Experts: In this step, it is consulted to the experts who have enough knowledge and experience about the problem in order to obtain consistent judgments.

Step 2 Determine Factors and Construct Fuzzy Scale: In this part, significant factors are ascertained in order to be analyzed and evaluated properly. Then, the linguistic variable is utilized with five scales (no influence, very low influence, low influence, high influence, and very high influence) according to the linguistic terms and fuzzy numbers. Thereafter, corresponding triangular fuzzy members are presented.

Step 3 Obtain Evaluation of the Group Decision Makers: The pairwise comparison is obtained in terms of linguistics variables. Furthermore, the fuzzy assessments are transformed into defuzzified and aggregated as a crisp value. As a result, the initial direct-relation fuzzy matrix ($\tilde{E}$) of group decision makers is constructed.

$$\tilde{E} = \begin{bmatrix} 0 & \cdots & \tilde{E}_{1n} \\ \vdots & \ddots & \vdots \\ \tilde{E}_{n1} & \cdots & 0 \end{bmatrix} \tag{7}$$

$$\tilde{e}_{ij} = \left(l_{ij}, m_{ij}, u_{ij}\right) \tag{8}$$

Step 4 Establish Normalized Direct-Relation Fuzzy Matrix: In the presence of the initial direct-relation matrix, normalized direct-relation fuzzy matrix is build up. In order to achieve that, firstly, it is considered $\tilde{\beta}_i$ and γ as triangular fuzzy numbers. The following calculations are done respectively.

$$xl_{ij}^k = \left(l_{ij}^k - \min l_{ij}^k\right) / \Delta_{\min}^{\max} \tag{9}$$

$$xm_{ij}^k = \left(m_{ij}^k - \min l_{ij}^k\right) / \Delta_{\min}^{\max} \tag{10}$$

$$xr_{ij}^k = \left(r_{ij}^k - \min xl_{ij}^k\right) / \Delta_{\min}^{\max} \tag{11}$$

Where

$$\Delta_{\min}^{\max} = \max r_{ij}^k - \min l_{ij}^k$$

Step 5 Compute Left (Ls) And Right (Rs) Normalized Value: After having established normalized direct-relation fuzzy matrix, a left (ls) and right (rs) normalized value are calculated as follows:

$$xls_{ij}^k = xm_{ij}^k / \left(1 + xm_{ij}^k - xl_{ij}^k\right) \tag{12}$$

$$xrs_{ij}^{k} = xr_{ij}^{k} / \left(1 + xr_{ij}^{k} - xm_{ij}^{k}\right) \tag{13}$$

Step 6 Compute the Total Normalized Crisp Values: After having left (ls) and right (rs) normalized value, the total normalized crisp values are calculated.

$$x_{ij}^{k} = \left[xls_{ij}^{k}\left(1 - xls_{ij}^{k}\right) + xrs_{ij}^{k} xrs_{ij}^{k}\right] / \left[1 - xls_{ij}^{k} + xrs_{ij}^{k}\right] \tag{14}$$

Step 7 Calculate the Crisp Values: The next process is the calculation of the crisp values as follows:

$$z_{ij}^{k} = \min l_{ij}^{k} + x_{ij}^{k} \Delta_{\min}^{\max} \tag{15}$$

Step 8 Integrate the Crisp Values: The crisp values are lastly integrated with the proposed approach. Z is the initial direct-relation matrix that is used in the process of DEMATEL. After obtaining the Z matrix, the all process is applied as in the classical DEMATEL approach. Then the total-relation matrix is calculated. The sum of rows and the sum of columns are separately denoted as r_i and c_j, within the total-relation matrix.

$$z_{ij}^{k} = \frac{1}{p}\left(z_{ij}^{1} + z_{ij}^{2} + \ldots + z_{ij}^{p}\right)$$

CASE STUDY

As the first phase of the case study, hospital service quality evaluation criteria are derived from the relevant literature (Chang, 2014; Akdag et al. 2014; Taşkın et al. 2015). We used the criteria of Yucesan and Gul (2020)'s study. In that study, 6 main criteria and 32 sub-criteria are considered. These criteria are described as follows:

Hospital equipment (C1): There are four sub-criteria under this main criterion.

- **C11:** Medical equipment level of the hospital
- **C12:** Availability of marked signs in the hospital
- **C13:** Sufficiency of outpatient treatment areas
- **C14:** Usability of "Hospital Information Management System" in the hospital

Service attitude (C2): There are eight sub-criteria under this main criterion.

- **C21:** Tidy appearance of service staff
- **C22:** Service staff with good communication skills
- **C23:** The attitude of nurses and medical staff to patients
- **C24:** Cordial attitude of service staff
- **C25:** Consideration of individual needs of patients by medical staff
- **C26:** The attitude of ward staff to patients
- **C27:** Concern shown by medical staffs towards illness
- **C28:** Medical staff responding to patients' requests and complaints

Pharmacy and medical treatment (C3): There are five sub-criteria under this main criterion.

- **C31:** Taking the advice of medical staffs to patients staying at home
- **C32:** Pharmacists advice on medicine preservation
- **C33:** Confidence to provided medical services
- **C34:** Giving a detailed description of taking medicine and the ingredients of medicine
- **C35:** Detailed description of the patient's illness by the doctor

Professional competence (C4): There are three sub-criteria under this main criterion.

- **C41:** Medical staff with professional abilities
- **C42:** Trusted medical staff with professional competence of healthcare
- **C43:** Service personnel with immediate problem-solving abilities

Administrative policies (C5): There are six sub-criteria under this main criterion.

- **C51:** Being user-friendly of hospital appointment system
- **C52:** Patient flow procedures of emergency department
- **C53:** Patient meals services
- **C54:** Outpatient waiting time for medical treatment
- **C55:** Patient admission procedures
- **C56:** Being user friendly of hospital websites

Cleaning of hospital facility (C6): There are six sub-criteria under this main criterion.

- **C61:** The quality and cleanliness of the bed linen
- **C62:** Lighting condition of the ward
- **C63:** Ventilation and sanitation of the ward
- **C64:** Number and quality of the bathrooms available
- **C65:** Given information on facilities available when patients first come to the hospital
- **C66:** Cleanliness of the toilets

This study is performed under the evaluation of 22 experts. They determine priority orders of hospital service quality criteria by the using fuzzy DEMATEL method. The experts are being employed under the governmental medical department, hospital administration, quality deployment department, medical staff from emergency department, intensive care unit, audiometry, and other inpatient units (doctor, nurse, technician, etc.) and ward service provider. These evaluators are employers who are well-experienced in the healthcare delivery and workflow in the hospitals. The information about the expert team and corresponding working experience is set out in Table 2. Due to anonymity reasons, experts' identity has not been revealed herein, and therefore, they have been demonstrated as E1, E2, ... and E22.

Secondly, the 32 evaluation criteria for hospital service quality, as provided above in detail are assessed in terms of the relationship using the fuzzy linguistic scale of Table 1. According to the consensus of evaluators, Table 3 shows the linguistic assessments of evaluators' consensus on the hospital equipment (C1) criteria for hospital service quality evaluation. The results of FDEMATEL for this main criterion are only given in the paper due to space limitations. Accordingly, the initial direct-fuzzy matrix is calculated. After having established the initial direct-fuzzy matrix, the normalized direct-relation fuzzy matrix is constructed by using the Eqs. (9 - 11) respectively.

In the light of the above outcomes, the values of r_i, c_j, $r_i + c_j$ and $r_i + c_j$ can be obtained. Then, the cause-effect relation diagram is to build up. In the last stage, the cause and effect relationship diagram can be depicted based on the above outcomes.

Table 2. Expert group information

Expert ID	Experience (in Years)	Title
E1	16	Medical assistant
E2	25	Physiotherapist
E3	10	Assistant
E4	22	Nurse
E5	10	Chef.
E6	8	x-Ray technician
E7	24	Nurse
E8	7	Nurse
E9	3	Laboratory assistant
E10	18	Nurse
E11	1	Information technologies
E12	20	Chef.
E13	1	Audiologist
E14	15	Nurse
E15	25	Assistant manager
E16	4	Assistant manager
E17	7	Audiologist
E18	21	Assistant
E19	23	Assistant
E20	18	Coordinator
E21	4	Secretary
E22	18	Assistant manager

Table 3. Linguistic assessment of the consensus.

	C11	C12	C13	C14
C11	No	H	VL	L
C12	L	No	VL	H
C13	VL	VL	No	H
C14	VL	VH	L	No

RESULTS AND DISCUSSION

In order to evaluate the key performance indicators of hospital service quality evaluation, it is substantial to focus on the cause factors (key performance indicators), which are required more attention. In the view of Figure 3, C11 (Medical equipment level of the hospital) has the highest $r_i - c_j$ value (10.68) among all factors in the cause group. This means that C11 has more impact on the entire process.

Figure 3. Cause-effect relation diagram for hospital equipment

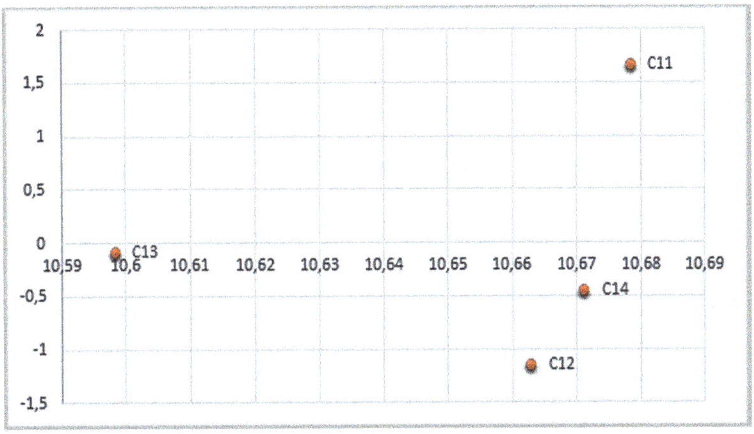

In the view of Figure 4, C23 (The attitude of nurses and medical staff to patients) has the highest $r_i - c_j$ value (19.36) among the all sub-key performance indicators of service attitude in cause group. If the service attitudes are considered, C23 has more impact on the entire process.

When the pharmacy and medical treatment is analyzed, the confidence to provided medical services (C33) and detailed description of the patient's illness by the doctor (C35) is under cause group (Figure 5). Since effect factors are simply impacted by the other key performance indicators, it may be essential to investigate effect factors that can become principal to thoughtful results in healthcare management. In the light of the cause-effect relation diagram, apparently, C32 (pharmacists' advice on medicine preservation) has the highest value (30.5) among the whole pharmacy and medical treatment.

In the view of Figure 6, C41 (medical staff with professional abilities) has the highest $r_i - c_j$ value (16.66) among the all sub-key performance indicators of Professional competence in cause group. It means that C41 has more impact on professional competence.

Figure 4. Cause-effect relation diagram for service attitude

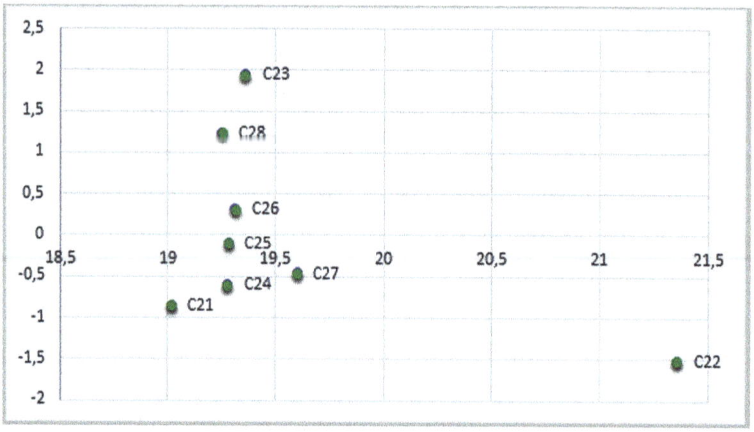

Figure 5. Cause-effect relation diagram for pharmacy and medical treatment

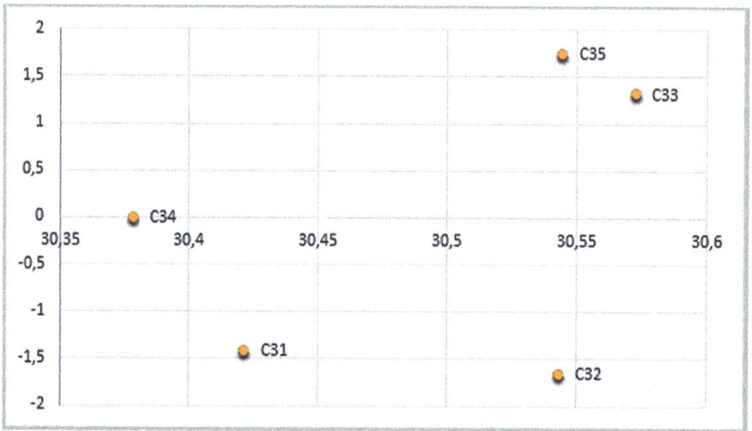

Figure 6. Cause-effect relation diagram for professional competence

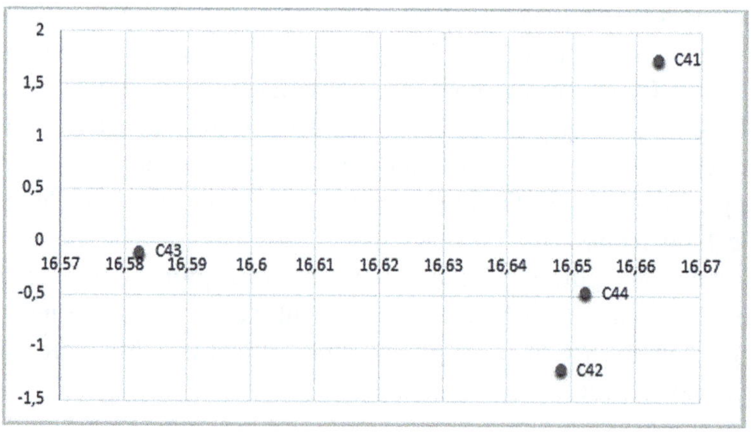

Figure 7. Cause-effect relation diagram for administrative policies

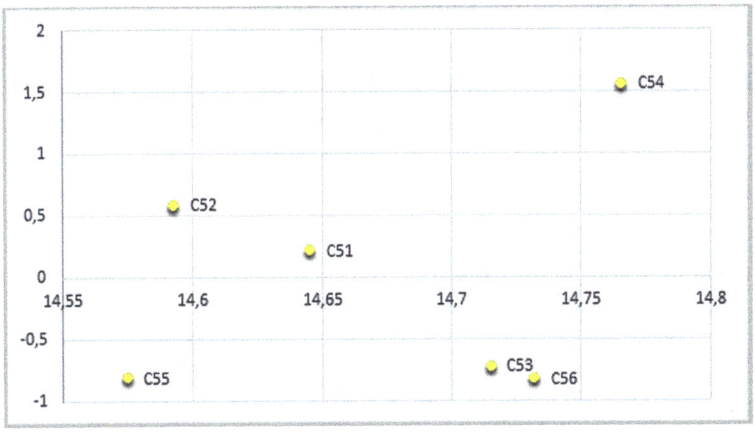

In administrative policies, C54 (Outpatient waiting time for medical treatment), C53 (Patient meals services), and C56 (Being user- friendly of hospital websites) should be analyzed in more detail (Figure 7). While C54 is under cause group, C53 and C56 are under effect group.

Figure 8. Cause-effect relation diagram for cleaning of hospital facility

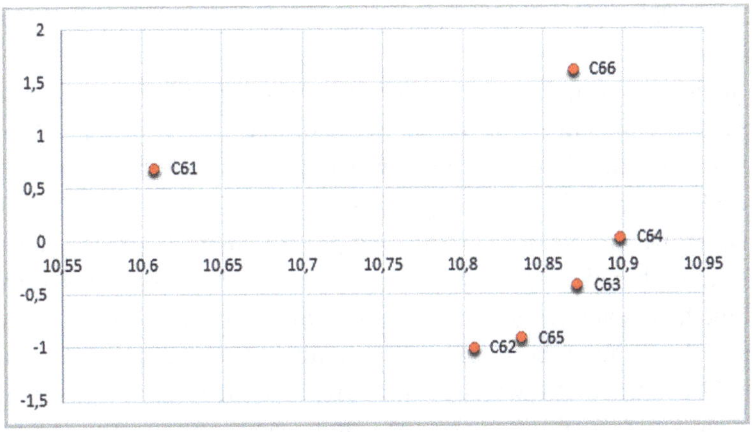

In the view of Figure 8, C64 (Number and quality of the bathrooms available) has the highest $r_i - c_j$ value (10.90) among the cleaning of a hospital facility in the cause group. This means that C64 has more impact on the cleaning of the hospital facility.

The Results of the study are then compared with Yucesan and Gul (2020)'s study. In the current study, C11 (Medical equipment level of the hospital) has more impact on the entire service quality as in the benchmark study. Yucesan and Gul (2020) obtain a global weight value of 0.145 for C11 criterion as it is the highest value of the C1 main criterion group. The remaining results are mostly consistent with Yucesan and Gul (2020), as shown in Table 4.

Table 4. Comparison of the results

Current Study			Yucesan and Gul (2020)		
The Most Important Criterion	**Weight Value (r-c Fuzzy DEMATEL Value)**	**Rank**	**The Most Important Criterion**	**Weight Value (Pythagorean Fuzzy AHP Score)**	**Rank**
C11	10.68	1	C11	0.696	1
C23	19.36	1	C23	0.168	1
C32	30.5	1	C35	0.393	1
C41	16.66	1	C41	0.449	1
C54	17.76	1	C54	0.254	1
C64	10.90	1	C66	0.335	1

CONCLUSION

Service quality has a major concern for private and public hospitals due to the importance and competition of the service industry. One of the most important challenges of our time is to measure service quality. Therefore, a multi-criteria decision-making model in evaluating hospital service quality criteria is proposed in this chapter. Due to the decision-making process involves vagueness of human judgments, a combination of fuzzy sets theory and DEMATEL method is used. The proposed method is applied to a case study to make better decisions and improve service quality. Six main hospital service quality criteria and 32 sub-criteria are interpreted by health experts, which includes employers from medical, administrative and auxiliary services, through the case study. According to the results of the approach, it contributes to hospital healthcare management in better providing healthcare services and as well as at a higher quality level. Results of the proposed approach are shared with hospital management to develop their service quality. As a result, the fuzzy DEMATEL method can be applied to similar operational processes in the different research areas. For future research, we plan to contribute to the methodological aspect of the study by developing new models like Best and Worst method, which requires less pairwise comparisons. For the application point of view, a multi-expert, multi-site (a group of hospitals), and a multi-criteria approach can be proposed.

REFERENCES

Afkham, L., Abdi, F., & Komijan, A. (2012). Evaluation of service quality by using fuzzy MCDM: A case study in Iranian health-care centers. *Management Science Letters*, *2*(1), 291–300. doi:10.5267/j.msl.2011.08.009

Akdag, H., Kalaycı, T., Karagöz, S., Zülfikar, H., & Giz, D. (2014). The evaluation of hospital service quality by fuzzy MCDM. *Applied Soft Computing*, *23*, 239–248. doi:10.1016/j.asoc.2014.06.033

Aktas, A., Cebi, S., & Temiz, I. (2015). A new evaluation model for service quality of health care systems based on AHP and information axiom. *Journal of Intelligent & Fuzzy Systems*, *28*(3), 1009–1021. doi:10.3233/IFS-141385

Akyuz, E., & Celik, E. (2015). A fuzzy DEMATEL method to evaluate critical operational hazards during gas freeing process in crude oil tankers. *Journal of Loss Prevention in the Process Industries*, *38*, 243–253. doi:10.1016/j.jlp.2015.10.006

Al-Neyadi, H. S., Abdallah, S., & Malik, M. (2018). Measuring patient's satisfaction of healthcare services in the UAE hospitals: Using SERVQUAL. *International Journal of Healthcare Management*, *11*(2), 96–105. doi:10.1080/20479700.2016.1266804

Ali, M., & Raza, S. A. (2017). Service quality perception and customer satisfaction in Islamic banks of Pakistan: The modified SERVQUAL model. *Total Quality Management & Business Excellence*, *28*(5-6), 559–577. doi:10.1080/14783363.2015.1100517

Ali, S. S., Basu, A., & Ware, N. (2018). Quality measurement of Indian commercial hospitals–using a SERVQUAL framework. *Benchmarking: an international journal*, *25*(3), 815-837.

Altuntas, S., Dereli, T., & Yilmaz, M. K. (2012). Multi-criteria decision-making methods based weighted SERVQUAL scales to measure perceived service quality in hospitals: A case study from Turkey. *Total Quality Management & Business Excellence*, *23*(11-12), 1379–1395. doi:10.1080/14783363.2012.661136

Balin, A., Demirel, H., Celik, E., & Alarcin, F. (2018). A fuzzy DEMATEL model proposal for the cause and effect of the fault occurrıng ın the auxılıary systems of the shıps' maın engıne. *International Journal of Maritime Engineering, 160*(A2), A141–A153. doi:10.3940/rina.ijme.2018.a2.465

Başhan, V., & Demirel, H. (2019). Application of fuzzy DEMATEL technique to assess most common critical operational faults of marine boilers. *Politeknik Dergisi, 22*(3), 545–555.

Behdioğlu, S., Acar, E., & Burhan, H. A. (2019). Evaluating service quality by fuzzy SERVQUAL: A case study in a physiotherapy and rehabilitation hospital. *Total Quality Management & Business Excellence, 30*(3-4), 301–319. doi:10.1080/14783363.2017.1302796

Celik, E., & Akyuz, E. (2016). Application of interval type-2 fuzzy sets DEMATEL methods in maritime transportation: the case of ship collision. *International Journal of Maritime Engineering, 158*(A 4), A359-A371.

Chakravarty, A. (2011). Evaluation of service quality of hospital outpatient department services. *Medical Journal, Armed Forces India, 67*(3), 221–224. doi:10.1016/S0377-1237(11)60045-2 PMID:27365810

Chang, T. H. (2014). Fuzzy VIKOR method: A case study of the hospital service evaluation in Taiwan. *Information Sciences, 271*, 196–212. doi:10.1016/j.ins.2014.02.118

Demir, P., Gul, M., & Guneri, A. F. (2018). Evaluating occupational health and safety service quality by SERVQUAL: A field survey study. *Total Quality Management & Business Excellence*, 1–18. doi:10.1080/14783363.2018.1433029

Demirer, Ö., & Bülbül, H. (2014). Kamu ve özel hastanelerde hizmet kalitesi, hasta tatmini ve tercihi arasındaki ilişki: Karşılaştırmalı bir analiz. *Amme Idaresi Dergisi, 47*(2), 95–119.

Gul, M., Celik, E., Aydin, N., Gumus, A. T., & Guneri, A. F. (2016). A state-of-the-art literature review of VIKOR and its fuzzy extensions on applications. *Applied Soft Computing, 46*, 60–89. doi:10.1016/j.asoc.2016.04.040

Gul, M., Guneri, A. F., & Derin, B. (2014). Evaluation of service quality criteria for a private medical center by using SERVQUAL and DEMATEL methods. *Sigma, 32*, 240–253.

Handayani, P. W., Hidayanto, A. N., Sandhyaduhita, P. I., & Ayuningtyas, D. (2015). Strategic hospital services quality analysis in Indonesia. *Expert Systems with Applications*, *42*(6), 3067–3078. doi:10.1016/j.eswa.2014.11.065

Kayapınar, S., & Erginel, N. (2017). Designing the airport service with fuzzy QFD based on SERVQUAL integrated with a fuzzy multi-objective decision model. *Total Quality Management & Business Excellence*, 1–20.

Kubler, S., Robert, J., Derigent, W., Voisin, A., & Le Traon, Y. (2016). A state-of the-art survey & testbed of fuzzy AHP (FAHP) applications. *Expert Systems with Applications*, *65*, 398–422. doi:10.1016/j.eswa.2016.08.064

Lee, H., Delene, L. M., Bunda, M. A., & Kim, C. (2000). Methods of measuring health-care service quality. *Journal of Business Research*, *48*(3), 233–246. doi:10.1016/S0148-2963(98)00089-7

Lin, Q. L., Liu, L., Liu, H. C., & Wang, D. J. (2013). Integrating hierarchical balanced scorecard with fuzzy linguistic for evaluating operating room performance in hospitals. *Expert Systems with Applications*, *40*(6), 1917–1924. doi:10.1016/j.eswa.2012.10.007

Liu, A., Guo, X., Liu, T., Zhang, Y., Tsai, S. B., Zhu, Q., & Hsu, C. F. (2019). A GRA-Based Method for Evaluating Medical Service Quality. *IEEE Access: Practical Innovations, Open Solutions*, *7*, 34252–34264. doi:10.1109/ACCESS.2019.2903684

Lupo, T. (2013). A fuzzy ServQual based method for reliable measurements of education quality in Italian higher education area. *Expert Systems with Applications*, *40*(17), 7096–7110. doi:10.1016/j.eswa.2013.06.045

Lupo, T. (2016). A fuzzy framework to evaluate service quality in the healthcare industry: An empirical case of public hospital service evaluation in Sicily. *Applied Soft Computing*, *40*, 468–478. doi:10.1016/j.asoc.2015.12.010

Ministry of Health in Republic of Turkey. (2017). Health Statistics Yearbook 2016. Republic of Turkey Ministry of Health General Directorate of Health Research, Ankara, Turkey.

Parasuraman, A., Zeithaml, V. A., & Berry, L. L. (1988). Servqual: A multiple-item scale for measuring consumer perc. *Journal of Retailing*, *64*(1), 12.

Pekkaya, M., Pulat İmamoğlu, Ö., & Koca, H. (2019). Evaluation of healthcare service quality via Servqual scale: An application on a hospital. *International Journal of Healthcare Management*, *12*(4), 340–347. doi:10.1080/20479700.2017.1389474

Raziei, Z., Torabi, S. A., Tabrizian, S., & Zahiri, B. (2018). A Hybrid GDM-SERVQUAL-QFD Approach for Service Quality Assessment in Hospitals. *Engineering Management Journal*, *30*(3), 179–190. doi:10.1080/10429247.2018.1443670

Roy, J., Adhikary, K., Kar, S., & Pamucar, D. (2018). A rough strength relational DEMATEL model for analysing the key success factors of hospital service quality. *Decision Making: Applications in Management and Engineering*, *1*(1), 121–142.

Shieh, J. I., Wu, H. H., & Huang, K. K. (2010). A DEMATEL method in identifying key success factors of hospital service quality. *Knowledge-Based Systems*, *23*(3), 277–282. doi:10.1016/j.knosys.2010.01.013

Singh, A., & Prasher, A. (2019). Measuring healthcare service quality from patients' perspective: Using Fuzzy AHP application. *Total Quality Management & Business Excellence*, *30*(3-4), 284–300. doi:10.1080/14783363.2017.1302794

Taşkin, H., Kahraman, Ü. A., & Kubat, C. (2015). Evaluation of the hospital service in Turkey using fuzzy decision-making approach. *Journal of Intelligent Manufacturing*, 1–12.

Teng, C. I., Ing, C. K., Chang, H. Y., & Chung, K. P. (2007). Development of service quality scale for surgical hospitalization. *Journal of the Formosan Medical Association*, *106*(6), 475–484. doi:10.1016/S0929-6646(09)60297-7 PMID:17588841

Tuzkaya, G., Sennaroglu, B., Kalender, Z. T., & Mutlu, M. (2019). Hospital service quality evaluation with IVIF-PROMETHEE and a case study. *Socio-Economic Planning Sciences*, *68*, 100705. doi:10.1016/j.seps.2019.04.002

Yucesan, M., & Gul, M. (2020). Hospital service quality evaluation: an integrated model based on Pythagorean fuzzy AHP and fuzzy TOPSIS. *Soft Computing*,1-19, 24, 3237-3255. doi:10.1007/s00500-019-04084-2.

Chapter 4
A Maximal Covering Location Model for the Organ Transplant Organization in Turkey

Barış Özkan
https://orcid.org/0000-0001-7767-4087
Ondokuz Mayıs University, Turkey

Eren Özceylan
https://orcid.org/0000-0002-5213-6335
Gaziantep University, Turkey

ABSTRACT

Transplantation of the organs is one of the principal treatment techniques for the people who have critical organ issues. One of the main steps of this treatment is getting the organ as quickly as possible to its recipient from a potential donor. To provide the aforementioned treatment, the spatial distributions of the organ transplant centers which maximize the donors/patients coverage become essential. In this chapter, the organ transplant process of Turkey which has 99 transplant centers (hospitals) in 81 cities is considered. The main goal of this study is to maximize the donor/patient coverage within the system constraints. As a potential demand source, 923 districts are determined using geographic information system (GIS). With the application of maximal covering location model, the number of covered donors/patients is maximized considering the cold ischemia time of organs. Optimal results are obtained for different scenarios based on heart, liver, and kidney.

DOI: 10.4018/978-1-7998-2581-4.ch004

INTRODUCTION

Organ donation is the process when a person allows an organ of their own to be removed and transplanted to another person, legally, either by consent while the donor is alive or dead. Donation may be for research or, more commonly, healthy transplantable organs and tissues may be donated to be transplanted into another person. Organ transplantation has transformed the survival and quality of life of patients with end-organ dysfunction. According to the U.S. Department of Health & Human Services, while every ten minutes, someone is added to the national transplant waiting list; approximately 22 people die each day waiting for a transplant in the United States. To solve this problem, organ transplantation has to remain its popularity. The total number of transplanted organ in world is continuously increasing since 2000 as shown in Figure 1. While 139,024 organs including kidney, liver, heart and etc. are transplanted in 2017, this number equals to 18.7 per million populations in the world.

Figure 1. Total number of transplanted organ in the world
(GODT, 2019)

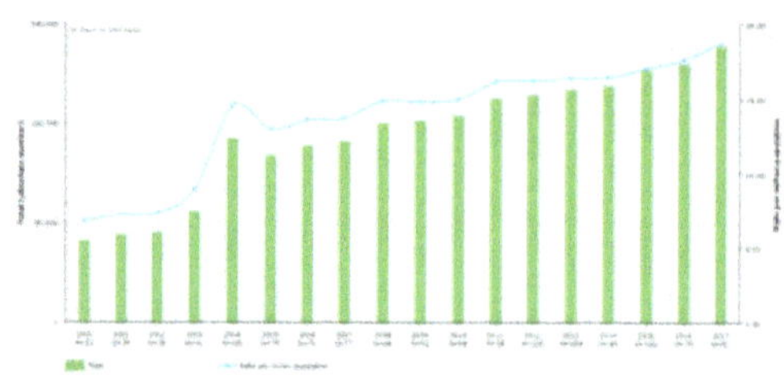

Living and cadaveric donors are the two main sources from whom organs are transplanted. While kidney and liver can be only donated by living donors; the process relies on cadavers for the hearts and lungs (Savaşer et al. 2009). Figures 2 and 3 show the number of worldwide deceased and living donors in 2017 for the top 20 countries, respectively (IRODaT, 2018). According to the Figures 2 and 3, while Spain ranks first by far in terms of number of deceased organ donors; Turkey is the top country in terms of number of living organ donors.

Figure 2. Worldwide deceased organ donors (pmp)
(IRODaT, 2018)

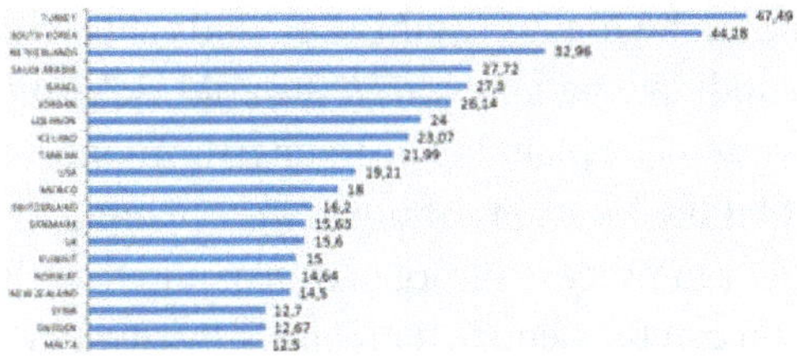

Figure 3. Worldwide living organ donors (pmp)
(IRODaT, 2018)

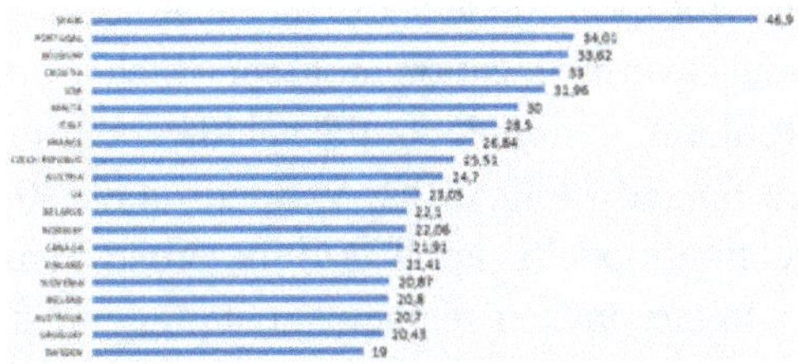

As shown in the aforementioned figures, organ transplantation is one of the important and successful treatment approaches for the people who have critical organ problems. A kidney transplant was the first ever organ transplantation in the world; and even in Turkey, the number of kidney transplants far exceeds those of other organs. In addition to kidney, heart, liver, pancreas and lungs are also needed in Turkey. One of the main steps of this treatment is getting the organ as quickly as possible to its recipient from the moment a potential donor is notified. The organ procurement organization should arrange the organs get ready for the patients when the donors are available. The scarcity of organ supply leads to life-challenging issues for the organ recipient. Therefore, the spatial distributions of organ transplant centers to maximize donor and patient coverage become essential (Rajmohan et al. 2017).

Organ transplantation procedures have both similarities and differences for each country. One of the basic process in organ transplantation system is the matching which is the process of finding the best recipient for the donated organ. There is a single waiting list within an entire country if the system is centralized. Here, priority can be given to the patients based on best match of organ or some other criteria such as tissue match, blood type, length of time on the waiting list, immune status, distance between the potential recipient and the donor and the degree of medical urgency (Savaşer et al. 2019). After removing the organs from the donor's body, the donated organs' life does not lead much. The life of the organ between donors and patients called as cold ischemia time. Therefore, the cold ischemia time also includes shipping time of the organs (Stahl et al. 2005). The donated organ should be operated into the candidate patient within the cold ischemia time bound of that organ. Therefore, the systematic planning of organs from donors to patients is needed.

It is a known fact that the locations of organ transplantation healthcare facilities have a noteworthy affect in process of organ transplantation. Because, the process of organ transplantation can be identified precisely by two key events: location and allocation. For this reason, the longest travel time between any pairs of donor and patient should not exceed the permitted transportation time for any organ. The most important goal is to maximize the number of covered donors/patients by assigning them to the hospitals under cold ischemia time. In literature, there are some papers which apply location-allocation models for the healthcare problems (Rais and Vianaa, 2011). Maximal covering location problem which is one of the well-known location-allocation problems is suitable for the healthcare problems including time or distance limits (see Fo and Mota, 2012; Valipour et al. 2013). In this paper, a maximal covering location model is applied to the organ transplantation problem of Turkey. To do so, a binary integer mathematical model is developed and tested with the real spatial data obtained by GIS. The aim is to find the best assignments of donor and patients in an available hospital considering cold ischemia time limit for any organ. All the spatial information of donors/patients (923 districts) and hospitals (99 organ transplant centers) are gathered and processed within ArcGIS software. The proposed study in this paper differs from the existing studies with several reasons (to the best knowledge of the authors): (*i*) application of a maximal covering model for an organ transplantation network and (*ii*) studying the real case of Turkey's organ transplantation problem including all actors.

This paper is divided into five parts. The second part presents a brief overview of the relevant literature. The third part describes the problem and the applied mathematical model. A real case with its data, application process and results are given in the fourth part, and finally, the fifth part contains the main conclusions of this study.

LITERATURE REVIEW

One of the main differentiations between the typical supply chain and the organ transplant one is perishability of the concerned products. As mentioned in the introduction section, each organ is constrained by a specific cold ischemia time defined as the maximum period the organ can be kept outside the body. This constraint forces and differentiates organ transplant models from the traditional logistics models.

Most work related to organ donations and organ transplants focuses on policies to allocate organs to recipients or to locate the healthcare facilities in a desired area. The existing literature related in this area is summarized below.

As a one of the earliest studies, Stahl et al. (2005) developed an integer programming model for determining optimal configurations of regions maximizing transplant allocation efficiency and geographic parity in USA. Their analysis indicated that liver transplantation may benefit through region reorganization. Later, Bruni et al. (2006) presented a mixed-integer linear programming (MILP) model to obtain an efficient system and equalize the waiting lists in Italy. Rogrilie and Shi (2007) focused on the USA network to produce a generic model of the interaction of the factors that affect the number of people on the wait list, the number of transplantations, and the length of wait time. In another study, Kong et al. (2010) utilized a branch-and-price approach aiming at the maximization of the efficiency of the liver allocation systems in the USA. The study benefits from clinical data for computational experiments. Belien et al. (2013) proposed a MILP model for defining the optimal location of transplant centers that minimizes the total weighted time as the objective function. They took five different organs (i.e., kidney, liver, lung, heart and pancreas) into consideration and linked them by a budget constraint. The model is then been applied to Belgium as a case study. Furthermore, Koizumi et al. (2013) applied a mathematical programming to construct alternative liver allocation boundaries that achieve more geographic equity in access to transplants than the current system in USA. The performance of the optimal boundaries was evaluated and compared to that of current allocation system using discrete event simulation.

To cope with the uncertainty in organ transplantation, Zahiri et al. (2014a; b) proposed a fuzzy multi-objective programming model for the design of an organ transplant transportation network. The model minimizes total cost and time, including waiting time in the queue for the transplant operation, while considering organs' priorities. Aghazadeh et al. (2017) developed a multi–objective mathematical model for an organ transplantation network. While the first objective function tries to minimize costs of opened centers, shipping organs, and allocations; the second objective function considers expected number of donors, coverage of other locations by taking into consideration the maximum remaining time for each organ out of body, and safety index. A credibility-based fuzzy common weights data envelopment analysis approach was applied by Ahmadvand and Pishvaee (2018) for kidney allocation. Verification and validation of the proposed approach were performed in two steps using a real case study from the Iranian kidney allocation system. Caruso and Daniele (2018) aimed at presenting a mathematical model, based on networks, which allows them to minimize the total costs associated with organ transplants. They found the related optimality conditions and the variational inequality formulation. Ghane and Tavakkoli-Moghaddam (2018) proposed a mixed-integer nonlinear programming model for minimizing the total transportation time and the maximizing shortage of organ simultaneously. A scenario-based stochastic approach is used in order to model the problem. In one of the recent studies, maximizing the potential compatible donor–recipient matches within the cold ischemia time bounds is addressed by Savaşer et al. (2019). They analyzed Turkey's organ transplantation logistics structure based on its dynamics and provide new mathematical models for maximizing potential-weighted intra-regional organ transplantation flow via evaluating different types of transportation modes while meeting the specified time bounds. Rabbani and Talebi (2019) proposed a bi-objective nonlinear mathematical programming model which includes uncertain cost and transport time parameters. The ε-constraint method had been used to solve the organ transportation problem and Iran was considered as a case study.

In literature, although there have been a lot of papers on maximal covering models, majority of these focus on traditional facility location problems (Cordeau et al. 2019). A few papers applied maximal covering location models for healthcare problems. For example, maximal covering location and the p-median methods are used by Shariff et al. (2010; 2012) to analyze accessibility of public health facilities in Malaysia. Elkady and Abdelsalam (2016a; b) proposed a modified particle swarm optimization algorithm to solve a modified capacitated maximal covering location problem. Røislien et al. (2017) estimated optimal air ambulance base locations in Norway. To do so, the maximal covering location problem was used to find the optimal helicopter base locations for time thresholds 30 and 45 min. Finally, Pouraliakbari et al. (2018) shed light onto the formulation and the solution of a probabilistic maximal covering location model for determining the optimal location of facilities in congested healthcare systems with referral hierarchical structure. To solve the model, two meta-heuristic algorithms, including simulated annealing and ant colony optimization had been executed.

When looking at the broader organ transplant literature above, we observe that the maximal covering is not commonly used and also the Turkey case is not studied widely. To fill this gap, a binary integer programming model is applied to the case of Turkey which includes 923 donors/patients and 99 hospitals. The scenarios based on the most three required organs, namely kidney, heart and liver are considered.

METHODOLOGY AND PROBLEM

In this chapter, the mathematical formulation of the maximal covering location model is presented. Later, the organ transplantation organization in Turkey is described.

Maximal Covering Location Model

The service distance concept in location problems appears in set covering location problem first. This problem identifies the minimal number and the location of facilities, which ensures that no demand point will be farther than the maximal service distance from a facility. However, in some cases which include health or safety issues, the covered population is more important than the cost of the facilities (Daskin, 2008). If there is such a situation, the decision maker may shift his/her attention to concern with the total population covered within a service distance. The maximal covering location problem seeks the maximum population which can be served within a pre-known service distance or time given a limited number of facilities (Toregas et al. 1971). As can be seen from the definition, maximal covering location model is a proper tool for the organ transplant organization. While the donor/patients may be considered as demand sources, the organ transplant centers may be considered as source nodes and the cold ischemia time may be considered as time/distance constraint. A mathematical formulation of this problem can be stated as follows (Mete et al. 2018):

Decision variables

$$y_k = \begin{cases} 1, & if\ organ\ transpant\ center\ (hospital)\ is\ selected\ (\forall k \in K) \\ 0, & otherwise \end{cases}$$

$$z_i = \begin{cases} 1, & if\ demand\ node\ (donor\ /\ patient)\ i\ is\ covered\ (\forall i \in I) \\ 0, & otherwise \end{cases}$$

Objective function

$$MaxZ = \sum_{i \in I} w_i z_i \tag{1}$$

Subject to

$$\sum_{k \in K} y_k = P \tag{2}$$

$$z_i \leq \sum_{k \in K} a_{ik} y_k \ \forall i \in I \tag{3}$$

$$z_i, y_i \in \{0,1\} \ \forall i \in I, \forall k \in K \tag{4}$$

The objective function (1) maximizes the number of covered demands where demand at location *i* is represented by w_i. Cons. (2) shows that *P* amount hospitals are to be located. Cons. (3) ensures link coverage variables and the location, and last one (4) is binary restriction constraint. Here, a_{ik} is a parameter:

$$a_{ik} = \begin{cases} 1, & if\ a\ demand\ node\ i\ can\ be\ reached\ by\ a\ hospital\ k\ in\ a\ cold\ ischemia\ time \left(\forall i \in I, \forall k \in K\right) \\ 0, & otherwise \end{cases}$$

Organ Transplant Organization in Turkey

In the Turkish organ transplantation organization, all operations are coordinated by the Transplantation Coordination Center (NCC) of the Ministry of Health in Turkey. This center also coordinates 9 Regional Coordination Centers (RCC) in Turkey (Figure 4). While the strategic and tactical decisions belong to the NCC, the operational decisions such as the organ transplantation between the nodes are in

Figure 4. NCC and 9 RCCs
(Savaşer et al. 2019)

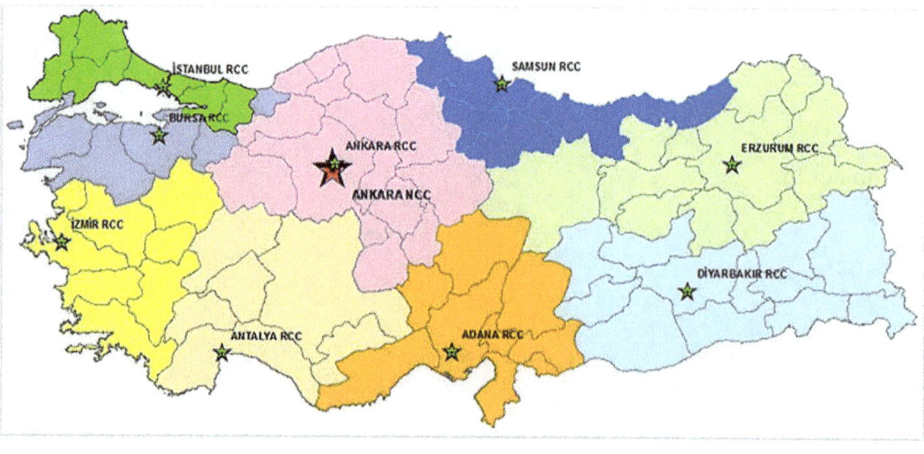

Table 1. Covered cities by the RCCs

RCCs	Covered Cities	# of Cities	# of Transplant Centers
Adana	Adana; Gaziantep; Hatay; Kahramanmaraş; Kayseri; Kilis; Mersin; Niğde; Osmaniye	9	9
Ankara	Aksaray; Ankara; Bartın; Bolu; Çankırı; Çorum; Eskişehir; Karabük; Kastamonu; Kırıkkale; Kırşehir; Nevşehir; Yozgat; Zonguldak	14	15
Antalya	Afyon; Antalya; Burdur; Isparta; Karaman; Konya	6	6
Bursa	Balıkesir; Bilecik; Bursa; Çanakkale; Düzce; Yalova	6	5
Diyarbakır	Adıyaman; Batman; Bitlis; Diyarbakır; Elazığ; Hakkari; Malatya; Mardin; Siirt; Şanlıurfa; Şırnak; Van	12	6
Erzurum	Ağrı; Ardahan; Artvin; Bayburt; Bingöl; Erzincan; Erzurum; Gümüşhane; Iğdır; Kars; Muş; Sivas; Tunceli	13	2
İstanbul	Edirne; İstanbul; Kırklareli; Kocaeli; Sakarya; Tekirdağ	6	43
İzmir	Aydın; Denizli; İzmir; Kütahya; Manisa; Muğla; Uşak	7	11
Samsun	Amasya; Giresun; Ordu; Rize; Samsun; Sinop; Tokat; Trabzon	8	2
Total		81	99

(Organ, 2019)

charge of RCCs. All the cities in Turkey are covered by and assigned to one RCC. The name of the cities with their RCCs is given in Table 1.

Hospitals with special equipment can only manage the organ transplantation process. A hospital which has specialized operating rooms, intensive care units and specialized doctors, should be an organ transplantation hospital. There are 99 transplant centers (hospitals) in 81 cities of Turkey. However, the spatial distribution of the RCCs is not balanced. For example, while there are 48 transplant centers in Marmara region, it is only two in Black Sea Region. In Turkey, while 4,571 organs were transplanted in 2018, there exist 24,935 people waiting for a suitable organ as of January 2018. The number of transplanted heart, liver and kidney between 2007 and 2018 are illustrated in Figure 5. On the other hand, the number of patients who are waiting for heart, liver and kidney based on RCC is given in Figure 6. When the Figures 5 and 6 are compared, it is easy to see that there is a mismatch between the number of transplanted organ and patients who are waiting for an organ.

The most needed organs in Turkey are kidney, liver and heart, respectively. As mentioned before, the donated organ should be placed into the patient who needs in the cold ischemia time limit. Otherwise, the organ becomes functionless. The cold ischemia time of three most needed organs are given in Table 2. It is clear to see from Table 2 that the longest ischemia time in minutes belongs to kidney and

Figure 5. Number of transplanted organs (heart, liver and kidney)
(Organ, 2019)

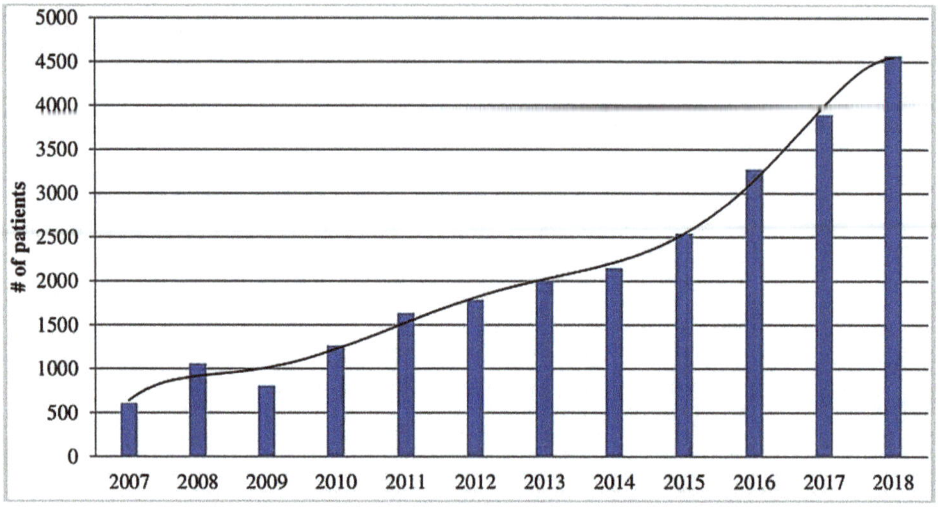

Figure 6. Distribution of patients who are waiting for heart, liver and kidney
(Organ, 2019)

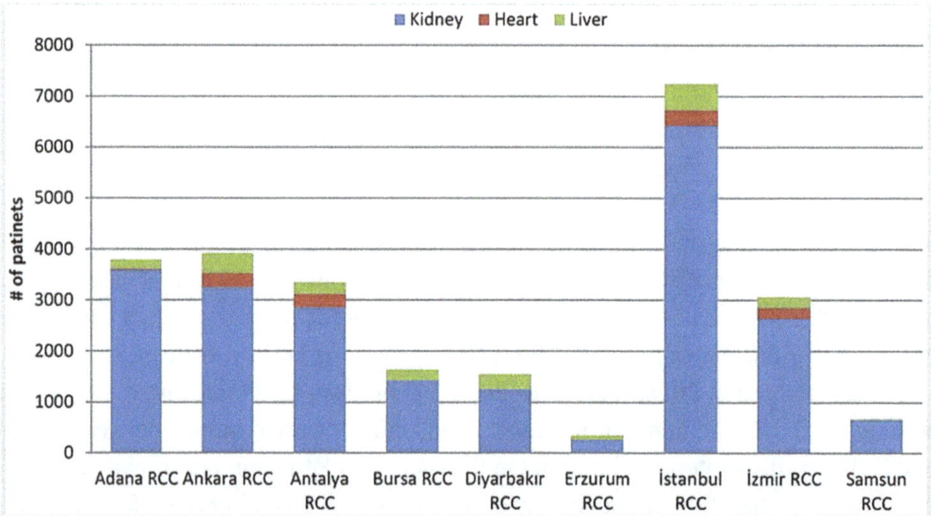

the shortest ischemia time belongs to heart. The shadow row in Table 2 shows the required time for transportation of organs which is used in our model. Depending upon the aforementioned time limits, the spatial distribution of the hospitals and the assignments of potential donors/patients to these hospitals become significantly essential.

Table 2. Cold ischemia time for three operations in three organs transplantation

Operations	Heart	Liver	Kidney
Surgery time for organ removal (*min*)	10	45	60
Time for transportation (*min*)	220	405	570
Surgery time for organ implementation (*min*)	70	270	450
Total (*min*)	300	720	1080

(Savaşer et al. 2019)

APPLICATION OF THE MODEL

In this section, the mathematical formulation described in third section is applied to the organ transplant case of Turkey. All run experiments were conducted on a server 1.8 GHz processor with 4 GB of RAM. The problem is solved with the GAMS-CPLEX and the computation time is required less than 2 CPU seconds. As mentioned before, 99 hospitals which are capable for organ transplant are chosen as a source node. The locations of 99 hospitals are illustrated in Figure 7.

Figure 7. 99 transplant centers (hospitals)
(Organ, 2019)

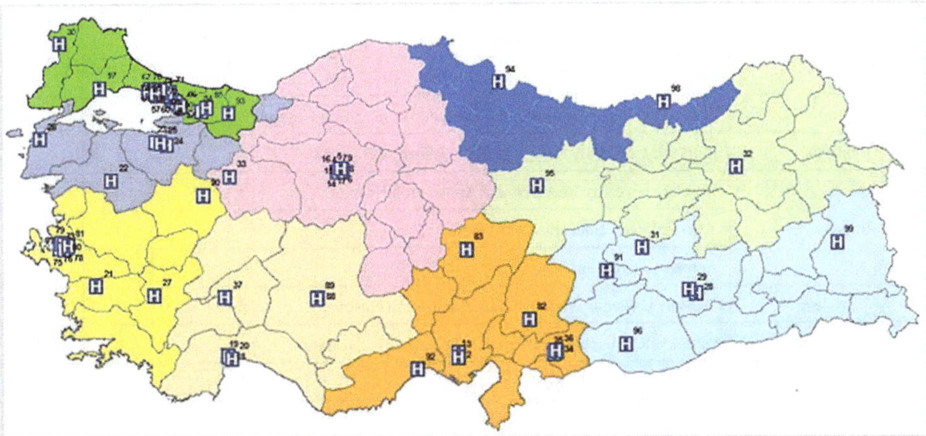

The list of 99 hospitals is given in Table 3 with their city name and the organ transplant capability. If there is a "+" in the relate cell, it means that the organ can be transplanted in that hospital. As can be seen from Table 3, while all the hospitals are capable of kidney transplantation, 23 and 42 of them are capable of heart and liver transplantation, respectively (Figures 8 and 9).

Table 3. List of transplant centers with their organ transplant capabilities

#	City	Transplant Center	Heart	Liver	Kidney
1	Adana	Başkent University Research and Application Hospital	+	+	+
2		Çukurova University Balcalı Education and Research Hospital	+	+	+
3		Numune Education and Research Hospital	-	-	+
4	Ankara	Atatürk Education and Research Hospital	-	-	+
5		Dışkapı Yıldırım Beyazıt Education and Research Hospital	-	-	+
6		Gazi University Research and Application Hospital	+	+	+
7		Hacettepe University Hospital	+	+	+
8		Numune Education and Research Hospital	-	-	+
9		Yıldırım Beyazıt University Yenimahalle Education and Research Hospital	-	+	+
10		Türkiye Yüksek İhtisas Education and Research Hospital	+	+	+
11		Ufuk University Dr. Rıdvan Ege Research and Application Hospital	-	-	+
12		İbni Sina Research and Application Hospital	+	+	+
13		Ankara University Cebeci Research and Application Hospital	+	-	+
14		Başkent University Research and Application Hospital	+	+	+
15		Ankara Güven Hospital	-	-	+
16		Medicana International Hospital	-	+	+
17		Gülhane Education and Research Hospital	+	+	+
18	Antalya	Akdeniz University Hospital	+	+	+
19		Antalya Education and Research Hospital	-	+	+
20		Medicalpark Hospital	-	-	+
21	Aydın	Adnan Menderes University Research and Application Hospital	-	+	+
22	Balıkesir	Balıkesir University Research and Application Hospital	-	+	+
23	Bursa	Uludağ University Research and Application Hospital	-	+	+
24		Yüksek Ihtisas Education and Research Hospital	-	-	+
25		Acibadem Hospital	-	+	+
26	Çanakkale	18 Mart University Research and Application Hospital	-	-	+
27	Denizli	Pamukkale University Research and Application Hospital	-	+	+
28	Diyarbakır	Dicle University Hospital	-	-	+
29		Gazi Yaşargil Education and Research Hospital	-	-	+
30	Edirne	Trakya University Hospital	-	-	+
31	Elazığ	Fırat University Research and Application Hospital	-	+	+
32	Erzurum	Atatürk University Research and Application Hospital	-	+	+
33	Eskişehir	Osmangazi University Research and Application Hospital	+	+	+

continued on following page

Table 3 continued

#	City	Transplant Center	Heart	Liver	Kidney
34	Gaziantep	Dr. Ersin Arslan Education and Research Hospital	+	+	+
35		Gaziantep University Şahinbey Hospital	-	+	+
36		Sani Konukoğlu Hospital	-	-	+
37	Isparta	Süleyman Demirel University Research and Application Hospital	-	-	+
38	İstanbul	Bakırköy Dr. Sadi Konuk Education and Research Hospital	-	-	+
39		Aydın University Research and Application Hospital	+	-	+
40		Başkent University Research and Application Hospital	-	+	+
41		Bezmialem University Hospital	-	-	+
42		Dr. Siyami Ersek Education and Research Hospital	+	-	+
43		Haydarpaşa Numune Education and Research Hospital	-	+	+
44		İstinye University Research and Application Hospital	-	-	+
45		Dr. Lütfi Kırdar Education and Research Hospital	-	-	+
46		Koç University Education and Application Hospital	-	+	+
47		Koşuyolu Yüksek İhtisas Education and Research Hospital	+	+	+
48		Mehmet Akif Ersoy Education and Research Hospital	-	+	+
49		Okan University Research and Application Hospital	-	-	+
50		Memorial Hospital	-	+	+
51		Medeniyet University Education and Research Hospital	-	-	+
52		Marmara University Education and Research Hospital	-	-	+
53		Süreyyapaşa Education and Research Hospital	+	-	+
54		Şişli Hamidiye Etfal Education and Research Hospital	-	-	+
55		Ümraniye Education and Research Hospital	+	+	+
56		İstanbul University Cerrahpaşa Hospital	+	+	+
57		İstanbul University Hospital	+	+	+
58		İstanbul Yedikule Education and Research Hospital	-	-	+
59		Yeditepe University Hospital	+	+	+
60		Acıbadem Altunizade Hospital	-	-	+
61		Acıbadem Atakent Hospital	-	-	+
62		Acıbadem International Hospital	-	-	+

continued on following page

Table 3 continued

#	City	Transplant Center	Heart	Liver	Kidney
63	Istanbul	Aile Bahçelievler Hospital	-	+	+
64		Kadıköy Florence Nightingale Hospital	-	+	+
65		Medical Park Göztepe Hospital	-	-	+
66		Medicana Bahçelievler Hospital	-	-	+
67		Medicana Çamlıca Hospital	-	-	+
68		Medicana International Istanbul Hospital	-	-	+
69		Medipol Mega Hospital	-	-	+
70		Memorial Ataşehir Hospital	-	+	+
71		Memorial Şişli Hospital	-	+	+
72		Şişli Florence Nightingale Hospital	-	-	+
73		Universal Çamlica Hospital	-	-	+
74		Yeni Yüzyıl University Gaziosmanpaşa Hospital	-	-	+
75	İzmir	Dokuz Eylül University Hospital	+	+	+
76		Ege University Hospital	+	+	+
77		Katip Çelebi University Education and Research Hospital	-	-	+
78		İzmir Tepecik Hospital	-	-	+
79		Kent Hospital	-	-	+
80		Medical Park Hospital	-	-	+
81		Bozyaka Education and Research Hospital	-	-	+
82		İzmir Tepecik Education and Research Hospital	-	-	+
83	Kahramanmaraş	Sütçü İmam University Research and Application Hospital	-	-	+
84	Kayseri	Erciyes University Hospital	-	+	+
85	Kocaeli	Anadolu Hospital	-	+	+
86		Kocaeli University Research and Application Hospital	-	-	+
87		Derince Education and Research Hospital	-	-	+
88	Konya	Başkent University Research and Application Hospital	-	-	+
89		Necmettin Erbakan University Meram Hospital	-	-	+
90	Kütahya	Dumlupınar University Education and Research Hospital	-	-	+
91	Malatya	İnönü University Hospital	-	+	+
92	Mersin	Mersin University Research and Application Hospital	-	+	+
93	Sakarya	Sakarya University Education and Research Hospital	-	-	+
94	Samsun	19 Mayıs University Research and Application Hospital	-	-	+
95	Sivas	Cumhuriyet University Research and Application Hospital	-	-	+
96	Şanlıurfa	Harran University Research and Application Hospital	-	-	+
97	Tekirdağ	Namık Kemal Univ. Research and Application Hospital	-	-	+

continued on following page

Table 3 continued

#	City	Transplant Center	Heart	Liver	Kidney
98	Trabzon	Karadeniz Teknik University Farabi Hospital	-	-	+
99	Van	Yüzüncü Yıl University Hospital	+	-	+

(Organ, 2019)

Figure 8. 23 hospitals with heart transplant capability

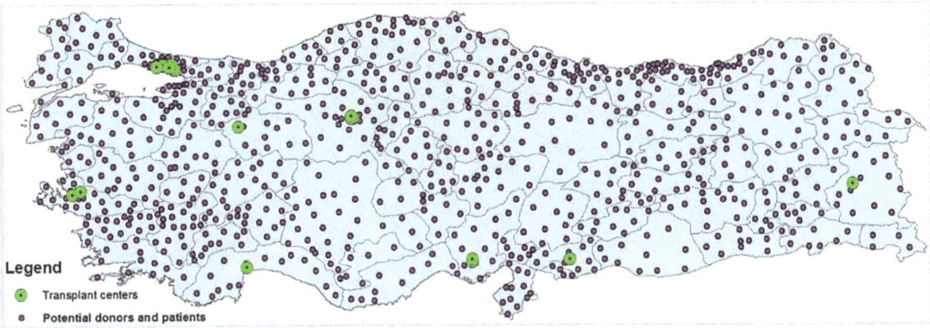

Figure 9. 42 hospitals with liver transplant capability

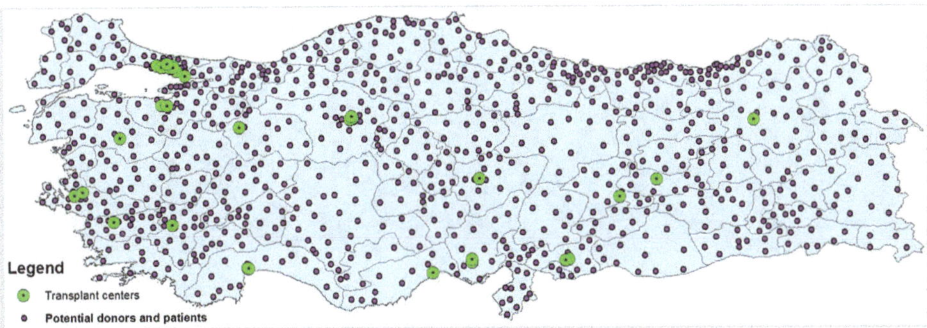

923 districts in Turkey are considered as a donor/patient source. The locations of districts are shown in Figure 10. To calculate the real road distance between hospitals and donor/patient nodes, road map of Turkey is gathered using GIS (Figure 11).

In the model, the demand of patients or supply of donors is (w_i) fixed as 1. Maximal covering location model are solved totally in three times for kidney, heart and liver, respectively. The cold ischemia times of three organs (Table 2) are used as a predetermined time limit in the models. The average speed of the ambulance is set to 100km/hour which means maximum 367km, 675km and 950km coverage is permitted for heart, liver and kidney transportation, respectively.

Figure 10. Total potential 923 donors/patients

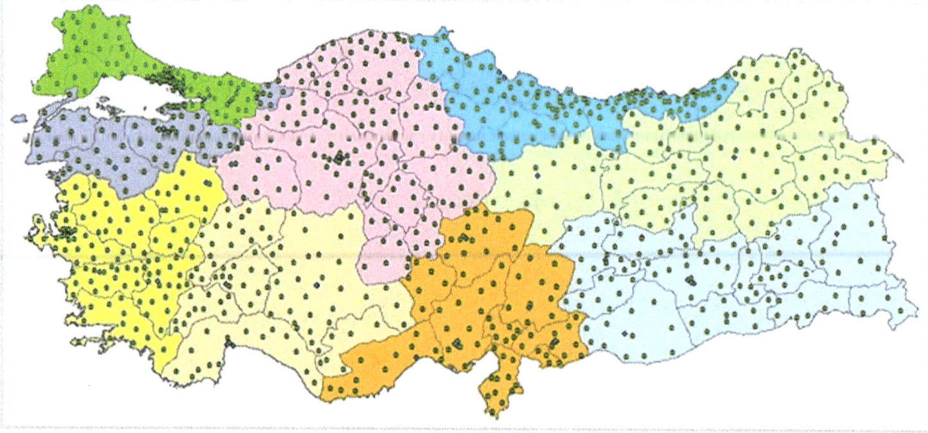

Figure 11. Highway map of Turkey

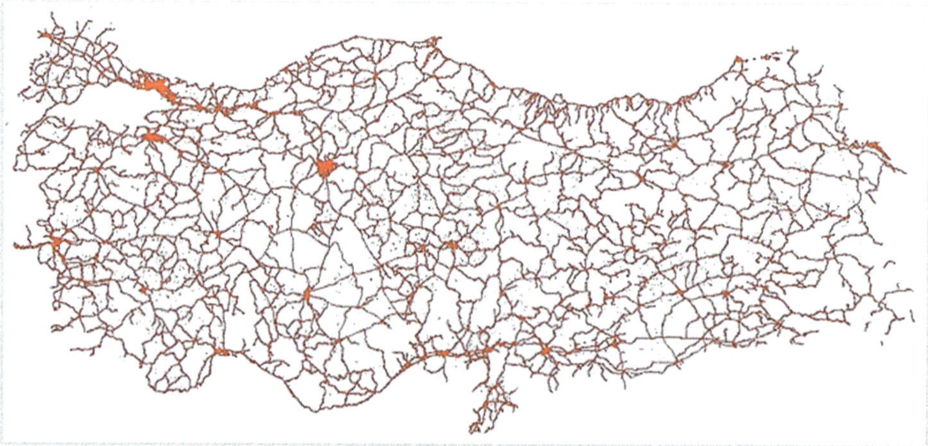

Results of the Kidney Case

The maximal covering location model is solved for the kidney case. In this case, there are 99 hospitals and 923 districts. The coverage limit is set to 950km. Due to high number of available hospitals and long coverage limit; only two hospitals are enough to cover all 923 donors/patients. 71st and 99th hospitals are opened and all donors/patients can reach to them in 950km (Figure 12). Different *P* values are tested and maximum demand is covered when *P* equals to 2.

Figure 12. Optimal solution of maximal covering location model for the kidney case

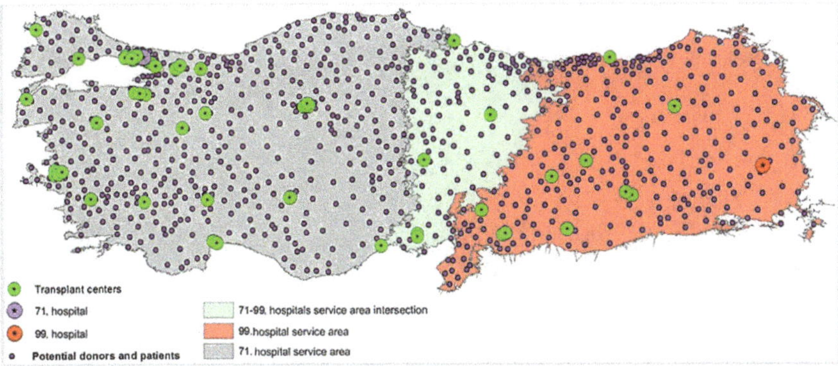

To see the effects of coverage limit on the objective function, different distances ranging from 50 to 350km are tested on the kidney case. Figure 13 indicates the relationship between coverage limit and number of covered donors/patients. According to the Figure 13, 350km coverage distance which is lower than kidney cold ischemia time meets all the demand. However, decreasing the coverage limit from 350km to 50km, the number of covered people decreases by 77%.

Figure 13. Number of covered people based on different distance limits

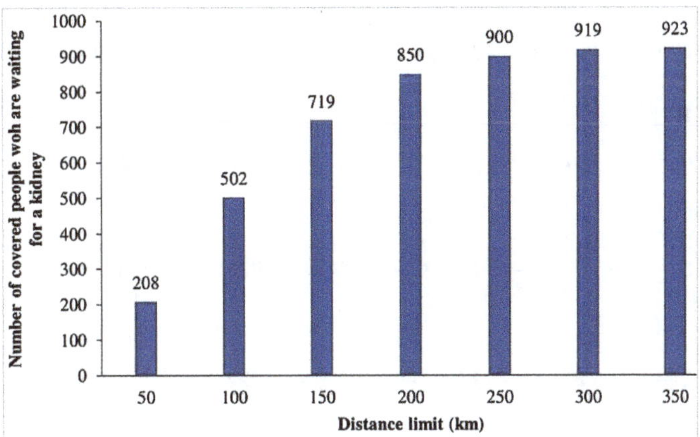

Figure 14. Optimal solution of maximal covering location model for the liver case

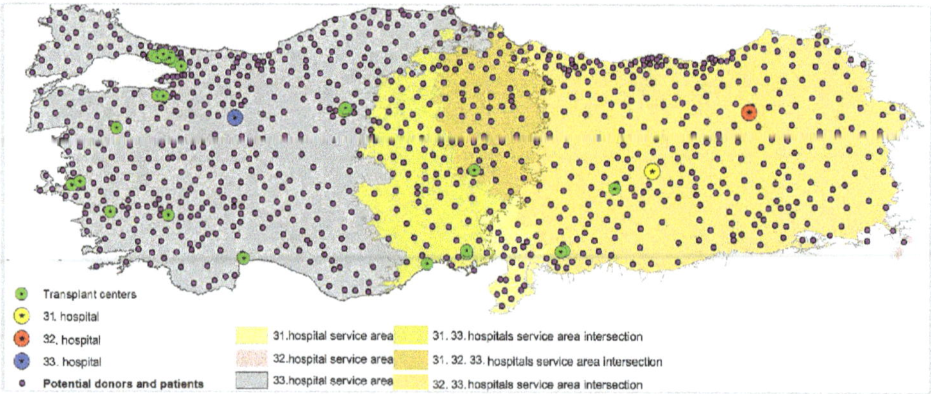

Results of the Liver Case

The maximal covering location model is also solved for the liver case. In this case, there are 42 hospitals and 923 districts. The coverage limit is set to 675km. As in the kidney case, due to high number of available hospitals and long coverage limit; three hospitals are enough to cover all 923 donors/patients. 31st, 32nd and 33th hospitals are opened and all donors/patients can reach to them in 675km (Figure 14). Different *P* values are tested and maximum demand is covered when *P* equals to 3.

Figure 15. Number of covered people who are waiting for a liver

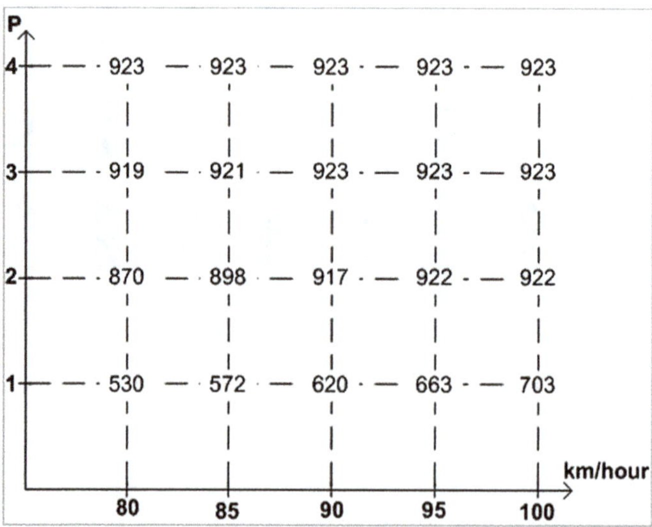

Figure 15 illustrates the number of covered people who are waiting for a liver based on different parameter combinations. As expected, when the speed of ambulance and number of hospital increases, the number of covered people who are waiting for a liver also increases. All people can be covered when the average speed is 90km/hour and the number of opened hospitals is 3.

Results of the Heart Case

The maximal covering location model is also solved for the heart case. In this case, there are 23 hospitals and 923 districts. The coverage limit is set to 367km due to cold ischemia time of the heart. Different from the kidney and liver cases, only 767 demand sources (83% of total demand) are covered with 23 hospitals within cold ischemia time of the heart. The covered and uncovered areas are illustrated in Figure 16. Figure 16 indicates that East Black sea Region and the west part of East Anatolia Region are not covered fully.

Figure 16. Optimal solution of maximal covering location model for the heart case

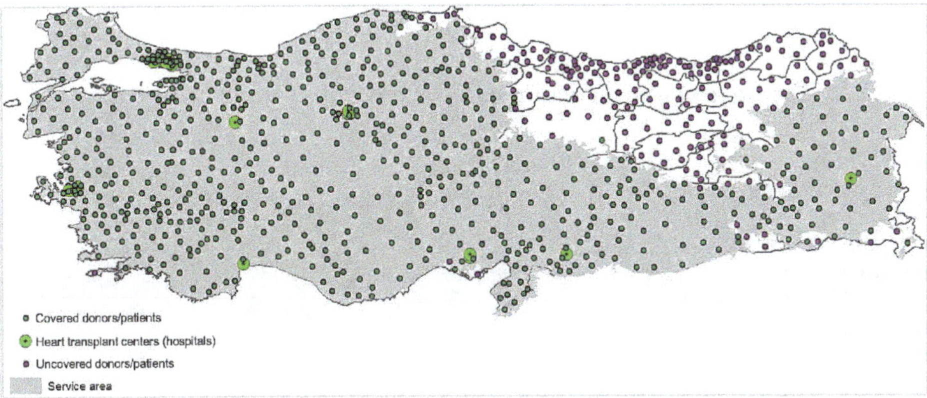

There are possible two reasons for this uncovered situation. While one of them is short cold ischemia time of the heart, the other one is the unbalanced distribution of the 23 heart transplant hospitals. To cope with the first reason, different average speed values of the organ transportation vehicles are tested. In the current solution, the average speed was 100km/hour. To see the effects of average speed, the current value is increased from 100km/hour to 190km/hour, in increments of 10km/hour.

According to the Figure 17, if the average speeds of the vehicle is increased from 100km/hour to 190km/hour; all the donors/patients are covered. In other words, an increment in the average speed by 90% also increases the number of covered people by 17%.

Figure 17. Number of covered people after the speed increments

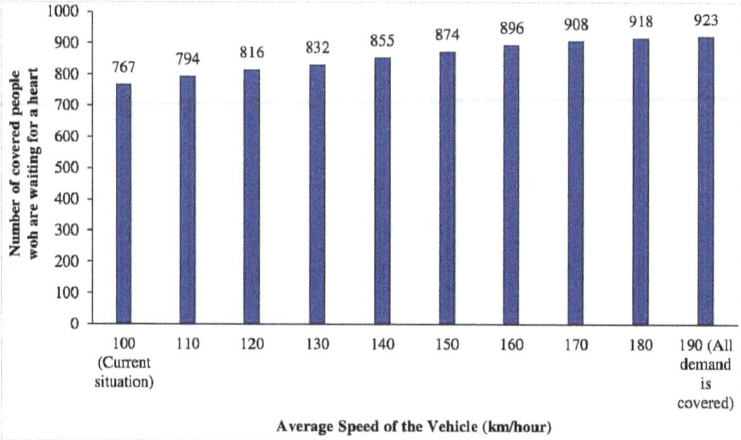

Figure 18. Coverage map with additional four hospitals for the heart case

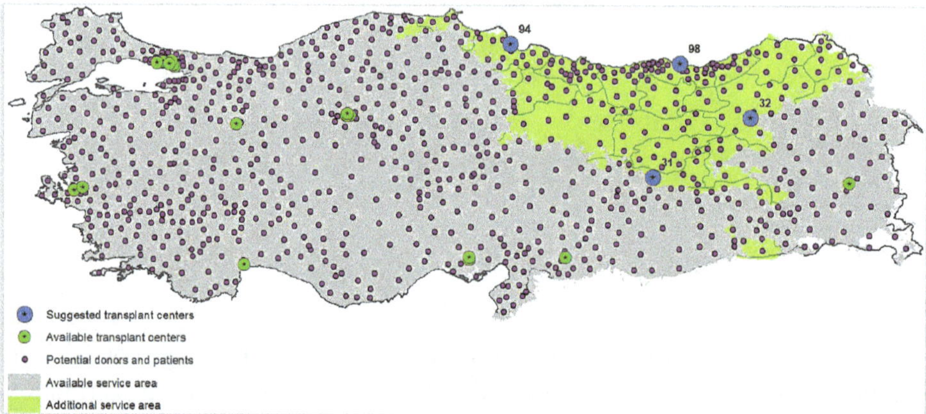

In addition to changing the speed value, adding more hospitals is also investigated while the average speed is fixed to 100km/hour. Normally 23 of 99 transplant centers have heart transplant capability. To increase the coverage, more hospitals, especially in East Black Sea Region, are needed. In the model, P is increased from 23 in increments of 1. When P=27, 923 donors/patients are covered fully. Added four hospitals are shown in Figure 18 with their numbers. It means that if 31st, 32nd, 94th and 98th hospitals have heart transplant capability, all potential patients who are waiting for a heart will be covered.

CONCLUSION

The organ transplant process is a typical example of a supply chain. However, instead of inventory or capacity in the traditional supply chain systems, there is an important constraint which is called as cold ischemia-time (the maximal time the organ can be kept outside the body) in organ transplant process. Therefore, the spatial distribution of the demand sources (patients) and hospitals (transplant centers) has to be investigated considering the cold ischemia time of the organs.

The contribution proposed in this paper was basically motivated by the observation that the current system of organ allocation (not only in Turkey, but in most of the developed countries) is hampered primarily by geographic inequalities in waiting times among various areas of the country. The model developed in this paper aims at maximizing the coverage of donors/patients by considering the cold ischemia time of organs and the locations of hospitals. To do so, a maximal covering location model is proposed for the Turkey case. The case of Turkey including 99 hospitals and 923 districts is solved. The most required three organs namely heart, liver and kidney cases are considered with different scenarios. As a result, the current organ transplant system for kidney and liver seems proper and covers all the patients. However, patients who are waiting for a heart are not fully covered by the suitable hospitals within the heart cold ischemia time. To increase the coverage for the heart case, different speed values of the vehicles and spatial distribution of the hospitals are analyzed. There are some limitations and weaknesses of the proposed paper. The centers of the districts are considered demand points in this paper. However, exact positions of donors/patients should be taken into considerations. Another limitation of the paper is considering only the road as a transportation mode.

Regarding to the limitations of the study, the paper can be enhanced on a few points: (*i*) a web-based decision support system should be developed to see the instant changes in organ transplant process; (*ii*) the uncertainty in the donors' process should be taken into account with fuzzy or stochastic approaches and finally, (*iii*) other location-allocation models such as set covering, P-median and etc. should be applied.

REFERENCES

Aghazadeh, S. M., Mohammadi, M., & Naderi, B. (2017). Multi objective organ transplant supply chain with effective location and time consideration. *Journal of Industrial and Systems Engineering*, *10*(4), 158–176.

Ahmadvand, S., & Pishvaee, M. S. (2018). An efficient method for kidney allocation problem: A credibility-based fuzzy common weights data envelopment analysis approach. *Health Care Management Science*, *21*(4), 587–603. doi:10.100710729-017-9414-6 PMID:28795254

Beliën, J., De Boeck, L., Colpaert, J., Devesse, S., & Van den Bossche, F. (2013). Optimizing the facility location design of organ transplant centers. *Decision Support Systems*, *54*(4), 1568–1579. doi:10.1016/j.dss.2012.05.059

Bruni, M. E., Conforti, D., Sicilia, N., & Trotta, S. (2006). A new organ transplantation location–allocation policy: A case study of Italy. *Health Care Management Science*, *9*(2), 125–142. doi:10.100710729-006-7661-z PMID:16895308

Caruso, V., & Daniele, P. (2018). A network model for minimizing the total organ transplant costs. *European Journal of Operational Research*, *266*(2), 652–662. doi:10.1016/j.ejor.2017.09.040

Cordeau, J.-F., Furini, F., & Ljubić, I. (2019). Benders decomposition for very large-scale partial set covering and maximal covering location problems. *European Journal of Operational Research*, *275*(3), 882–896. doi:10.1016/j.ejor.2018.12.021

Daskin, M. S. (2008). What you should know about location modeling. *Naval Research Logistics*, *55*(4), 283–294. doi:10.1002/nav.20284

Elkady, S. K., & Abdelsalam, H. M. (2016). A modified multi-objective particle swarm optimisation algorithm for healthcare facility planning. *International Journal of Business and Systems Research*, *10*(1), 1–22. doi:10.1504/IJBSR.2016.073685

Elkady, S. K., & Abdelsalam, H. M. (2016a). A modified particle swarm optimization algorithm for solving capacitated maximal covering location problem in healthcare systems. *Intelligent Systems Reference Library*, *96*, 117–133. doi:10.1007/978-3-319-21212-8_5

Fo, A. R. A. V., & Mota, I. S. (2012). Optimization models in the location of healthcare facilities: A real case in Brazil. *Journal of Applied Operational Research*, *4*(1), 37–50.

Ghane, M., & Tavakkoli-Moghaddam, R. (2018). A stochastic optimization approach to a location-allocation problem of organ transplant centers. *Journal of Optimization in Industrial Engineering*, *11*(1), 103–111.

GODT. (2019). Global Observatory on Donation and Transplantation. Retrieved from http://www.transplant-observatory.org/data-charts-and-tables/chart/, Access date: 22.10.2019.

IRODaT. (2018). International Registry in Organ Donation and Transplantation. Retrieved from http://www.irodat.org/img/database/pdf/IRODaT%20Newsletter%20 2017.pdf, Access date: 22.10.2019.

Koizumi, N., Ganesan, R., Gentili, M., Chen, C. H., Waters, N., & Das Gupta, D. (2013). Redesigning organ allocation boundaries for liver transplantation in the United States. *Proceedings of the International Conference On Health Care Systems Engineering* (pp. 15–27).

Kong, N., Schaefer, A. J., Hunsaker, B., & Roberts, M. S. (2010). Maximizing the efficiency of the US liver allocation system through region design. *Management Science*, *56*(12), 2111–2122. doi:10.1287/mnsc.1100.1249

Mete, S., Cil, Z. A., & Özceylan, E. (2018). Location and coverage analysis of bike-sharing stations in university campus. *Business Systems Research*, *9*(2), 80–95. doi:10.2478/bsrj-2018-0021

Organ. (2019). *Turkey organ transplant statistics*. Retrieved from https://organ.saglik.gov.tr

Pouraliakbari, M., Mohammadi, M., & Mirzazadeh, A. (2018). Analysis of maximal covering location-allocation model for congested healthcare systems in user choice environment. *International Journal of Industrial and Systems Engineering*, *28*(2), 240–274. doi:10.1504/IJISE.2018.089139

Rabbani, M., & Talebi, E. (2019). A comprehensive mathematical model for designing an organ transplant supply chain network under uncertainty. *International Journal of Engineering*, *32*(6), 835–841.

Rais, A., & Vianaa, A. (2011). Operations research in healthcare: A survey. *International Transactions in Operational Research*, *18*(1), 1–31. doi:10.1111/j.1475-3995.2010.00767.x

Rajmohan, M., Theophilus, C., Sumalatha, M. R., & Saravanakumar, S. (2017). Facility location of organ procurement organizations in Indian health care supply chain management. *South African Journal of Industrial Engineering*, *28*(1), 90–102. doi:10.7166/28-1-1508

Rogrilie, M., & Shi, A. W. P. (2007). Optimizing the effectiveness of organ allocation. *Academic Journal, 28*(2), 1–17.

Røislien, J., van den Berg, P. L., Lindner, T., Zakariassen, E., Aardal, K., & van Essen, J. T. (2017). Exploring optimal air ambulance base locations in Norway using advanced mathematical modeling. *Injury Prevention, 23*(1), 10–15. doi:10.1136/injuryprev-2016-041973 PMID:27325670

Savaşer, S., Kınay, Ö. B., Kara, B. Y., & Cay, P. (2019). Organ transplantation logistics: A case for Turkey. *OR-Spektrum, 41*(2), 327–356. doi:10.100700291-018-0538-y

Shariff, S. S. R., Moin, N. H., & Omar, M. (2012). Location allocation modeling for healthcare facility planning in Malaysia. *Computers & Industrial Engineering, 62*(4), 1000–1010. doi:10.1016/j.cie.2011.12.026

Shariff, S. S. R., Omar, M., Moin, N. H., & Smith, D. K. (2010). Locational analysis of public health facilities: A case study of Telok Panglima Garang, Selangor, Malaysia. *Malaysian Journal of Science, 29*(2), 98–118. doi:10.22452/mjs.vol29no2.2

Stahl, J. E., Kong, N., Shechter, S. M., Schaefer, A. J., & Roberts, M. S. (2005). A methodological framework for optimally reorganizing liver transplant regions. *Medical Decision Making, 25*(1), 35–46. doi:10.1177/0272989X04273137 PMID:15673580

Toregas, C., Swain, R., ReVelle, C., & Bergman, L. (1971). The location of emergency service facilities. *Operations Research, 19*(6), 1259–1551. doi:10.1287/opre.19.6.1363

Valipour, M. T., Nedjati, A., & Kazemi, R. (2013). Solving health care facility location problems with new heuristic algorithm method. *International Journal of Modeling and Optimization, 3*(1), 12–14. doi:10.7763/IJMO.2013.V3.225

Zahiri, B., Tavakkoli-Moghaddam, R., Mohammadi, M., & Julab, P. (2014a). Multi-objective design of an organ transplant network under uncertainty. *Transportation Research Part E, Logistics and Transportation Review, 72*, 101–124. doi:10.1016/j.tre.2014.09.007

Zahiri, B., Tavakkoli-Moghaddam, R., & Pishvaee, M. S. (2014b). A robust possibilistic programming approach to multi–period location–allocation of organ transplant centers under uncertainty. *Computers & Industrial Engineering, 74*, 139–148. doi:10.1016/j.cie.2014.05.008

Chapter 5
Computational Intelligence Approach for Classification of Diabetes Mellitus Using Decision Tree

Engin Pekel
Hitit University, Turkey

Ebru Pekel Özmen
Ondokuz Mayıs University, Turkey

ABSTRACT

Diabetes mellitus (DM) is a group of metabolic disorders with one common manifestation: elevated blood sugar or hyperglycemia. The diagnosis of diabetes is the most crucial point due to chronic hyperglycemia. This chapter improves the performance of the Classification and Regression Trees (CART) algorithm because the accurate classification of diabetes depends on the algorithm efficiency. Authors use the accuracy rate for the objective function in the prediction process by Genetic Algorithm (GA). The proposed GA-CART algorithm provides the best performance at 96.05%.

DOI: 10.4018/978-1-7998-2581-4.ch005

INTRODUCTION

Diabetes mellitus (DM) is a group of metabolic disorders with one common manifestation: elevated blood sugar or hyperglycemia. The diagnosis of diabetes is the most crucial point because of chronic hyperglycemia. It causes permanent damages to the eye, kidney, nerves, heart, and blood vessels. This contingency makes the diagnosis of diabetes important. The traditional diagnosis methods may be more painful and slower such as blood analysis. A physician commonly determines decisions by testing the current blood analysis results of a patient. Therefore, the diagnosis of diabetes for the physicians and the patient is a very difficult matter. A lot of the intelligent diagnosis systems for diabetes have evolved by inspiring human-being biological constructors. These evolved methods predict whether the probable patient suffers from DM including no surgeon progress. The application of the most suitable hybrid methods is essential for gaining the best results. The artificial intelligent technique provides to increase diagnostic accuracy and reduces costs and human resources.

DM is a major public health problem all over the world and especially in developing countries. According to data from the International Diabetes Federation (IDF), there are approximately 463 million adults with diabetes around the world in 2019 and the researchers expect this number to reach 628 million by 2045. Just under half a billion people are living with diabetes worldwide and the number is projected to increase by 25% in 2030 and 51% in 2045 (Saeedi et al.). Early and accurate diagnosis of diabetes is critical for the prevention of disease and the selection of treatment. Researchers have used several statistical methods and machine learning models to predict and diagnose diabetes. The papers for medical diagnosis have widely performed classification algorithms (Samant and Agarwal, 2018). In the literature, many studies exist for the early and accurate diagnosis of DM using classification algorithms. Kannadasan et al. (2018) aim to classify the Pima Indians diabetes dataset with better performance with the Deep Neural Network (DNN). They achieved a classification accuracy of 86.26%. Sisodia and Sisodia (2018) compared three machine learning classification algorithms namely Decision Tree, SVM and Naive Bayes to detect diabetes at an early stage on Pima Indians Diabetes Database that is sourced from UCI machine learning repository. The performances of all the three algorithms are evaluated and Naive Bayes outperforms with the highest accuracy of 76.30% comparatively other used algorithms. Davi et al. (2019) proposed an integrated approach of the Farthest First (FF) clustering algorithm and Sequential Minimal Optimization (SMO) classifier algorithm for diagnosing diabetes mellitus. Their proposed integrated approach achieved 99.4% classification accuracy. Swapna et al. (2018) presented a methodology for the classification of diabetic and normal HRV signals using deep learning architectures that are named long short-term memory (LSTM), convolutional neural network (CNN) and its combinations (CNN-LSTM).

Table 1 summarizes some classification studies and performance values used in the literature.

Table 1. Studies in diabetes mellitus classification

Study	Approach	Validation Method	Accuracy (%)
Carpenter and Markuzon, 1998	ARTMAP-IC	Hold-out (75% train-25% test)	81.00
Chang and Lilly, 2004	VISIT-GA	Hold-out (52.1% train-47.9% test)	78.20
Gonçalves et al., 2006	$HNFB^{-1}$	Hold-out (50% train-50% test)	78.26
Srinivasa et al., 2007	SAMGA	Cross-validation (10-fold)	73.00
Ghazavi and Liao, 2008	ANFIS	Cross-validation (5-fold)	77.65
Kahramanli and Allahverdi, 2008	Hybrid NN	Cross-validation (10-fold)	84.24
Polat et al., 2008	LS-SVM	Cross-validation (10-fold)	78.21
Polat et al., 2008	GDA-LS-SVM	Cross-validation (10-fold)	82.05
Li et al., 2011	Fuzzy based transformation-PCA-SVM	Hold-out (Different scenarios)	76.84
Luukka, 2011	Fuzzy entropy-based feature selection -similarity classifier	Hold-out (50% train-50% test)	75.97
Isa and Mamat, 2011	Clustered-HMLP	Hold-out (80% train-20% test)	93.33
Seera and Lim, 2014	FMM-CART-RF	Cross-validation (10-fold)	78.39
Shen et al., 2016	SVM	Cross-validation (10-fold)	77.46

Decision trees have a well-documented history in supporting diagnosis in the medical field. The method fits for particularly diagnosis owing to the transparency of the decision rules determined by the algorithm. In obesity, researchers have performed decision trees to classify patients who are at risk for metabolic syndrome, in which behaviors lead to long-term success in bariatric surgery patients, and predicting childhood obesity from early age factors. Unlike methods such as neural networks, the thresholds and subsequent class predictions determined by decision trees often have a practical interpretation that may draw logical medical conclusions to support clinical decisions. Specifically, the categorical thresholds that dictate splits between predicted classifications provide intuitive decision-making rules for clinicians.

The decision tree is one of the algorithms that perform to classify the DM types. Decision trees are a technique that can stimulate trees for classifying both categorical and real-valued targets, and hence it may provide decent performance for classification. The decision tree performs the classification of DM because it offers some advantages addressed in the following.

- The flexibility to overcome a broad range of response types such as categorical, numeric data.
- Simple to understand and to evaluate the structure of the tree.
- Decision tree regression enables to validate a model using statistical tests. That points out the decision tree regression as a reliable model.
- The ability to overcome missing values in explanatory and response variables.
- The ability to overcome multi-output variables.

Although the decision tree offers many advantages, some disadvantages exist. Some of them are as follows:

- The decision tree can be unsteady because small variations in the data may result in a different tree. An ideal validation method may avoid variations in experiments.
- The overfitting problem may take place in the decision tree. To avoid this problem, the parameters of the decision tree require to be tuned.

The decision tree performs classification for the DM types by using its advantages and avoiding its disadvantages. Somehow, there are various types of decision tree such as ID3, CD.5. While C4.5 uses gain ratio for splitting, ID3 uses information gain. In this paper, we use CART that is an alternative decision tree-building algorithm. CART can handle both classification and regression tasks, unlike other decision trees algorithms. This algorithm uses a metric named Gini index to create decision points for classification tasks.

MATERIAL AND METHOD

DM is the inability of the pancreas to produce sufficient levels of insulin hormone or the situation not to produce insulin hormone healthily. A classification problem deals with the diabetes status of patients who give medical and demographic information. This research uses the data titled as Pima Indian Diabetes taken from UCI Machine Learning Repository database site. Report of 500 healthy women and 268 diabetes women over 21-year-old exist in the dataset. The dataset includes 768 instances, eight input variables, and one output variable. The following describes the variables briefly.

- **The Number of Pregnancy:** The deficiency of insulin in pregnant women is higher than in non-pregnant women. The requirement of insulin increases after the first three months of pregnancy in diabetic pregnant women. To balance the increased deficiency of glucose and insulin in the organism is crucial for both mother and child in diabetic pregnant women.
- **Plasma Glucose Concentration a 2-h in Oral Glucose Tolerance:** The glucose tolerance test, also known as the oral glucose tolerance test, measures the reaction of the body for glucose and is used to diagnosis for type 2 diabetes.
- **Diastolic Blood Pressure:** Hypertension develops within a few years from the beginning of the disease in type 1 diabetes patients, usually as a symptom of diabetic nephropathy. It often exists at the time of diagnosis or even before the diagnosis in type 2 diabetes patients.
- **Triceps Skin Folds Thickness:** Skinfold thickness measurements aim to determine the size of the subcutaneous fat reservoir and to calculate the total body fat. These measures are associated with diabetes status directly.
- **2 h Serum Insulin:** The researches in the literature show the relationship between 2 h serum insulin and diabetes (McKeigue et al., 1991).
- **Body Mass Index:** The body mass index alone may not be a crucial parameter in the diagnosis of diabetes (Bays et al., 2007). However, it is meaningful if the other parameters consider it.
- **Diabetes Pedigree Function:** The researches show that there is a close relationship between diabetes pedigree history and diabetes condition of the individual (Deo et al., 2006).
- **Age:** The variable of age is also available as demographic information in the data set. The decision tree offers the opportunity to classify the DM types by considering variables.

CART

Decision Trees (DTs) is one of the supervised learning algorithms that is widely used in classification problems. Decision trees learn and train themselves from training data and predict the class label of new data. Decision trees work on both categorical and continuous input and output variables. x is the input variable, and y is the output variable known as classes in Eq (1). It is one of the most widely used and practical methods for inductive inference(Wang et al., 2011).

$$(x, Y) = (x_1, x_2, x_3, \ldots, Y) \tag{1}$$

Figure 1. Decision trees structure

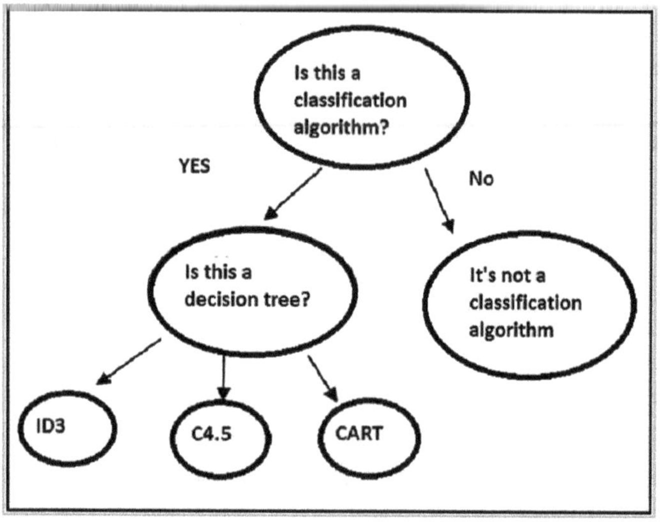

Each branch node represents a choice between several alternatives. Each leaf node represents a decision as seen in Figure 1. In DTs, there have been some measures that can help us in selecting the best choice such as entropy, gained information or Gini index (Quinlan, 1986). This research performs the CART algorithm because it is a newer algorithm by comparing it with other traditional decision trees and it is more suitable for a binary classification problem. The CART algorithm uses the Gini index to construct a decision tree (Han et al., 2011). Therefore, the researcher calls it a Gini algorithm. CART comprises the principle of dividing the tree into two branches from each decision node. The parent node is decided by considering the Gini index value. The Gini index value is the ratio of the objects in the data set. If the Gini value of the two objects is the same, the result distribution is the same (Rutkowski et al., 2014).

Let be *D* set of training tuples, the Gini value is obtained as follows (Han et al., 2011).

$$Gini(D) = 1 - \sum_{i=1}^{t} \left[\frac{C_{i,D}}{D} \right]^2 \tag{2}$$

In Equation (2),t denotes the number of class labels and $C_{i,D}$ denotes the number of the tuple in D belongs to *the* i^{th} class.

Attributes are a kind of parameter used to estimate the class of data. For instance, the foreign language level, graduation score, and resume are the main criteria for a job position. The prediction uses the attributes of the job to recruit a person. On the other hand, this research paper uses eight attributes to predict diabetes.

If the dataset has a binary split, there will be two different Gini index as D_1 and D_2 in each attribute A.

$$Gini_A(D) = \frac{|D_1|}{|D|} Gini(D_1) + \frac{|D_2|}{|D|} Gini(D_2) \tag{3}$$

This research chooses the attribute that has the maximum of the reduction in impurity as the splitting attribute (next parent node). Equation (4) provides the opportunity to get a reduction in impurity.

$$\Delta Gini(A) = Gini(D) - Gini_A(D) \tag{4}$$

GA-CART

If the tree architecture of decision trees includes all attributes, there may be inaccurate results for some samples in the test stage. Herewith, not every attribute requires a branching process when creating a decision tree. Otherwise, overfitting occurs, and this results in a decrease in the accuracy of the model.

The data are weighted before processing in the CART-GA approach, to meaningfully enhance the clearness in computations and the accuracy of the model as seen in Equation (5). In this approach, the data are updated with optimal weight values by GA. Then, the updated data are included in the decision tree model to set up the decision tree again.

$$(x, Y) = (w_1x_1, w_2x_2, w_3x_3, \ldots, Y) \tag{5}$$

The weight of each input is obtained using GA in the proposed CART-GA approach, while the weights of all input variables equal to 1 in the traditional decision tree algorithm. The acquired input weights are used to establish a decision tree.

When t and t + 1 stated the current iteration and the next iteration consecutively, the pseudocode of the proposed CART-GA approach is as seen in Table 2.

Table 2. The pseudo-code of CART-GA

```
Initialize initial weights ( w_0 )
t←1;
accuracy_(0) = 0;
While not_terminated() do
update data with w_i
configure the tree structure
accuracy_(t)←compute the model accuracy
improvement←accuracy_(t)- accuracy_(t-1)
generate w_i by ga
t←t+1;
end while
```

PERFORMANCE MEASURES

In classification problems, the crucial step in data preprocessing is to allocate dataset as training and test data. The most frequently used as validation methods are hold-out and k-cross-validation method.

The hold-out is a method that divides the dataset into two parts: training and testing. Classification models use the training data to produce outputs by using extracted rules in the testing dataset. Afterward, the model uses the testing data to interpret how healthy the training process continues. Many research articles choose the 80/20 ratio in the literature. The training and the testing process use 80% and 20% of the dataset in this research paper, respectively. It is also possible to see the ratios 70/30 and 60/40 in the literature (Crowther and Cox, 2005).

There is also a popular method called k-fold cross-validation. The k parameter states the number of parts separated into the data set. Parameter k provides to conduct the classification process up to its k value. The testing and training process allocate one different part and the rest (k-1) in each classification process to the testing and training, respectively. The average for the k-results provides the ultimate result of all classification process (Reitermanov, 2010).

The confusion matrix is a two by two table that contains four outcomes produced by a binary classifier. The confusion matrix derives various measures such as error-rate, accuracy, specificity, sensitivity, precision, and F-measure. Table 3 shows the structure of the confusion matrix.

Table 3. Confusion matrix

<table>
<tr><th></th><th colspan="4">Predicted Value</th></tr>
<tr><td rowspan="4">Actual Value</td><td></td><td>p</td><td>n</td><td>Total</td></tr>
<tr><td>p’</td><td>True Positive (TP)</td><td>False Negative (FP)</td><td>P’</td></tr>
<tr><td>n’</td><td>False Positive (FP)</td><td>True Negative (TN)</td><td>N’</td></tr>
<tr><td>Total</td><td>P</td><td>N</td><td></td></tr>
</table>

(Batista et al., 2004)

Several different measures are used to evaluate the performance of classification algorithms(Wang et al., 2011). The most popular measure is the accuracy rate of the classification model. The accuracy rate is the ratio of the number of true classified samples (TP + TN) to the total number of samples (TP + TN + FP + FN).

$$Accuracy = \frac{TP + TN}{TP + TN + FN + FP} \tag{6}$$

Precision is the ratio of the number of True Positives (TP) samples predicted as class 1 to the total number of samples (TP + FP) predicted as class 1.

$$Precision = \frac{TP}{TP + FP} \tag{7}$$

Sensitivity is the ratio of the number of correctly classified positive samples (TP) to the total number of positive samples (TP + FN).

$$Sensitivity = \frac{TP}{TP + FN} \tag{8}$$

Precision and sensitivity metrics alone are not enough to make a meaningful comparison in the application comprised of a few machine-learning algorithms. Both criteria together offer a better comparison to evaluate the results. Therefore, this research paper uses F-measure (F) to compare the algorithms. The F-criterion is the harmonic mean of the precision (P) and the sensitivity (S).

$$F\text{-}measure = \frac{2 * P * S}{P + S} \tag{9}$$

Specificity is described as the ratio of actual negatives, which got predicted as the negative (or true negative).

$$Specificity = \frac{TN}{\left(TN + FP\right)} \tag{10}$$

RESULTS

This research paper analyzes the CART-GA approach to the dataset of diabetes. The performance measures in the previous section are used to evaluate the performance of the proposed algorithms. The proposed approach s coded in Matlab 2018b. Performance measures are calculated separately in both test and training datasets. 80/20 split and 10-fold cross-validation methods are employed as a validation method because these are the most commonly used validation methods in the literature. Moreover, both validation methods calculate the performance measures again. It represents that the efficiency of classification is better during the precision value is close to 1. Experimental results show that the proposed hybrid CART-GA approach outperforms the CART algorithm in terms of performance measures by considering accuracy rate, sensitivity, precision, specificity, F-measure.

$$I = \frac{Accuracy_{CART-GA} - Accuracy_{CART}}{Accuracy_{CART}} \tag{11}$$

Traditional machine learning algorithms may present good results in training data, even in their simplest form because algorithms usually train the model with the training data. The improvements carried out in more or less all performance measures seen from Table 4-5 and are calculated as in Eq.11. Improvements more obviously appear in the test data. In this analysis, the traditional CART model presents a 90.42% and 92.07% accuracy rate for 80/20 split and 10-fold cross-validation, respectively. However, it will not perform the same in the test data. The accuracy rate increases 94% in the training data with the optimization of the CART algorithm with GA. According to these results, the improvements in both split and 10-fold validation methods are 4% and 3%, respectively. These ratios may not seem quite large, but as previously mentioned, the traditional CART method has already performed quite well.

Table 4. The performance measures of the conducted approaches for training data

Validation Method	%80 Training-%20 Test		10-Fold Cross	
Method	**CART**	**GA-CART**	**CART**	**GA-CART**
Accuracy	0.9042	**0.9414**	0.9207	**0.9493**
Precision	0.9429	**0.9501**	0.9427	**0.9711**
Sensitivity	0.9135	**0.9597**	0.934	**0.9521**
F-Measure	0.928	**0.9549**	0.9385	**0.9615**
Specificity	0.885	**0.9078**	0.8941	**0.944**

Table 5. The performance measures of the conducted approaches for test data

Validation Method	%80 Training-%20 Test		10-Fold Cross	
Method	**CART**	**GA-CART**	**CART**	**GA-CART**
Accuracy	0.6818	**0.9605**	0.7013	**0.9605**
Precision	0.7308	**0.9545**	0.78	**0.98**
Sensitivity	0.7835	**0.9767**	0.7647	**0.9608**
F-Measure	0.7562	**0.9655**	0.7723	**0.9703**
Specificity	0.5088	**0.9394**	0.5769	**0.96**

The investigation of the test data reveals the real performance of the model. GA determines weights, which are most suitable for the dataset, in the training data and form a proper tree structure in the GA-CART. Later, GA-CART applies the proper tree structure to the test data.

Precision shows what proportion of Positive Identifications is correct. While the CART algorithm alone provides 73.08% precision, the GA-CART algorithm improves the precision considerably, and it offers 95.45% precision in the split validation. This indicates that almost all of the data predicted as positive output is positive.

The precisions of GA-CART and CART algorithms equal to 98% and 78% in the 10-fold validation, respectively. This indicates that almost all of the data predicted as positive output is positive. Sensitivity, also known as recall, shows how accurate the proposed algorithm predicts positive situations. This indicates that the proposed algorithm predicts another proportion of actual positive situations incorrectly (the false negative).

While the sensitivity of the CART algorithm is 78.35%, the sensitivity of the GA-CART algorithm increases to 97.67% in the split validation. The sensitivity of the GA-CART algorithm equals to 96.08%, and the CART algorithm provides 76.47% the sensitivity in the 10-fold validation. The higher sensitivity means a higher value of the true positive and lower value of false negative. The healthcare sector desires high sensitivity because of its requisite importance.

Specificity is the proportion of people not suffering from the disease and it shows a correct prediction in terms of the ones not suffering from the disease. The positive state is the situation suffering from the disease unlike the logic in real life. While the CART algorithm alone obtains 50.88% specificity, the GA-CART algorithm improves the specificity and reaches 93.94% specificity in the split validation. Besides GA-CART and the CART algorithm find 96% and 57.69% specificity in the 10-fold validation, respectively. The proposed model provides higher sensitivity and specificity values compared to the traditional model. The F-measure value of the proposed model is expected to be higher because of higher sensitivity and specificity values.

Figure 2. The accuracy rates of the approaches for training data

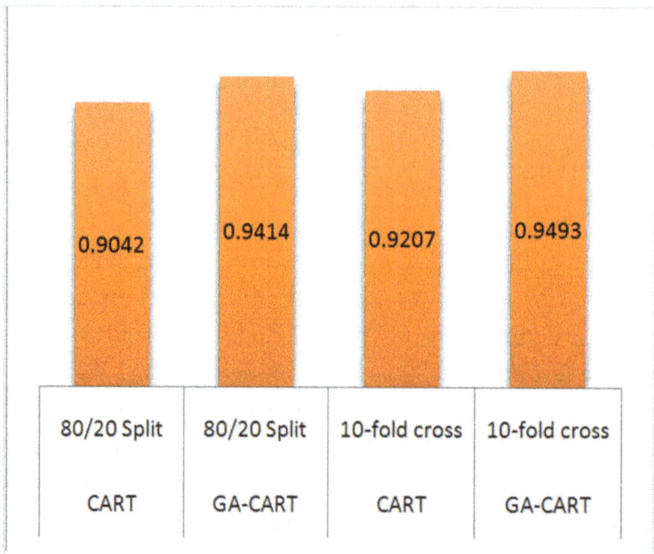

Figure 3. The accuracy rates of the approaches for test data

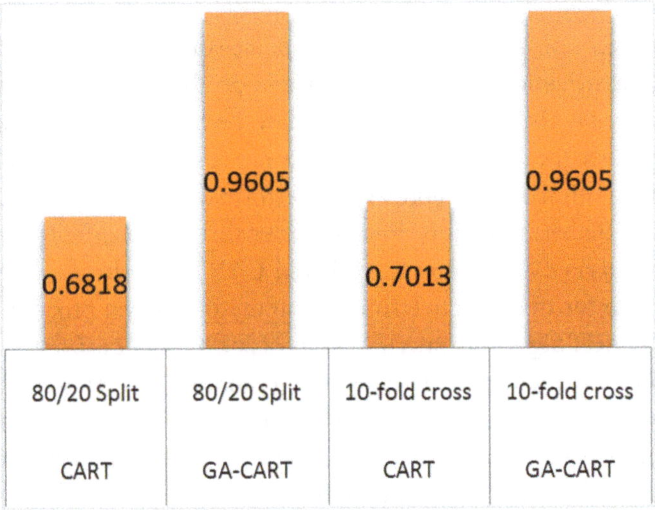

Table 6. Improvement in performance measurements

Dataset	Validation Method	Accuracy	Precision	Sensitivity	F-Measure	Specificity
Training	Split(80/20)	4.11%	0.76%	5.06%	2.90%	2.58%
	10-fold cross	3.11%	3.01%	1.94%	2.45%	5.58%
Test	Split(80/20)	**40.88%**	**30.61%**	24.66%	**27.68%**	**84.63%**
	10-fold cross	36.96%	25.64%	**25.64%**	25.64%	66.41%

The most common performance criterion is the accuracy rate in the literature. This research paper considers the accuracy rate of the objective function in the stage of generating weights with GA. The change in accuracy rate is important to evaluate the effectiveness of the proposed algorithm because of the objection function. The CART algorithm finds 68.18% and 70.13% accuracy rate in split validation and 10-fold validation methods, respectively. GA-CART algorithm finds a 96.05% accuracy rate in the split and 10-fold validation methods. Thus, the application of split and 10-cross validation provides 40.88% and 37% improvement, respectively. Table 6 presents the improvement rates in all other performance criteria.

CONCLUSION

This research paper aims to improve the performance of the CART algorithm because the accurate classification of diabetes depends on the algorithm efficiency. The CART is a common classification algorithm in the literature and it does not offer decent performance for this dataset. The paper proposes a hybrid model GA-CART because the integration of GA improves the performance of the CART algorithm for the diagnosis of diabetes mellitus. Precision, sensitivity, specificity and f-measure performance criteria evaluate GA-CART and CART algorithms. The paper uses the accuracy rate for the objective function in the prediction process by GA. The proposed GA-CART algorithm provides the best performance at 96.05%. The CART algorithm achieves to reach an improvement of almost 40% on accuracy rate.

Robust decisions are necessary to provide both accurate information and transform information into correct and useful inferences. This research paper uses Pima Indian diabetes dataset and the proposed algorithm obtains a decent classification performance in Pima Indian dataset.

Nowadays, machine learning has progressed further with deep learning. Its applicability seems to be quite reasonable especially in the field of health. Besides, deep learning has self-learning structures. For future research, the researcher may explore whether the effectiveness of deep learning can outweigh the effectiveness of machine learning algorithms in health researches.

REFERENCES

Batista, G. E., Prati, R. C., & Monard, M. C. (2004). A study of the behavior of several methods for balancing machine learning training data. ACM SIGKDD explorations newsletter, 6(1), 20-29.

Bays, H. E., Chapman, R. H., & Grandy, S.SHIELD Investigators' Group. (2007). The relationship of body mass index to diabetes mellitus, hypertension, and dyslipidaemia: Comparison of data from two national surveys. *International Journal of Clinical Practice*, *61*(5), 737–747. doi:10.1111/j.1742-1241.2007.01336.x PMID:17493087

Carpenter, G. A., & Markuzon, N. (1998). ARTMAP-IC and medical diagnosis: Instance counting and inconsistent cases. *Neural Networks*, *11*(2), 323–336. doi:10.1016/S0893-6080(97)00067-1 PMID:12662841

Chang, X., & Lilly, J. H. (2004). Evolutionary design of a fuzzy classifier from data. *IEEE Transactions on Systems, Man, and Cybernetics. Part B, Cybernetics*, *34*(4), 1894–1906. doi:10.1109/TSMCB.2004.831160 PMID:15462454

Crowther, P. S., & Cox, R. J. (2005, September). A method for optimal division of data sets for use in neural networks. *Proceedings International Conference on Knowledge-Based and Intelligent Information and Engineering Systems* (pp. 1-7). Berlin, Germany: Springer. 10.1007/11554028_1

Deo, S. S., Gore, S. D., Deobagkar, D. N., & Deobagkar, D. D. (2006). Study of inheritance of diabetes mellitus in Western Indian population by pedigree analysis. *JAPI*, *54*, 441–443. PMID:16909690

Devi, R. D. H., Bai, A., & Nagarajan, N. (2019). A Novel Hybrid Approach for Diagnosing Diabetes Mellitus using Farthest First and Support Vector Machine Algorithms. Obesity Medicine, 100152.

Ghazavi, S. N., & Liao, T. W. (2008). Medical data mining by fuzzy modeling with selected features. *Artificial Intelligence in Medicine*, *43*(3), 195–206. doi:10.1016/j.artmed.2008.04.004 PMID:18534831

Gonçalves, L. B., Vellasco, M. M. B. R., Pacheco, M. A. C., & de Souza, F. J. (2006). Inverted hierarchical neuro-fuzzy BSP system: A novel neuro-fuzzy model for pattern classification and rule extraction in databases. *IEEE Transactions on Systems, Man and Cybernetics. Part C, Applications and Reviews*, *36*(2), 236–248. doi:10.1109/TSMCC.2004.843220

Han, J., Pei, J., & Kamber, M. (2011). *Data mining: concepts and techniques*. Elsevier.

Isa, N. A. M., & Mamat, W. M. F. W. (2011). Clustered-hybrid multilayer perceptron network for pattern recognition application. *Applied Soft Computing*, *11*(1), 1457–1466. doi:10.1016/j.asoc.2010.04.017

Kahramanli, H., & Allahverdi, N. (2008). Design of a hybrid system for the diabetes and heart diseases. *Expert Systems with Applications*, *35*(1-2), 82–89. doi:10.1016/j.eswa.2007.06.004

Kannadasan, K., Edla, D. R., & Kuppili, V. (2018). *Type 2 diabetes data classification using stacked autoencoders in deep neural networks*. Clinical Epidemiology and Global Health.

Li, D. C., Liu, C. W., & Hu, S. C. (2011). A fuzzy-based data transformation for feature extraction to increase classification performance with small medical data sets. *Artificial Intelligence in Medicine*, *52*(1), 45–52. doi:10.1016/j.artmed.2011.02.001 PMID:21493051

Luukka, P. (2011). Feature selection using fuzzy entropy measures with similarity classifier. *Expert Systems with Applications*, *38*(4), 4600–4607. doi:10.1016/j.eswa.2010.09.133

Luukka, P., & Leppälampi, T. (2006). Similarity classifier with generalized mean applied to medical data. *Computers in Biology and Medicine*, *36*(9), 1026–1040. doi:10.1016/j.compbiomed.2005.05.008 PMID:16159657

McKeigue, P. M., Shah, B., & Marmot, M. G. (1991). Relation of central obesity and insulin resistance with high diabetes prevalence and cardiovascular risk in South Asians. *Lancet*, *337*(8738), 382–386. doi:10.1016/0140-6736(91)91164-P PMID:1671422

Polat, K., Güneş, S., & Arslan, A. (2008). A cascade learning system for classification of diabetes disease: Generalized discriminant analysis and least square support vector machine. *Expert Systems with Applications*, *34*(1), 482–487. doi:10.1016/j.eswa.2006.09.012

Quinlan, J. R. (1986). Induction of decision trees. *Machine Learning*, *1*(1), 81–106. doi:10.1007/BF00116251

Reitermanov, Z. (2010). Data splitting. *WDS'10 Proceedings of Contributed Papers, Part I,* 31–36.

Rutkowski, L., Jaworski, M., Pietruczuk, L., & Duda, P. (2014). The CART decision tree for mining data streams. *Information Sciences*, *266*, 1–15. doi:10.1016/j.ins.2013.12.060

Saeedi, P., Petersohn, I., Salpea, P., Malanda, B., Karuranga, S., Unwin, N., ... Shaw, J. E. (2019). WITHDRAWN: Global and regional diabetes prevalence estimates for 2019 and projections for 2030 and 2045: results from the International Diabetes Federation Diabetes Atlas. *Diabetes Research and Clinical Practice*. doi:10.1016/j.diabres.2019.107843 PMID:31518657

Samant, P., & Agarwal, R. (2018). Machine learning techniques for medical diagnosis of diabetes using iris images. *Computer Methods and Programs in Biomedicine*, *157*, 121–128. doi:10.1016/j.cmpb.2018.01.004 PMID:29477420

Seera, M., & Lim, C. P. (2014). A hybrid intelligent system for medical data classification. *Expert Systems with Applications*, *41*(5), 2239–2249. doi:10.1016/j.eswa.2013.09.022

Shen, L., Chen, H., Yu, Z., Kang, W., Zhang, B., Li, H., ... Liu, D. (2016). Evolving support vector machines using fruit fly optimization for medical data classification. *Knowledge-Based Systems*, *96*, 61–75. doi:10.1016/j.knosys.2016.01.002

Sisodia, D., & Sisodia, D. S. (2018). Prediction of diabetes using classification algorithms. *Procedia Computer Science*, *132*, 1578–1585. doi:10.1016/j.procs.2018.05.122

Srinivasa, K. G., Venugopal, K. R., & Patnaik, L. M. (2007). A self-adaptive migration model genetic algorithm for data mining applications. *Information Sciences*, *177*(20), 4295–4313. doi:10.1016/j.ins.2007.05.008

Swapna, G., Vinayakumar, R., & Soman, K. P. (2018). Diabetes detection using deep learning algorithms. *ICT Express*, *4*(4), 243–246. doi:10.1016/j.icte.2018.10.005

Wang, Y., Chen, W., Zhang, J., Dong, T., Shan, G., & Chi, X. (2011). Efficient volume exploration using the gaussian mixture model. *IEEE Transactions on Visualization and Computer Graphics*, *17*(11), 1560–1573. doi:10.1109/TVCG.2011.97 PMID:21670489

Chapter 6
Machine Learning Applications for Classification Emergency and Non-Emergency Patients

Zeynel Abidin Çil
https://orcid.org/0000-0002-7270-9321
İzmir Demokrasi University, Turkey

Abdullah Caliskan
https://orcid.org/0000-0002-9265-6335
Iskenderun Technical University, Turkey

ABSTRACT

Emergency departments of hospitals are busy. In recent years, patient arrivals have significantly risen at emergency departments in Turkey like other countries in the world. The main important features of emergency services are uninterrupted service, providing services in a short time, and priority to emergency patients. However, patients who do not need immediate treatment can sometimes apply to this department due to several reasons like working time and short waiting time. This situation can reduce efficiency and effectiveness at emergency departments. On the other hand, computers solve complex classification problems by using machine learning methods. The methods have a wide range of applications, such as computational biology and computer vision. Therefore, classification of emergency and non-emergency patients is vital to increase productivity of the department. This chapter tries to find the best classifier for detection of emergency patients by utilizing a data set.

DOI: 10.4018/978-1-7998-2581-4.ch006

INTRODUCTION

The healthcare management system encounters some difficulties since demand has increased significantly in recent years. The primary purpose of the efficient healthcare management system is to improve quality, to reduce total cost, and increase the satisfaction of patients. One of the main problems in the hospital is to manage emergency departments (ED) because it has a highly dynamic structure. The ED encounters high patients demand during peak hours because the ED is more complex and uncertain than other units of hospitals. Therefore, prolonged waiting times in the department lead to dissatisfaction with patients (Gul & Guneri, 2012.; Xu, Wong, & Chin, 2013). One of the primary purposes in the ED is to minimize the waiting time of patients. Therefore, the patients must be classified according to non-emergency and emergency patients to reduce the waiting time because non-emergency patients cause to increase in the total number of patients significantly and waiting times of emergency patients. In this way, non-emergency patients can be forward to another unit of the hospital using this classification.

Concerning healthcare management literature, Wrenn, Jones, Lanaghan, Congdon, & Aronsky (2005) provide an artificial neural network to forecast the length of ED stay of patients. The data feature contains several variables form age to laboratory exams. Gul & Guneri (2012) work a computer simulation of an ED in a hospital to develop a resource utilization rate to decrease patient waiting time. Li, Tian, Liu, Shu, & Liang (2013) present a type of neural network to build a prediction model to estimate the length of hospital stay. In their case, data contains 921 patients, and the model gives 80% accuracy. On the other hand, Xu et al. (2013) are also interested in the classification of emergency and non-emergency patients. They use an artificial neural network to model the problem, and it is compared with the non-linear least square regression (NLLSR) and multiple linear regression (MLR) in terms of mean average percentage error. Gul and Guneri (2015a) provide a model to estimate the length of ED stays in hospitals with the use of an artificial neural network technique. The model is built based on ED medical personnel. The data includes 1500 ED patients with 21 features, such as categorical and numerical variables. A recent review paper by Gül & Güneri (2015b) can be analyzed for detail information about healthcare management about applications for regular and disaster conditions.

Machine learning methods are efficient tools which can improve diagnostic accuracy in several diseases (Bala & Goyal, 1998; Baştürk, Badem, Caliskan, & Yüksel, 2019; Caliskan & Yuksel, 2017; Safavian & Landgrebe, 1990; Tomioka, Aihara, & Müller, 2007). Compared to sophisticated diagnoses techniques which required highly educated experts, machine learning methods are a very affordable and useful tool to support experts (Bishop, 2006; Çetin, Temurtaş, & Gülgönül, 2015, Caliskan 2017). Therefore, machine learning methods can be used in any country where people cannot reach suitable medical services. On the other hand, these techniques can be used all over the world to help experts whose number is minimal.

In light of the literature mentioned above, the purpose of this study is to classify emergency and non-emergency patients using machine learning methods, including decision tree (DT), support vector machines (SVM), K-nearest neighbour algorithm (KNN) and logistic regression (LR). The data is obtained from Gül & Güneri (2015a). Although original data contains 1500 samples, there is a significant imbalance between the emergency and non-emergency classes. The equal number of data is selected for each class to eliminate imbalance data. In the end, the data set has 22 features with 368 samples and two classes.

The rest of the paper is organized as follows. In Section 2, the machine learning methods and performance metrics are proposed. In Section 3, the computational study is presented to compare the performance of the proposed methods. Conclusions, directions for future research and managerial impacts are argued in the last section.

METHOD

Computers are utilized to solve complex classification problems by using machine learning methods, which are beneficial and practical techniques. Machine learning methods have a wide range of applications, computational biology, natural language processing, computer vision, signal classification, and so on (Caliskan, Badem, Basturk, & Yuksel, 2017; Caliskan, Yuksel, Badem, & Basturk, 2017; LeCun, Bengio, & Hinton, 2015). One of the most critical advantages of machine learning methods is not necessarily being explicitly programmed. Since, they generally have black-box models, which attempts to learn connections and relations between input and output data.

There exist several machine learning techniques to classify a data set, such as SVM and DT. These methods have more or less some drawbacks over each other. Unfortunately, there is not a systematic way to decide which method is more successful than another for classification problems. However, there is an opportunity to gain the practical ability to quickly and powerfully apply these methods into new problems (Caliskan 2017).

Classification Problem

Classification is utilized in many areas of science and industrial applications (Bishop, 2006; Boser, Guyon, & Vapnik, 1992; Fan, Chang, Hsieh, Wang, & Lin, 2008; Xu et al., 2013). The classification problem is to determine the class of a new observation using a historical data set (Bishop, 2006). For example, the classification is used to estimate the probability of a second heart attack of a patient who has had a heart attack before based on some clinical findings. If there is a high possibility of a second heart attack, the patient can be kept under observation. In another example, classification can be used to determine the diagnosis of diabetes or to predict whether the patient will have diabetes within a few years by looking at the patient's age, weight, blood sugar levels, and so on (Caliskan 2017).

Classification is a standard set of basic sciences such as statistics, artificial intelligence, machine learning methods, and data mining. Although the classification is considered from different perspectives in each of these disciplines, they all serve the same purpose. Classification is the process of labelling elements in a given data set according to their properties. For example, different types of fruits may be labelled according to their appearance, colour, taste and many more features. As another example, it is possible to determine whether the person sees a real face or a meaningless face from the MEG signals. (Caliskan, et al., 2017).

An appropriate model is created using a classifier based on the available data (Bishop, 2006; Gul & Guneri, 2012). While certain classifiers are customized to differentiate different classes according to their statistical characteristics, some are designed to find a sample based on an example. All classifiers are designed to provide a good understanding of the relationship between the input and output of the data set (Bishop, 2006; Gul & Guneri, 2012).

Preliminary Operations on Raw Data

Raw data obtained from a process, model, or patient is often unsuitable for sending directly to the classifier. Therefore, the data must be pre-processed before sending the classifier (Bishop, 2006; Gul & Guneri, 2012). These operations consist mainly of three steps. The first of these steps is dimension reduction, the second is the calculation of the Z-score, and the last one is normalization. The order of these steps may vary depending on the classifier. For example, in most of dimension reduction techniques, the Z-score of the data is calculated if necessary and then normalization is performed. The aim of calculating the Z-score is to provide a coherent comparison between the scores by showing how many units deviate from the average of the scores taken on any scale or test. For example, a data set with two attributes called A and B is considered. One of these features change between -200 and 200 for A, and between -0.1 and 0.1 for B. A reasonable result is often not possible with these two attributes because value ranges of the features are very different. However, the two features have numerical values ranging from approximately -3 to 3 using Z-score. It is seen from Figure 1, the numerical values of the two features are close to each other. Also, the Z-score is calculated according to the standard normal distribution whose mean value is 0, and the standard deviation is 1. The purpose of this process is to better handle the information into the classifier (Caliskan 2017).

Figure 1. Status of A and B feature after calculating Z-scores

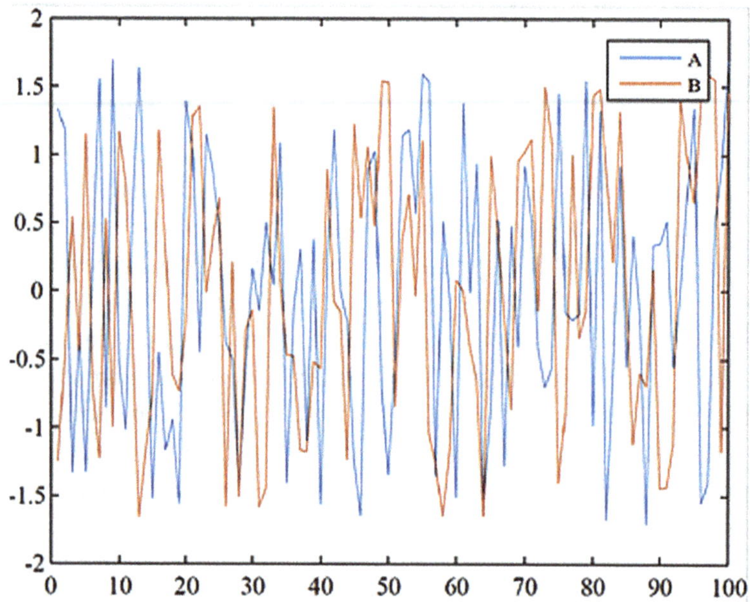

The normalization process allows adjustment of the available data to a certain value range. This is necessary to maintain the balance between the features of the data. If the data is applied directly to the classifier without the normalization process, the results are unlikely to be as expected.

Classifiers

In this chapter, the authors try to find the best classifier for the detection of the emergency patient by utilizing a data collected by Gül & Güneri (2015a). The data set has 22 features, with 368 samples and 2 classes. Of these samples, 184 samples were emergencies, and the remaining samples were non-emergency situations. The input of the data set structured as follows:

$$X = \left[x_1 x_2 x_3 \ldots x_n \right] \tag{1}$$

where $x_1, x_2, x_3 \ldots x_n$ feature vectors with m dimensional. In our case $n = 22, m = 368$. The output of the data set can be given as:

$$y = \left[y_1 y_2 y_3 \cdots y_m\right]^T \tag{2}$$

where y_1, y_2, y_3 *and* y_m are labels related to each input samples and *T* shows transpose of a vector **y**. In our case y_i can be $0\, or\, 1$.

The data set is generally divided into two sections, training data set $\{X_{train}, y_{train}\}$ and testing data set $\{X_{test}, y_{test}\}$ which are structured as X and y defined in Equation 1 and 2, respectively. The classification of a data set is achieved by utilizing a model whose parameters tuned by an appropriate technique.

The main framework in classification problem can be summarized in Figures 2 and 3. In Figure 2, the training process of a model attempts to decrease the total error between and . In Figure 3, the performance of the trained model is measured by the testing data set. The output of the trained model is compared with by using some metrics, such as accuracy, sensitivity, and specificity.

Classification is an essential procedure for every field in science. The different kinds of classifiers are proposed to separate different objects or situations concerning some attributes related to these objects or situations (Bishop, 2006). For example, a classifier can be designed to detect cats and dogs from pictures by using pixels as attributes or features. There are several classifiers designed for different aims and data sets. The most common classifiers are support vector machine (SVM), decision tree (DT), logistic regression (LR) and k-nearest neighbor algorithm (KNN).

Figure 2. Training Process of a Model

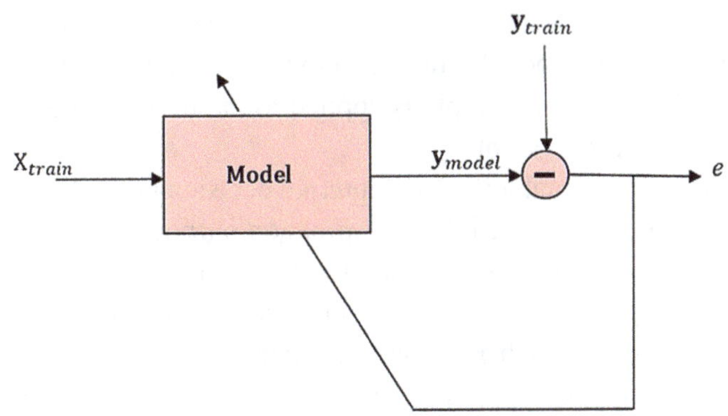

Figure 3. Testing process of a model

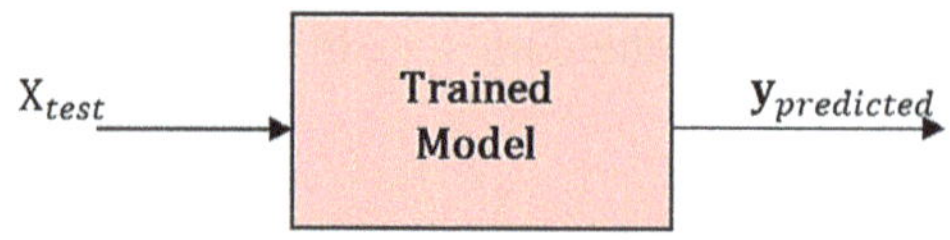

Support Vector Machine (SVM)

SVM is used to solve many classification problems in both industrial and academic fields. SVM is one of the most important classifiers. It produces the suitable hyperplanes that separates two classes by maximizing distances between two classes of samples. The aim of SVM is to differentiate the classes of data with optimal hyperplanes. A designed objective function, which control the location of the hyperplanes in a space, is handled in order to find local minimum of this function. Hyperplanes can be selected as the linear kernel for data sets that can be separated linearly. On the other hand, thanks to the flexible structure of the SVM, the hyperplanes can also be selected in a non-linear kernel provided that the data set is not linear. The location and shape of hyperplanes are evaluated by using an appropriate optimization technique concerning data samples. The optimum line shape can be chosen for the nature of the data sets. Having this feature makes SVM a fast and practical method for different kind of data set (Suykens & Vandewalle, 1999).

Decision Tree (DT)

There are different types of DT based classifiers, which use a model based on tree structures (Safavian & Landgrebe, 1990). The tree structure is based on if-then rules. The structure is divided into various branches based on features. Each branch is ended with a leaf node. The main aim of DT evaluates the optimum path from roots to Leaf Nodes by using if-then rules. In other words, a model is formed according to the training data in the form of a tree structure consisting of decision nodes and leaf nodes. In overall, this model is designed to learn the relationship between data input and label. When a new sample is applied to the trained model, it is easy to determine the class of this sample.

DT consisting of terminal leaves and internal decision nodes has a hierarchical structure. If the DT is to be used for classification purposes, each leaf represents a class. However, if the DT is to be used for regression purposes, the leaves are customized to carry fixed numbers. The input vector is defined as . In the canonical constant binary DT model, each decision node is applied to to select the next subtree. is a binary tree structure created by a subtree with a root of m. and will have two outputs as defined in the following equation to represent the right and left subtree designed.

$$F_m(x) = \begin{cases} F_m^L(x) & if\ g_m(x) > 0 \\ F_m^R(x) & otherwise \end{cases}.$$

In response to an input sent from the root node, each internal node is divided into two branches. This process continues recursively until a leaf node encounters a class. The architecture in which DT is constructed depends on how $g_m(x)$ is selected. These architectures are modified according to the nature of the data in order to generate to more effective results. The major disadvantage of DT is that it cannot be used effectively in over-learning problems. Besides, the DT does not perform well on large scale data sets. Worse classification performance can be observed when there are too many differences in the number of instances of classes in the discriminant data (Caliskan 2017).

K-Nearest Neighbours Algorithm (KNN)

KNN is one of the oldest classification methods, and also it is a well-known classifier. It measures distances of samples to each other. It is often preferred because it is extremely fast and easily applied to many problems. The classification process is carried out by deciding which class belongs to a sample by using a group of data sets with certain classes. For example, when a new sample is added in the training data, the class of new members is decided by using the following steps: *(i)* if the nearest *k* neighbour of the new sample is a member of the same group, the new sample will be included the same group. (Bala & Goyal, 1998).

The distances between the samples are calculated based on lengths Euclid, Hamming and so on. The classification performance of the KNN algorithm depends on the distance method and the number of neighbours. In Figure 4, the KNN is summarized in more detail. According to Figure 4, two classes, one marked in red and one in green are shown. Two new samples marked with blue and black are added to the data set. The blue element is included in the red because the location of the nearest three (k = 3) neighbours is closer to the red group. On the other hand, the black sample is included in the group of greens since it is closer to the greens neighbours (Caliskan 2017).

Figure 4. KNN algorithm sample representation

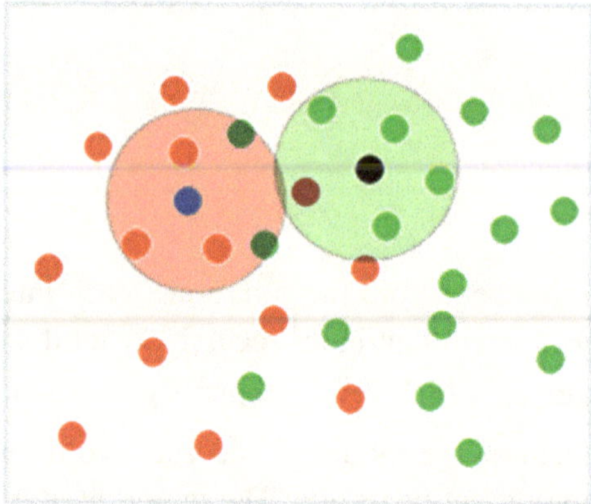

Logistic Regression (LR)

LR is a classifier model that uses a similar technique with linear regression. It proposes a model that learns the hierarchy between input and output of the data set. The model tries to decrease the error between the output of the model and labels by using a convenient optimization algorithm such as gradient descent (Tomioka et al., 2007). LR is an essential and efficient classifier for linearly separable data sets. LR attempts to learn the hierarchy between n dimensional m input feature column vectors ($x_1, x_2, \ldots, x_m$) and m scaler labels $(y_1, y_2, \ldots, y_m)$ and $y \in \{0,1\}$. Following equation is minimized in order to make a connection between the input vectors and output labels.

$$J(\theta) = \frac{1}{m}\sum_{i=1}^{m}\left[-y_i \log\left(h_\theta\left(x_i\right)\right) - \left(1 - y_i\right)\log\left(1 - h_\theta\left(x_i\right)\right)\right]$$

$J(\theta)$ is a function, which depends on $\theta = \left[\theta_0 \theta_1 \ldots \theta_n\right]^T$. $h_\theta(x)$ is known as logistic regression hypothesis, which given as:

$$h_\theta(x) = g\left(\theta^T x\right)$$

where g is a sigmoid activation function. This activation function can be defined as:

$$g(z) = \frac{1}{1+e^{-z}}$$

As z approaches to positive infinite, the output of the function approaches one. As z approaches to negative infinite, the output of the function approaches zero. Therefore, the output of the sigmoid function is between zero and one. Logistic regression is not useful for large data sets with a high number of features (for example 100). It makes that the optimization process becomes more complicated. Because LR is not efficient to learn nonlinear relationships among the features, however, LR can classify the data set, which is linearly separable and has a low or moderate dimension.

Evaluating a Classifier

The descriptions of the most common performance evaluators (Gul & Guneri, 2012) are given as follows:

If the situation of a patient is a proven emergency, the model also indicates the presence of the emergency, the results of the model are considered true positive (TP). Similarly, if a situation of a patient is not proven emergency, the model suggests the presence of not emergency as well, the model result is true negative (TN). Both TP and TN indicate a consistent result between the model and the reel condition.

However, no model is perfect to learn the relationship between input and output. If the model indicates the presence of an emergency patient whose situation is not an emergency, the model result is false positive (FP). Similarly, if the model suggests that the emergency is absent for a patient with an emergency for sure, the model result is a false negative (FN). Both FP and FN indicate that the model results are opposite to the reel condition.

1. **Accuracy** is the ratio of correct prediction performed by a model in Equation (3). It is defined as follows:

$$Accuracy = \frac{TN + TP}{TN + TP + FN + FP} \tag{3}$$

2. **Sensitivity** also is known as recall which measures how much a model can detect emergency situations in Equation (4).

$$Sensitivity = \frac{TP}{TP + FN} \tag{4}$$

3. **Specificity** measures how much a model can detect no emergencies.

$$Specificity = \frac{TN}{TN + FP} \tag{5}$$

4. **Precision** is the ratio of predicted positive examples which are emergencies.

$$Precision = \frac{TP}{TP + FP} \tag{6}$$

5. **F-measure** is the harmonic mean of precision and sensitivity [1].

$$F\text{-}measure = \frac{Sensitivity * Precision}{Sensitivity + Precision} \tag{7}$$

6. **G-mean** is the geometric mean of specificity and sensitivity [1]

$$G\text{-}mean = \sqrt{(specificity * sensitivity)} \tag{8}$$

In addition to these performance metrics, A receiver operating characteristic curve, or ROC curve demonstrates the performance of a classifier.

Cross-Validation Technique

Different methods are available to measure the performance of the classifier. In the most basic of these methods, data is divided into two parts as training and testing. Usually, 70% of the data set is organized for training and 30% of the data set is used for testing. In the second method, the data set is divided into three parts: training, validation, and testing. A classifier is trained with training data set. The performance of the classifier is checked with the validation set. Whenever the difference between the classification performances of the training set and the validation data set begins to unfold, the training is stopped at that time. After that, the performance of the classifier is measured by using test data. In this process, 70% of the data set is usually used for training, 15% of the data set for validation and the remaining 15% of the data set is used for testing the classifier. However, all classifiers are not suitable for this method.

The cross-validation technique is useful to validate the proposed model. The cross-validation technique prevents disadvantages due to tests or training data distributions. Since, in some cases, challenging samples can be used in training sets. Therefore, this may make the proposed classifier seems better or worse than it is. In Figure 5, 10 cross-validation technique is summarized. The data set is divided into 10 parts, one of them is used as the test part, the remain parts are utilized to train the classifiers. After the training process, the test part is used to evaluate the classifier performance for the first part. This process is repeated until each part is used as the test part. The obtained accuracy rate from each part is averaged to find the classifier performance. The same procedure can be applied to the other evaluations' metrics, including sensitivity, specificity, precision, F-measure, and G-mean.

Figure 5. Cross-validation technique

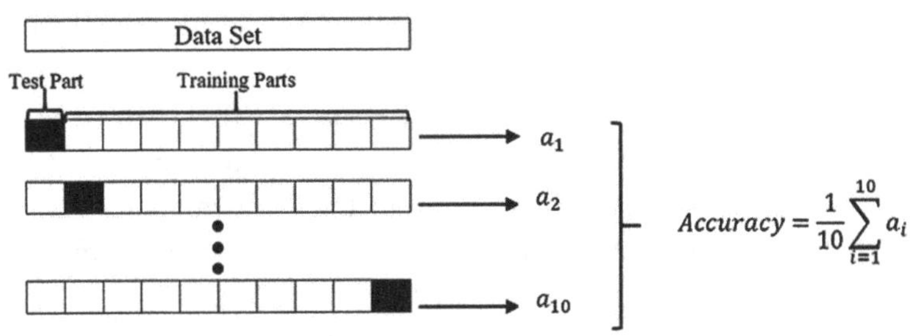

EXPERIMENTAL RESULTS AND DISCUSSIONS

In this chapter, four different classifier models are introduced to determine emergency by utilizing a data set. Several experiments have been conducted to verify the efficacy of these frameworks in terms of eight performance metrics, including, accuracy, sensitivity, specificity, precision, F-measure, g-mean and AUC. For sake of fair comparison, the simulations are repeated 30 times with 10 cross-validation technique to reveal the performance of the classifiers on the emergency data set.

The comparison results can be seen in Table 1. In overall, the DT outperforms other classifiers in terms of all metrics used in this chapter. Also, the KNN algorithm is the best performing algorithm after the DT algorithm. The performance of the SVM is relatively weak in this problem due to the nature of the data set, although it has superior performance in many classification problems.

In detail, the DT algorithm provides the highest sensitivity. It means that the probability of the positive test given that the emergency patients is 0.87 for DT classifier. In addition, specificity measures the rate of correctly identified non-emergency patients. Thus, the probability of the negative test given that the non-emergency situation is 0.76 for the DT classifier. On the other hand, the precision evaluates that the probability of the emergency given that the positive is 0.81 for the DT classifier. The DT is the best classifier in terms of all metrics; precision, sensitivity and specificity rates. Therefore, the DT can be used to detect an emergency.

In some cases, F-measure and G-mean are also essential metrics to measure the performance of the classifier because both metrics can measure the effect of sensitivity and precision. According to result, the DT algorithm has also better classification performance than KNN, SVM, and LR in terms of F-measure and G-mean.

In addition to these comments, Figure 6 provides a visual comparison of the DT, KNN, LR, and SVM concerning ROC (Receiver Operating Characteristics) curves. When the area under the curve is equal to one, the performance of the classifier approach is ideal, which predicts all labels without error. Figure 6 shows that the DT has the most significant area among the other classifiers. The DT has superior performance to predict both emergency satiation and non-emergency patients.

The confusion matrix shows some numerical results for all classifiers. We can observe the behaviour of the DT, KNN, LR and SVM classifiers by using the confusion matrix from Figure 7. We know that the total true value (emergency patients) is 164. 124 out of 164 samples are detected as emergencies and remain 40 samples are detected as non-emergency patients, which are emergencies. Similarly, we know that total false value (non-emergency patients) 204. 171 out of 204 samples are detected as non-emergency situations, and other 33 samples are detected as emergency patients, which are non-emergencies. Compared to SVM, KNN, and LR, we observe from figure 7 that the DT has an efficient ability to detect emergency and non-emergency patients. On the other hand, SVM is successful in identifying emergencies patients, but non-emergency patients cannot be detected effectively.

Table 1. Comparison performance of DT, KNN, LR and SVM in terms of different performance metrics

	Accuracy	Sensitivity	Specificity	Precision	F-Measure	Gmean	AUC
DT	**0.82**	**0.87**	**0.76**	**0.82**	**0.84**	**0.81**	**0.81**
KNN	0.66	0.72	0.59	0.69	0.7	0.65	0.66
LR	0.58	0.52	0.65	0.65	0.58	0.58	0.59
SVM	0.57	0.43	0.76	0.69	0.53	0.57	0.6

Figure 6. Receiver Operating Characteristics of DT, KNN, LR and SVM classifiers

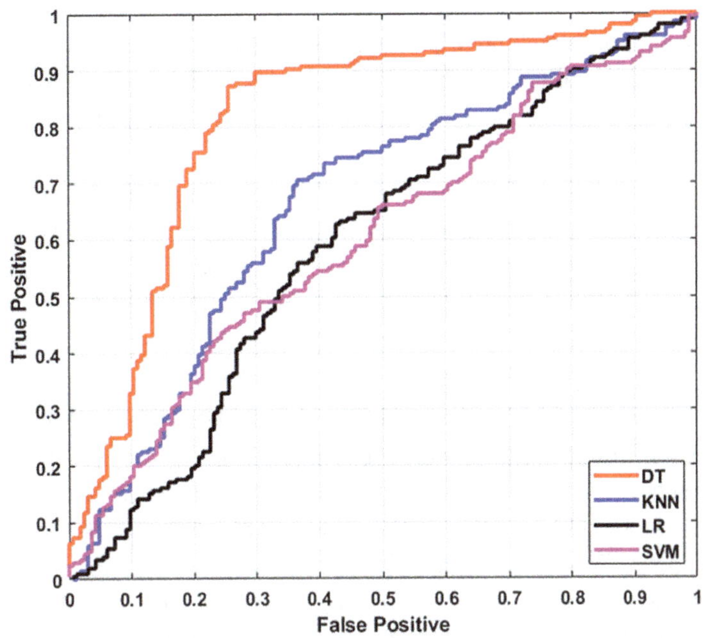

Figure 7. Confusion matrix of DT, KNN, LR and SVM classifiers

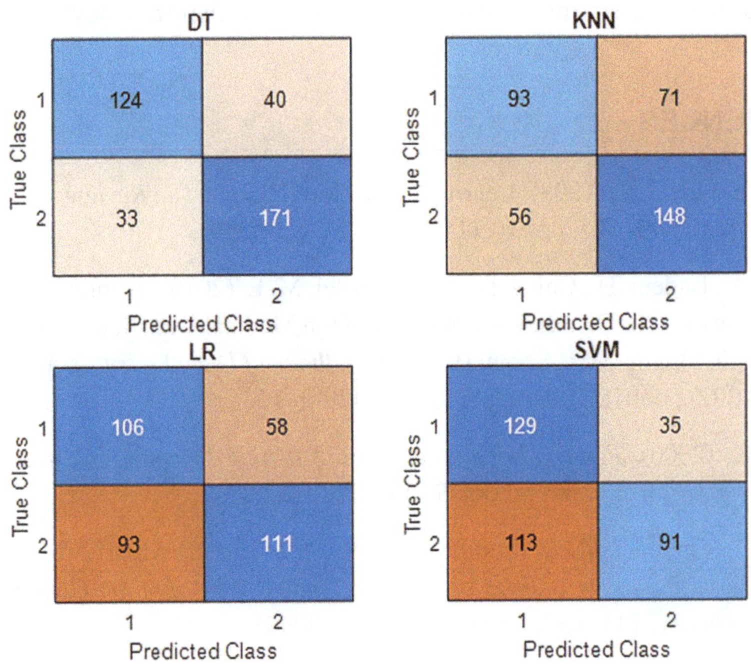

CONCLUSION

Machine learning techniques have been applied to a large number of areas from varied from computational biology to computer vision. All of the mentioned classifiers are designed to handle even the most complex data sets. Different solutions are proposed so that each of these methods can be used in all kinds of data sets. For example, classification performance may be improved in selecting different cores in SVM, changing the number of neighbourhoods or choosing the method of calculating the distance between samples in KNN, using different models in DT according to the nature of the data. However, despite all these measures, a classifier does not show the same performance in different data sets. Notably, the classification performance of traditional methods can decrease significantly when the size of the data and the number of samples are increased. In this paper, different machine learning techniques are used to determine emergency and non-emergency patients in the ED department in the hospital because non-emergency patients can cause to increase waiting length of patient stay and to reduce intervention time emergency patients. Considering all the reasons above, the classification of the patients applying to the ED department can be one of the vital problems in the healthcare management system. A case study obtained form Gul and Guneri (2015) is considered in the paper. The case includes 368 patients with 22 features. The DT provides a better result than SVM, LR, and KNN for detection emergency or non-emergency patients. As far as managerial impact is concerned, after the detection of non-emergency patients, they can be forward to another department in the hospital to increase the efficiency of the system.

REFERENCES

Bala, V., & Goyal, S. (1998). Learning from Neighbours. *The Review of Economic Studies*, *65*(3), 595–621. doi:10.1111/1467-937X.00059

Baştürk, A., Badem, H., Caliskan, A., & Yüksel, M. E. (2019). Application of Deep Neural Networks for Disease Diagnosis Through Medical Data Sets. In V. E. Balas, S. S. Roy, D. Sharma, & P. Samui (Eds.), *Handbook of Deep Learning Applications* (pp. 259–292)., doi:10.1007/978-3-030-11479-4_12

Bishop, C. (2006). *Pattern Recognition and Machine Learning*. Retrieved from https://www.springer.com/gp/book/9780387310732

Boser, B. E., Guyon, I. M., & Vapnik, V. N. (1992). A Training Algorithm for Optimal Margin Classifiers. *Proceedings of the Fifth Annual Workshop on Computational Learning Theory*, 144–152. 10.1145/130385.130401

Caliskan, A. (2017). *Derin sinir ağının sınıflandırma başarımının artırılması için yeni bir eğitim stratejisi geliştirilmesi ve biyomedikal veri setleri üzerinde test edilmesi*. Erciyes Üniversitesi Fen Bilimleri Enstitüsü Biyomedikal Mühendisliği Anabilim Dalı, Doktora Tezi.

Caliskan, A., Badem, H., Basturk, A., & Yuksel, M. E. (2017). Diagnosıs of the Parkınson dısease by usıng deep neural network classıfıer. *Istanbul University - Journal of Electrical and Electronics Engineering (Oradea)*, *17*(2), 3311–3318.

Caliskan, A., & Yuksel, M. E. (2017). Classification of coronary artery disease data sets by using a deep neural network. *The EuroBiotech Journal*, *1*(4), 271–277. doi:10.24190/ISSN2564-615X/2017/04.03

Caliskan, A., Yuksel, M. E., Badem, H., & Basturk, A. (2017). A Deep Neural Network Classifier for Decoding Human Brain Activity Based on Magnetoencephalography. *Elektronika ir Elektrotechnika*, *23*(2), 63–67. doi:10.5755/j01.eie.23.2.18002

Çetin, O., Temurtaş, F., & Gülgönül, Ş. (2015). An application of multilayer neural network on hepatitis disease diagnosis using approximations of sigmoid activation function. *Dicle Medical Journal / Dicle Tip Dergisi*, *42*(2). doi:10.5798/diclemedj.0921.2015.02.0550

Fan, R.-E., Chang, K.-W., Hsieh, C.-J., Wang, X.-R., & Lin, C.-J. (2008). LIBLINEAR: A Library for Large Linear Classification. *Journal of Machine Learning Research*, *9*(Aug), 1871–1874.

Gul, M., & Guneri, A. F. (2012). *A computer sımulatıon model to reduce patıent length of stay and to ımprove resource utılızatıon rate ın an emergency department servıce system*. 12.

Gül, M., & Güneri, A. F. (2015a). Forecastıng patıent length of stay ın an emergency department by artıfıcıal neural networks. *Journal of Aeronautics and Space Technologies*, *8*(2), 43–48.

Gül, M., & Güneri, A. F. (2015b). A comprehensive review of emergency department simulation applications for normal and disaster conditions. *Computers & Industrial Engineering*, *83*, 327–344. doi:10.1016/j.cie.2015.02.018

LeCun, Y., Bengio, Y., & Hinton, G. (2015). Deep Learning. *Nature*, *521*(7553), 436–444. doi:10.1038/nature14539 PMID:26017442

Li, J.-S., Tian, Y., Liu, Y.-F., Shu, T., & Liang, M.-H. (2013). Applying a BP Neural Network Model to Predict the Length of Hospital Stay. In G. Huang, X. Liu, J. He, F. Klawonn, & G. Yao (Eds.), Health Information Science (pp. 18–29). Berlin, Germany: Springer. doi:10.1007/978-3-642-37899-7_2

Safavian, S. R., & Landgrebe, D. A. (1990). *A Survey of Decision Tree Classifier Methodology*. Retrieved from https://books.google.com.tr/books?id=Y0G2SgAACAAJ

Suykens, J. A. K., & Vandewalle, J. (1999). Least Squares Support Vector Machine Classifiers. *Neural Processing Letters*, *9*(3), 293–300. doi:10.1023/A:1018628609742

Tomioka, R., Aihara, K., & Müller, K.-R. (2007). Logistic Regression for Single Trial EEG Classification. In B. Schölkopf, J. C. Platt, & T. Hoffman (Eds.), Advances in Neural Information Processing Systems, Retrieved from http://papers.nips.cc/paper/3134-logistic-regression-for-single-trial-eeg-classification.pdf

Wrenn, J., Jones, I., Lanaghan, K., Congdon, C. B., & Aronsky, D. (2005). Estimating patient's length of stay in the Emergency Department with an artificial neural network. *AMIA ... Annual Symposium Proceedings. AMIA Symposium*, *2005*, 1155–1155.

Xu, M., Wong, T. C., & Chin, K. S. (2013). Modeling daily patient arrivals at Emergency Department and quantifying the relative importance of contributing variables using artificial neural network. *Decision Support Systems*, *54*(3), 1488–1498. doi:10.1016/j.dss.2012.12.019

Chapter 7
Fuzzy Logic in Health Services:
Integrated Fuzzy Method for Multi-Criteria Inventory Classification

Nihan Kabadayi
Istanbul University, Turkey

Sündüs Dağ
Istanbul University, Turkey

ABSTRACT

Healthcare inventory management is a complex task which contains critical decision phases. One of the efficient ways of healthcare inventory management is to classify inventory items into predefined categories in terms of their significant features. This chapter proposes a guideline to healthcare decision makers to implement appropriate inventory control methods. The proposed method combines Fuzzy AHP (Analytical Hierarchy Process), TOPSIS (Technique for Order of Preference by Similarity to Ideal Solution) and ABC (Always Better Control) analysis methods to determine the priority of inventory items. The corresponding method, which takes into account multiple criteria in the classification of inventory items, cope with the limits of the classical ABC method. It also helps to reduce the uncertainty in the inventory classification problem as the proposed method is based on the fuzzy logic approach. A real-life case study is conducted in a hospital laboratory to test the proposed method.

DOI: 10.4018/978-1-7998-2581-4.ch007

INTRODUCTION

Nowadays, firms need to focus on their supply chain success in order to gain competitive advantage. Supply chain management is the organization of activities between independent companies; from raw material suppliers to the end customers. The main objective of supply chain management is to decrease total supply chain costs while increasing the customer service level. Both inventory and distribution costs are the major costs in the supply chain. It is important to have a well-managed inventory and distribution system to minimize the total costs of supply chain.

Hospitals are one of the most crucial institutions offering health services to the public. The primary purpose of hospitals is to provide the highest-quality healthcare services using their resources effectively and efficiently. Healthcare supply chain management is an important tool to control healthcare costs and improve the service quality in healthcare. According to the results of Kwon et al. (2016), the logistics costs in healthcare accounted for 38% of total costs, while it is 5% in the retail industry and 2% in the electronics industry. One of the reasons for the high logistics costs in healthcare is the lack of successful healthcare supply chain management applications.

The purpose of hospital inventory management is to minimize the cost of inventory while ensuring that necessary medicines and health supplies are available when needed. The inventory management department is responsible for efficient use of drugs and medical supplies, which are important resources of hospitals. However, hospital inventory management is a complex task due to the wide variety of inventory items and the availability of inventory items with different levels of importance. For this reason, it needs to be considered systematically.

Inventory classification is one of the effective ways to manage hospital inventory. Traditional ABC analysis is a well-known and useful method for inventory classification. However, this method classifies inventory items only in terms of one criterion: mostly annual usage values of inventory items. This is not enough for obtaining accurate classification of inventory items in practice. The ABC classification method is significantly affected by other criteria such as inventory holding unit cost, criticality, lead time, substitutability, scarcity, and durability. Therefore, traditional classification cannot give reliable results (Guvenir & Erel, 1998, p. 30). Based on the type and attribute of the company, the number of criteria, which are needed in order to manage inventory items, can vary. In the food industry, for example, expiry date may be the most important criterion in deciding importance of inventory items. On the other hand, in the health sector, lead time may be the most critical criterion due to the human life. For this reason, more than one evaluating criterion should be considered to classify or rank inventory items. Analyzing the criteria in multi-criteria context may improve inventory management and contribute toward the productivity of the company.

This chapter is organized as follows: Firstly, a brief overview on the literature dealing with the main approaches to the multi-criteria inventory classification problem is presented. Secondly, under the main topic of the chapter, importance of the healthcare supply chain management and inventory management are emphasized. Thirdly, the solution methodology, which contains both the Fuzzy AHP and TOPSIS methods, is described. Finally, future research directions and conclusions were discussed.

BACKGROUND

In the literature, multi-criteria inventory classification is considered in different ways. Classification of inventory items according to their cost and vital importance using the ABC and VED analyses is generally studied in the related literature. The ABC-VED analysis, which classifies inventory items according to the cost and vital importance criteria, is the most studied method in the related literature. Yeşilyurt et al. (2015) proposed a stock classification method, which is based on the ABC-VED analysis for a state hospital in Turkey. According to the findings, they pointed out that monitoring and analyzing medical materials and drugs have a significant role in order to manage hospital costs. Kumar and Chakravarty (2015) showed the benefit of the inventory classifying techniques in a tertiary care hospital using the ABC-VED analysis. Millstein et al. (2014) developed an ABC analysis method, which optimized the number of inventory groups according to their service level and stock-keeping units. Antonoglou et al. (2017) conducted an ABC-VED analysis in a military hospital to highlight the most crucial medical-technological items. Fitriana et al. (2018) applied the ABC-VED method in the pharmacy store of veterinary hospital, Indonesia. They showed the main principle of effective inventory management. Also, they provided information on decision making in purchasing and distributing specific drug items.

Guvenir and Erel (1998) presented a model based on the genetic algorithm to learn criteria weight vector and cut-off points between groups A and B and groups B and C. Partovi and Anandarajan (2002) applied an artificial neural network for the ABC classification of inventory items in a pharmaceutical company. Two learning methods, the back propagation and genetic algorithms, were utilized. The results were compared with the multiple discriminate analyses. Tsai and Yeh (2008) proposed a particle swarm optimization approach for the inventory classification problem. A speciðc objective and multiple objectives were used to classify inventory items in this model.

Ng (2007) improved a simple and useful model for multi-criteria inventory classiðcation that is named as Ng-model in this study. Zhou and Fan (2007) extended the R-model for multi-criteria inventory classiðcation that is referred to as ZF-model. Park et al. (2014) suggested a cross-evaluation-based weighted linear optimization model for multi-criteria inventory classiðcation. Hadi-Vencheh (2010) extended the Ng-model and used the weighted linear optimization model for multi-criteria classification of inventory items. This model does not only associate multi-criteria but also moves the effect of weights to the final solution.

Some studies also consider multiple criteria in order to classify inventory items. Firstly, Flores and Whybark (1986) suggested some extensions to the traditional ABC analysis. They used the joint criteria matrix for only two criteria, but there is no way with their methods to extend the method to more than two criteria. Then, Cohen and Ernst (1988) advised the cluster analysis method to group similar items.

The multi-criteria decision-making methods (MCDM) such as AHP, TOPSIS, and ANP were applied to solve multi-criteria inventory classification problems. These methods provide opportunity to take into accounts both qualitative and quantitative criteria. Ramanathan (2006) advised a basic ABC-based classiðcation model using weighted linear optimization that is referred to as R-model. The proposed model is easy to implement and can be easily understood by the inventory staff and managers. Partovi and Burton (1993) presented a model based on the AHP for multi-criteria inventory classification problems, and a real-life application was conducted. The results showed that the proposed model can improve the company's inventory control system. Ozdemir and Ozveri (2004) performed a multi-criteria ABC analysis using the AHP method for the inventory items of a generator company. According to the results of their study, it may be more advantageous for the firm to decide based on the AHP analysis, which takes into account the different criteria except for the cost and demand. The results were compared with each other in terms of the cost criterion. Tanrıverdi (2010) and Ertugrul (2013) applied the ABC and AHP methods for classifying inventory items in a textile company. They mentioned that using the AHP analysis for inventory classification is better than the classical ABC method when the total inventory costs considered. Cakir and Canbolat (2008) integrated inventory classification with fuzzy concepts and designed a new decision support system for inventory classification problem. They proposed the AHP method to prioritize the inventory classification criteria. Bhattacharya et al. (2007) used the distance-based multi-criteria framework based on the TOPSIS method for the ABC analysis. The proposed methodology is a significant tool for classifying items and contributes to the average inventory investment. Fu et al. (2016) extended the Ng-model multi-criteria ABC inventory classification model by utilizing distance-based decision-making method. They used three different criteria, namely annual dollar usage, average unit cost, and lead-time, for classification of inventory items. The contribution of the proposed method is to improve the Ng-model by obtaining the common weights for all criteria importance sequences. Begik et al. (2017) compared the ABC analysis with the ANP method in classifying the inventory items. The results indicated that the ANP method gives lower total inventory cost when compared with the ABC method.

Nag and Helal (2018) presented a study on multi-criteria inventory classifying for diabetes drugs. They compared the results of the AHP and Fuzzy AHP methods. Results showed that the Fuzzy AHP model which can cope with the uncertainties was able to eliminate some unnecessary criteria.

Kilic et al. (2013) used the AHP and TOPSIS methods for inventory classification and then compared these model with the classical ABC method. Based on the results of the evaluations, it has been shown that the AHP-TOPSIS method gives more effective results. Citak (2013) proposed the ABC-AHP-TOPSIS integration approach for multi-criteria inventory classification in an electronic firm. The traditional ABC analysis and the proposed method were compared with each other and figured out that the proposed method provides better results in terms of total inventory cost. Soylu and Akyol (2014) applied two types of utility function on the inventory classification problem. They evaluated classification methods for inventory cost and fill rate. Then, the results were compared with the other algorithms in the literature. Ladhari et al. (2016) evolved a new procedure, which is named as the constructive order classification algorithm (COCA), to obtain a consensus classification that reduces the discrepancy among different methods.

MAIN FOCUS OF THE CHAPTER

The main objective of this chapter is to propose a practical and efficient model for healthcare professionals. Since inventory management is a vital task for healthcare operations, effective and efficient mathematical methods should be used to solve problems related to this issue. In the healthcare industry, a vast amount of items such as specialized equipment, materials, and medications are used. To track and organize this complex system, inventory classification is a very useful tool. The traditional ABC method is a simple and effective method for inventory classification. However, this method can be inadequate for classifying healthcare inventory items since it only considers one criterion while there are some other important criteria needed to be considered for healthcare inventory item classification such as vital criticality, expiration date, availability of substitute drugs, etc. Hence, multi-criteria inventory classification methods that take into account multiple criteria are more suitable for healthcare inventory classification. According to the literature, the Fuzzy AHP and TOPSIS methods are efficient and simple methods for multi-criteria inventory classification problem. Also, there are a limited number of studies about the related issues in the healthcare industry. Therefore, in this study, an integrated method that combines the Fuzzy AHP and TOPSIS methods is used to solve the multi-criteria inventory classification problem in the healthcare industry. In addition, the results of the model are also compared with the traditional ABC method in order to analyze the performance of the proposed method.

HEALTHCARE SUPPLY CHAIN MANAGEMENT

Recently, healthcare supply chain management has gained importance due to the increasing competition conditions and high costs in the health sector. The main objective in the healthcare supply chain is to optimize efficiency and effectiveness of the treatment provided (Arora & Gigras, 2018, p. 101). One of the most important issues in the healthcare supply chain is to provide adequate, accurate, and on-time medical supply according to the patient's needs. In addition, it is important to optimize operation costs while ensuring a high level of service quality in order to increase patient satisfaction in the healthcare service.

Healthcare supply chain management differs from traditional supply chain management in various ways. Since the main product in the healthcare supply chain is medical service and since the production process starts only when an order is placed by the consumer, it may be considered as a service supply chain. Since it is not possible to hold service inventory throughout the supply chain, service supply chains are more complex than the traditional supply chains. In addition to this, demand forecasting in the healthcare supply chain is a difficult task due to the lack of precise consumption data. One of the reasons is that physicians prefer the drugs to be used in their operations according to their personal preferences (Mustaffa & Potter, 2009, p. 235). On the other hand, healthcare supply chain management may be considered as a critical task because it is vitally important in human life. For this reason, each operational task in the healthcare supply chain has a critical role. All parties in the supply chain must be organized so that they work in harmony to maintain a flawless service stream along the chain. In the traditional supply chain, the main objective is to manage the three main flows: physical product, information, and financial. The healthcare supply chain differs from the other supply chains because financial and information flows are the key components of the supply chain design (Samuel et al., 2010, p. 634). Pharmaceutical products are one of the most important components of the healthcare supply chain. It can be expensive to purchase and distribute pharmaceutical items in the chain. In addition, the shortage or misuse of some critical drugs can be life-threatening (Uthayakumar & Priya, 2013, p. 52).

Inventory and distribution management in the supply chain are the most important decision processes that affect the total supply chain costs. Successful inventory management could be a necessity for healthcare supply chains for many reasons.

One of the main reasons is that holding inventory in a healthcare organization can be costly. It was proven that an effective inventory control of expensive drugs can reduce total hospital costs by 20%. These results indicate that inventory control has a significant impact on the total costs of healthcare supply chain (Dwivedi & Kothiyal, 2012, p. 125). Inventory management is, therefore, one of the important tools for cost management in the healthcare supply chain. Another critical point about healthcare inventory management is that it has vital importance for human life. A basic responsibility of the inventory management department is to establish a system to track and control inventory items. This system should include a classification method for inventory items because of two important reasons. The first is to minimize holding costs and shortage costs. Reducing these types of inventory costs provides competition power for hospitals. The other is to define the importance level of inventory items. Detecting the vital level inventory items is significant for hospitals to maintain high service quality.

Another critical issue about healthcare inventory management is the product perishability. Outdated or expired pharmaceutical items are one of the most important reasons for the waste of resources in the healthcare supply chain. According to a survey in 2003, the estimated cost of the expiration of products in pharmacies and supermarkets is over $500 million. Beyond that, the usage of expired drugs may have potentially dangerous effects on human life (Uthayakumar & Priya, 2013, p. 53). Therefore, inventory management is important for the healthcare supply chain in terms of cost management and safety.

One of the most difficult issues regarding healthcare inventory management is that healthcare personnel who do not have any related education are responsible for this duty. However, this is not an efficient situation for operation management and patient's health. For this reason, the simplicity of inventory control methods has critical importance in healthcare. The proposed methods should therefore be easy to implement and understand by health professionals. On the other hand, it is more appropriate to consider multiple criteria while classifying healthcare inventory items. Multi-criteria inventory classification methods are suitable for healthcare inventory management for the sake of their simplicity and capability of considering multiple criteria simultaneously.

Inventory Management

Due to the globalization and rising competition, companies strive to manage their business processes efficiently in order to compete with the other firms and maintain their presence in the market. One of these processes is the establishment of an inventory management system that enables company inventories to be planned to meet customers' changing demands.

Inventory management is a business function that aims to increase the service level of companies and create customer satisfaction by balancing demand and supply. The primary activity of the inventory management is to determine inventory policies and procedures to make some decisions on inventories of companies. These decisions are realized with coordination of several departments in the company such as production, planning, purchasing, and warehouse. The accurate and reliable information flow between these departments contributes to efficiently carrying out inventory management.

The purpose of inventory management is to provide the necessary materials (raw materials, semi-finished products, and final products) and equipment for customer/production at the desired time and quantity. Besides, inventory management focuses on expenses arising from excess inventory and losses due to insufficient inventory to increase the profitability and decrease the inventory costs (Heizer & Render, 2005, p. 490). In order to ensure efficiency in inventory management, it is an obligation to check inventory items regularly and systematically. One of the most significant ways to succeed in business activities is to observe movements of the inventory items and share the necessary information with the related department correctly.

Inventory control is to determine the quantity-time factors and to monitor and coordinate the storage conditions in order to strike a balance between sale and order of the inventory items. Through the inventory control techniques, inventory managers can meet customers' demands on time or prevent interruptions in manufacturing and decrease inventory holding cost. Therefore, using inventory control techniques regularly helps manage inventories successfully. There are some questions to be answered while performing inventory management:

- Which inventory items are necessary?
- How much inventory should you keep?
- Where are the right places to keep inventory items?
- How much equipment is needed to transport inventory items?

Using inventory control techniques, these questions can be answered correctly. Efficient and effective inventory control is very important for supply chain performance. Also, inventory control is a tool to help correctly carry out the processes in the supply chain.

Inventories may have both positive and negative effects on firms. Although keeping inventory is a burden, which costs firms much money, it ensures customer satisfaction by meeting customer demands on time. Inventory management aims to bring positive and negative effects of inventory to an optimum level thanks to the inventory control function. In other words, it tries to find balance advantages and disadvantages of inventory.

To monitor and control inventories has many benefits. The most important ones are explained as follows:

- To adapt to changing production, supply, and delivery conditions
- To eliminate customer dissatisfaction due to non-availability
- To reduce costs by preventing any unnecessary material
- To avoid inventory losses through periodic monitoring
- To minimize the waste and scrap rates
- To decrease the negative effects of demand changes

Today, companies apply various inventory control methods. These methods vary according to the type and characteristics of the business. No matter what type of business, all companies must maintain a certain level of inventory. The important point is to choose the inventory control methods that will determine the most appropriate inventory levels.

The most used inventory control techniques are briefly explained below.

- **Visual Control Method:** It is one of the oldest methods used for inventory control and mostly applied by small businesses. The designated officer reviews the inventory levels. The officer informs the relevant department of company. Although it is a cheap and practical method, it has a high margin of error because it depends on personal judgment (Kobu, 2006, p. 312).
- **Two-Bin Control Method:** The two-bin inventory control method is usually used for small or low-value items. Any type of inventory items is stored in a two-compartment bin. When items in the first bin are completely emptied, a new order is placed to refill the items. Sales are made from the second bin until the order arrives. The first bin has a minimum of inventory, and the second bin keeps reserve inventory (Kobu, 2017, p. 316).
- **Fixed-Order Quantity Method:** In this method, firstly, the maximum inventory level is determined for each inventory item. Then, fixed order quantity, which minimizes the total cost of inventory, is determined. Decreasing inventory levels are completed by placing orders up to the maximum inventory level. Order time varies for each period. This is a very difficult method to apply in a system that has many different inventory items (Demir & Gümüşoğlu, 2011, p. 623).
- **Fixed-Order Period Method:** In this method, firstly, the maximum inventory level is determined for each inventory item. Then, a certain period of time is determined for ordering the inventory. At the end of the period, the decreasing inventory levels are completed by placing orders up to the maximum inventory level (Demir & Gümüşoğlu, 2011, p. 623).

- **ABC Analysis:** The ABC control method is an inventory management principle that stands for Always Better Control (Gupta & Kant, 2000, pp. 14-16). It is based on the apparent majority-influential minority principle put forward by Italian economist Pareto. The ABC control method is used to identify the importance of each item of the inventory in terms of its value of annual consumption. This method divides the inventory items into three categories: A, B, and C; where A is the most important item and C the least valuable. Brief definitions about the groups are given below (Heizer & Render, 2005, p. 491).
    - **Group A:** Inventory items included in Group A constitute 15-20% of total inventory amount and 75-80% of total annual usage value. High-value inventory items are classified in this group. The company keeps strict and periodic control over these inventory items. It is recommended that these inventory items should be ordered less and that its records should be kept regularly. Focusing on this group of inventory item can reduce the total inventory cost of the firm.
    - **Group B:** Inventory items included in Group B constitutes 30-40% of the total inventory amount and 15% of the total annual usage value. It has relatively less value or has moderate importance. A reasonable control is enough on the B category inventory items.
    - **Group C:** Low-value inventory items are categorized as C. It constitutes 40-50% of the total inventory amount and 5-10% of the total annual usage value. It can be ordered in large quantities and simply followed without strict control.

In the ABC analysis, the annual consumption amount of each item is firstly determined. Consumption quantities are multiplied by unit prices, and annual consumption values are found. Items are ranked from the highest consumption value to the lowest value, and finally, the inventory items are classified according to their cumulative percentage. Inventory items are divided into three groups as A most important, B medium important, C least important. The general ABC graph is shown in Figure 1.

Figure 1. ABC graph

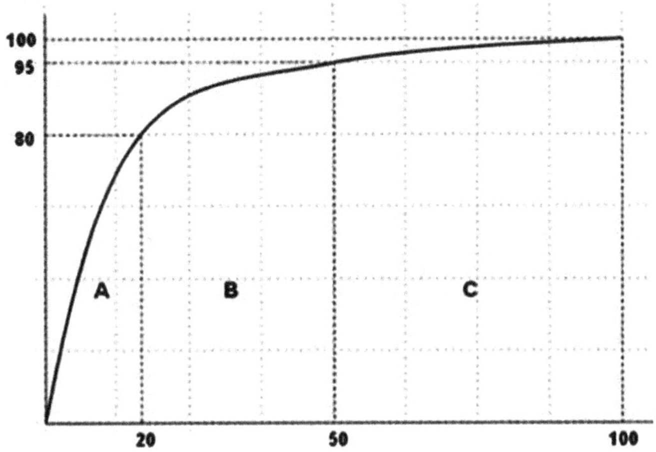

- **VED Analysis:** This method is used in the control of medicine and medical equipment in hospitals. VED analysis stands for Vital, Essential, and Desirable. The analysis classifies items on the basis of their criticality for the industry or company (Nigah & Gupta, 2010, p. 202).
- **Vital:** The items which are critically needed for the survival of the patients and must be available at all times were included in the vital category.
- **Essential:** The items with a lower criticality need and those that might be available in the hospital were included in the essential category.
- **Desirable:** The items with lowest criticality, the shortage of which would not be harmful to the health of the patients, were included in the desirable category. There is no obligation for the availability of these items.

The ABC analysis alone cannot effectively control inventory items. In a similar vein, the VED analysis alone would not be useful in order to classify inventory items in terms of criticality, essentiality, and desirability. Therefore, it is advised that the ABC and VED methods are combined to obtain more efficient and effective control results. Some of the examples about the ABC-VED analysis are given in the introduction of this study.

SOLUTION METHODOLOGY

MCDMs are efficient and simple methods widely used for solving multi-criteria inventory classification problems. For many years, the AHP and TOPSIS methods have successfully been applied to solve complicated decision-making problems. On the other hand, an inventory classification problem may include vagueness derived mainly from the evaluation of conflicting criteria. In the literature, it has been proved that the fuzzy logic approach is a powerful tool to handle vagueness. Therefore, in this chapter, an integrated fuzzy model is proposed to solve multi-criteria inventory classification problem.

Fuzzy Analytic Hierarchy Process

The AHP is a well-known MCDM. It is an effective and simple method to compare a set of alternatives with respect to a predefined target. It determines the relative importance weight of a set of alternatives by applying pair-wise comparisons. AHP has been applied to solve many different problems in the literature since it was developed by Saaty in 1980. The main advantage of this method is the incorporation of expert comments on the solution using pair-wise comparisons along with expert judgments. Thanks to this feature of this method, complicated real-life problems can be solved efficiently. The Fuzzy AHP is the extension of Saaty's theory and basically the combination of the fuzzy set theory and AHP methods. The fuzzy set theory is firstly developed by Zadeh in 1965. The main idea of the fuzzy theory is that the key elements in human thought are linguistic terms, not numbers, and can be measured using fuzzy set labels (Srichetta & Thurachon, 2012, p. 169). Therefore, an expert's ambiguous judgments can be represented by a fuzzy number. Thanks to being based on fuzzy set theory, the fuzzy AHP is an appropriate method to deal with the intangibility and uncertainty of real-life problems. The fuzzy AHP method has been used extensively in the literature since 1983 to solve various decision problems such as supplier selection, location selection, project selection, personnel selection, energy recourses selection, and machine selection (Kubler et al., 2016, p. 409). In the fuzzy AHP, the pairwise comparisons are conducted using well-known linguistic statements that can be represented by fuzzy numbers. Triangular fuzzy numbers (TFNs) are a special kind of fuzzy numbers that are frequently used in the literature due to its simplicity. There have been many TFNs developed in the literature. In this case, TFNs shown in Table 1 are used to convert the preferences scale of the crisp AHP.

Table 1. Triangular fuzzy conversion scale

Linguistic Scale	TFNs	Reciprocal TFNs
Equally important	(1,1,1)	(1,1,1)
Weakly more important	(2/3, 1, 3/2)	(2/3, 1, 3/2)
Strong more important	(3/2, 2, 5/2)	(2/5, 1/2, 2/3)
Very strong more important	(5/2, 3, 7/2)	(2/7, 1/3, 2/5)
Absolutely more important	(7/2, 4, 9/2)	(2/9, 1/4, 2/7)

The membership function of the TFNs is defined by three real numbers (l, m, u). The parameters l, m, and u respectively represent the smallest possible value, the most promising value, and the largest possible value that describe a fuzzy event. A TFN $\widetilde{M}$ is shown in Figure 2 and illustrated mathematically below (Vahidnia et al., 2009, p. 3050).

$$\mu_{M}(x) = \begin{cases} (x-l)/(m-l), & l \leq x \leq m \\ (u-x)/(u-m), & m \leq x \leq u \\ 0 & otherwise \end{cases}$$

Figure 2. TFN, $\tilde{M}$

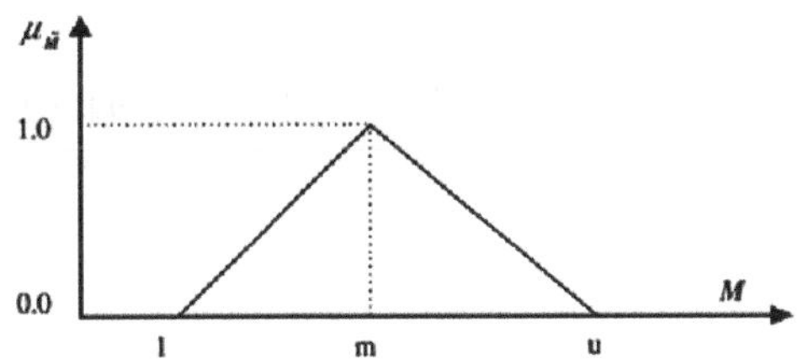

In the literature, the fuzzy AHP is first used in 1983 by Van Laarhoven and Pedrycz. Since then, a variety of different fuzzy AHP approaches were presented by various researchers. Among these, the extent analysis method developed by Chang (1996) is the most popular fuzzy AHP approach in the literature. Due to the simplicity of the approach, it has been widely used in the literature. However, Wang et al. (2008) reported that there are some weaknesses in this method. The most important of these weaknesses are as follows: The first is the removal of a valuable decision criterion from the solution by assigning zero weight, and the second is the inability of calculating the relative importance of the decision criteria or alternatives. Therefore, in this study, Chang's (1996) extent analysis method was adapted, and the total integral value method was applied (Liou & Wang, 1992) to rank fuzzy numbers to overcome the related disadvantages. Steps of the proposed fuzzy AHP method can be given as below (Kabir & Sumi, 2014, pp. 719-720; Sen & Cinar, 2010, p. 2045):

Step 1: Calculation of the fuzzy synthetic extent value of each pairwise comparison. Linguistic pairwise comparisons are transformed to the corresponding TFNs using the fuzzy scale presented in Table 1. The value of fuzzy synthetic extent S_i with respect to the ith element is computed as:

$$S_i = \sum_{j=1}^{m} M_{gi}^{j} \otimes \left[\sum_{i=1}^{n} \sum_{j=1}^{m} M_{gi}^{j} \right]^{-1} \quad (1)$$

Where the fuzzy addition operation of m extent analysis values for a particular matrix to derive $\sum_{j=1}^{m} M_{gi}^{j}$ is defined as:

$$\sum_{j=1}^{m} M_{gi}^{j} = \left(\sum_{j=1}^{m} l_j, \sum_{j=1}^{m} m_j, \sum_{j=1}^{m} u_j \right) \quad (2)$$

and the fuzzy addition operation of $M_{gi}^{j} \left(j = 1, 2, \ldots., m \right)$ values is performed to maintain $\left[\sum_{j=1}^{n} \sum_{j=1}^{m} M_{gi}^{j} \right]^{-1}$

$$\sum_{i=1}^{n} \sum_{j=1}^{m} M_{gi}^{j} = \left(\sum_{i=1}^{n} l_i, \sum_{i=1}^{n} m_i, \sum_{i=1}^{n} u_i \right) \quad (3)$$

$$\left[\sum_{j=1}^{n} \sum_{j=1}^{m} M_{gi}^{j} \right]^{-1} = \left(\frac{1}{\sum_{i=1}^{n} u_i}, \frac{1}{\sum_{i=1}^{n} m_i}, \frac{1}{\sum_{i=1}^{n} l_i} \right) \quad (4)$$

Step 2: Determination of fuzzy ranking value of $\widetilde{S}_i$. According to Chang (1996), while

$$M_1 = \left(l_1, m_1, u_1\right) and\, M_2 = \left(l_2, m_2, u_2\right)$$

are two TFNs, the degree of possibility of

$$M_2 = \left(l_2, m_2, u_2\right) \geq M_1 = \left(l_1, m_1, u_1\right)$$

is determined as:

$$V\left(M_2 \geq M_1\right) = \begin{cases} 1, & if\, m_2 \geq m_1 \\ 0, & if\, l_1 \geq u_2 \\ \dfrac{l_1 - u_2}{\left(m_2 - u_2\right) - \left(m_1 - l_1\right)} & otherwise \end{cases} \tag{5}$$

where *d* is the ordinate of the highest intersection between μ_{M1} and μ_{M2}. Thus, it can be represented as

$$V\left(M_2 \geq M_1\right) = hight\left(M_1 \cap M_2\right) = \mu_{M1}\left(d\right).$$

Additionally, both values of $V\left(M_2 \geq M_1\right)$ and $V\left(M_1 \geq M_2\right)$ are needed in order to compare M_1 with M_2.

However, according to Wang et al. (2008), the degree of possibility defined in this step is just an index for comparing two TFNs instead of an index for computing their relative importance. Therefore, the total integral value with index of optimism proposed by Liou and Wang (1992) is calculated using Eq. (6) in order to generate the priorities of the synthetic extent values:

$$I_T^{\alpha}\left(S_i\right) = \frac{1}{2}\alpha\left(m_i + u_i\right) + \frac{1}{2}\left(1 - \alpha\right)\left(l_i + m_i\right)$$

$$= \frac{1}{2}\left[\alpha u_i + m_i + \left(1-\alpha\right)l_i\right] \quad (6)$$

where α is index of optimism which represents degree of optimism for decision makers. When $\alpha = \left[0,1\right]$, if α approaches 1, decision makers are more optimistic, otherwise they are more pessimistic.

Step 3: Definition of the normalized importance weight vector $W = \left(w_1, w_2, \ldots\ldots, w_3\right)^T$ of the fuzzy judgment matrix A using Eq. (7)

$$w_x = \frac{I_T^\alpha\left(S_x\right)}{\sum_{k=1}^{n} I_T^\alpha\left(S_k\right)}; x = 1, \ldots..n. \quad (7)$$

where w_x is a non-fuzzy number.

TOPSIS Method

The TOPSIS method is one of the popular MCDMs, which is developed by Hwang and Yoon in 1981. This method is based on the main idea that the chosen alternative should have the shortest distance from the positive ideal solution and the farthest distance from the negative ideal solution. The positive ideal solution maximizes the benefit criteria and minimizes the cost criteria, while the negative ideal solution minimizes the benefit criteria and maximizes the cost criteria (Behzadian et al., 2012, p. 13052; Nyaoga et al., 2016, p. 435).

In the literature, TOPSIS has been applied to solve a wide range of real-life problems in many different fields. Supply chain management and logistics are the most popular topics in TOPSIS applications, whereas healthcare management is one of the recent topics that utilize the TOPSIS method (Behzadian et al., 2012, p. 13053).

Solution steps of the TOPSIS method is given below:

Step 1: Construction of Decision Matrix

Decision matrix $D = \left(x_{ij}\right)_{nxm}$, is the initial matrix in which decision makers evaluate each alternative i according to each criteria j.

$$D = \begin{bmatrix} \begin{pmatrix} x_{11} & x_{12} & \cdots & x_{1j} \\ x_{21} & x_{22} & \cdots & x_{2j} \\ \vdots & \vdots & \ddots & \vdots \\ x_{i1} & x_{i2} & \cdots & x_{ij} \end{pmatrix} \end{bmatrix} \quad (8)$$

Step 2: Normalization of the Decision Matrix

The decision matrix D is normalized using Eq. (9) as follows:

$$r_{ij} = \frac{x_{ij}}{\sqrt{\sum_{j=1}^{n} x_{ij}^{2}}} \quad (9)$$

Step 3: Construction of the Weighted Normalized Decision Matrix

The weighted normalized value v_{ij} is computed using Eq. (10) as follows:

$$v_{ij} = w_i x_{ij},\ j = 1,\ldots..,J; i = 1,\ldots.,n \quad (10)$$

where w_i is the weight of the ith attribute or criterion and $\sum_{i=1}^{n} w_i = 1$.

Step 4: Determination of the Positive and Negative Solution

In this step, positive-ideal solution S^+ and negative-ideal solution S^- are determined respectively as follows;

$$S^+ = \left\{x_1^+,\ldots..x_m^+\right\} = \left\{\left(maks_i x_{ij} \middle| j \in I\right), \left(\min_i x_{ij} \middle| j \in J\right)\right\} \quad (11)$$

$$S^- = \left\{x_1^-,\ldots..x_m^-\right\} = \left\{\left(\min_i x_{ij} \middle| j \in I\right), \left(maks_i x_{ij} \middle| j \in J\right)\right\} \quad (12)$$

where I is associated with the benefit criteria, and J is associated with the cost criteria.

Step 5: Calculation of the Separation Measures

The separation measures are calculated for each alternative using Euclidean distance.

μ_i^+ of each alternative from the positive-ideal solution is computed as follows:

$$\mu_i^+ = \sqrt{\sum_{j=1}^{m}\left(x_{ij} - x_j^+\right)^2}, i = 1,\ldots,n. \tag{13}$$

μ_i^- of each alternative from the negative-ideal solution is calculated as given below:

$$\mu_i^- = \sqrt{\sum_{j=1}^{m}\left(x_{ij} - x_j^-\right)^2}, i = 1,\ldots,n. \tag{14}$$

Step 6: Determination of the Closeness Coefficient T

The relative closeness to ideal solution is calculated with Eq. (15), and the ranking order of all alternatives is obtained.

$$T_i = \frac{\mu_i^-}{\mu_i^+ + \mu_i^-} \tag{15}$$

where $T_i = \left[0,1\right]$, and the larger the index value, the better the performance of the alternatives.

CASE STUDY

This study presents the outcome of applying a multi-criteria ABC analysis on inventory data of a state hospital Pharmacy in Turkey. There are 41 different types of antibiotic to be used for treating different diseases in the hospital pharmacy. This study focused on developing a classification model for only antibiotic groups used in the pharmacy. A real-life case study was conducted with the data which was obtained from a decision-making team consisting of one pharmacy warehouse manager, one supervisor, and three staff. The proposed model classifies a number of inventory items in the presence of both qualitative and quantitative criteria. The method takes into account discordant criteria which are like annual usage cost, warehouse space usage, expire date, availability of the substitute item, and criticality. The determined inventory classification criteria are presented and described in Table 2. Also, criticality criterion was classified into three classes using VED rules.

Table 2. Inventory classification criteria

Inventory Classification Criteria	Definition
Annual Usage Cost **(C1)**	Annual consumption value.
Vital Criticality **(C2)**	This criterion determines the criticality of the drug for human life.
Expire Date **(C3)**	This takes into account the duration of the shelf life of the drug.
Availability of the Substitute Item **(C4)**	This criterion indicates the availability of a substitute drug in case of absence of an original prescribed drug.
Warehouse Space Usage **(C5)**	The area which occupied by an inventory item in warehouse.

The proposed method has two stages. In the first stage, the Fuzzy AHP method which can cope with the uncertainty decisions was used to determine weight of the criteria, and then in the second stage, inventory items were ranked in categories A, B, and C using the TOPSIS method. Besides, the classical ABC inventory classification method was applied to analyze the performance of the proposed method. The schematic diagram of the proposed method is given in Figure 3.

Figure 3. Schematic framework of the proposed method

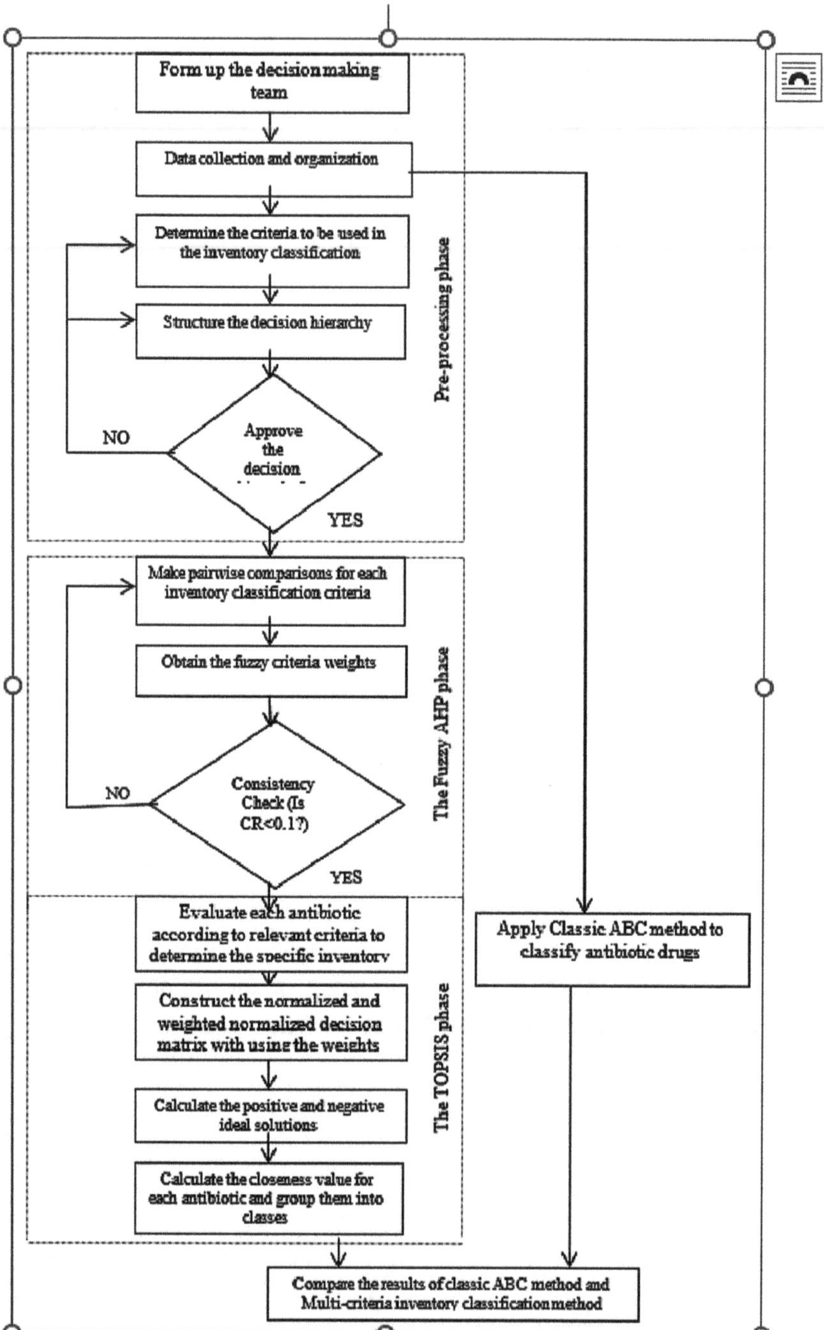

Since each inventory classification criterion does not have the same importance level for healthcare department, the relative importance value of each criterion ought to be calculated. The fuzzy AHP method was applied to calculate the criteria weights that indicate the relative importance of each criterion. Decision-making team members were asked to rate the importance of the selected criteria over each other using the linguistic scale given in Table 1. The aggregated fuzzy pairwise comparison matrix shown in Table 3 is provided by geometric mean. In the next step, the fuzzy synthetic extent value of each criterion was calculated as presented in Table 4.

Table 3. The aggregated fuzzy pair-wise comparison matrix

	C1	C2	C3	C4	C5
C1	(1,1,1)	(0.52, 0.71, 1)	(1.50, 2, 2.50)	(1.94, 2.45, 2.96)	(1.94, 2.45, 2.96)
C2	(1, 1.41, 1.94)	(1, 1, 1)	(2.50, 3, 3,50)	(2.50, 3, 3.50)	(2.50, 3, 3.50)
C3	(0.40, 0.50, 0.67)	(0.29, 0.33, 0.40)	(1, 1, 1)	(1.11, 1.41, 1.75)	(1.11, 1.41, 1.75)
C4	(0.32, 0.38, 0.47)	(0.29, 0.33, 0.40)	(0.57, 0.71, 0.90)	(1, 1, 1)	(0.90, 1, 1.11)
C5	(0.34,0.41, 0.52)	(0.29, 0.33, 0.40)	(0.57, 0.71, 0.90)	(0.90, 1, 1.11)	(1, 1, 1)

Table 4. Synthetic extent value of each criterion

Sc1	(0.19, 0.27, 0.39)
Sc2	(0.26, 0.36, 0.51)
Sc3	(0.10, 0.15, 0.21)
Sc4	(0.08, 0.11, 0.15)
Sc5	(0.08, 0.11, 0.15)

The integral values of these synthetic extent value was computed using Eq. (6) as given in Table 5. The optimism index α is taken as 0.80. Finally, the normalized importance weight of each criterion is obtained via normalization as shown in Table 6.

Table 5. Integral value of each criterion

Criteria	Integral Value
C1	0,31
C2	0,41
C3	0,17
C4	0,12
C5	0,12

Table 6. Normalized weight of each criterion

Criteria	Normalized Weight
C1	0,28
C2	0,36
C3	0,15
C4	0,11

To check the inconsistency of each comparison matrix, the consistency ratio (CR) was computed. Since all of the CR values are less than 0.1, the level of inconsistency in each comparison matrix is considered satisfactory. Fuzzy AHP application results revealed that *Vital Criticality (C2)* is the most important inventory classification criterion with %0.36 weightage followed by Annual Usage Cost (C1) with a weightage of %28. As can be seen in Table 4, vital criticality criteria that are not considered in the traditional ABC method have the highest importance for health inventory classification. Therefore, it is possible to claim that the proposed method is more suitable for healthcare inventory classification problems.

After determining the importance weight of criteria, each pharmacist was asked to evaluate each antibiotic according to the relevant criterion to determine the specific inventory class of a drug. The TOPSIS method was applied to classify antibiotic drugs. For the sake of the computational simplicity, numerical transformation scales were used to indicate intangible criteria that are drug criticality, availability of the substitute item, expire date limitation, and limitation of warehouse space. The transformation scale for each of these criteria is given in Table 7, Table 8, Table 9, and Table 10, respectively.

the list of drugs with respect to their criteria is presented in Table 11. TOPSIS method computation steps, explained in the previous section, are applied to this data. Firstly, the given data were normalized using Eq. (9), and then Eq. (10) was applied to compute weighted normalized decision matrix. Criteria weights derived by the Fuzzy AHP was used in this step. The weighted normalized decision matrix is given in Table 12.

Table 7. Transformation scale for drug criticality

Drug Criticality Levels	Scale
Vital (V)	5
Essential (E)	3
Desirable (D)	1

Table 8. Transformation scale for availability of the substitute item

Availability of the Substitute Item	Scale
No alternative drugs available	5
Alternative drugs available, can be recommended	3
Alternative drugs available of almost same composition	1

Table 9. Transformation scale for expire date limitation

Expire Date Limitation	Scale
Short	5
Medium	3
Long	1

Table 10. Transformation scale for limitation of warehouse space

Volume of Drug Package	Scale
Large	5
Medium	3
Small	1

Table 11. List of drugs with respect to their criteria

Drug	Annual Usage Amount	Unit Price (TL)	Annual Usage (TL)	Criticality	Expire Date Limitation	Limitation of Warehouse Space	Availability of the Substitute Item
EQICEFT	7.200,00	7,80	56.160,00	5	5	1	1
TARGOCID	324,00	51,10	16.556,40	5	3	1	5
LEFOX	504,00	2,50	1.260,00	5	5	1	5
INVANZ	360,00	67,10	24.156,00	5	1	1	5
SULZON	3.600,00	3,00	10.800,00	5	5	1	1
MOPEM	2.700,00	22,00	59.400,00	5	5	1	5
ZIDIM	192,00	3,28	629,76	5	5	1	5
VANCOTEK	4.200,00	10,83	45.486,00	5	5	1	5
CANDISEPT	4.200,00	2,77	11.634,00	3	5	1	5
UNACEFIN	7.200,00	5,55	39.960,00	5	5	1	1
CEFPERAZON	3.600,00	11,04	39.744,00	5	5	1	1
CIPROPOL	1.800,00	2,15	3.870,00	5	5	5	5
PNEMOX	720,00	3,15	2.268,00	5	3	5	1
TEZARACIN	2.880,00	19,79	56.995,20	5	3	1	5
IESEF	240,00	6,36	1.526,40	5	3	1	5
POLINOKSID	264,00	11,70	3.088,80	5	5	5	5
TIGEJECT	12,00	18,17	218,04	5	5	1	5
ZOVIRAX	48,00	7,66	367,68	1	1	1	1
ASIRAX	48,00	7,83	375,84	1	5	1	1
COLISOD	900,00	16,88	15.192,00	1	5	1	5
MOXSACIN	720,00	5,62	4.046,40	5	5	1	1
AMIZECSIN	1.200,00	1,07	1.284,00	5	5	1	5
AMOKLAVIN	12,00	4,20	50,40	5	1	1	5
PENBISIN	60,00	3,62	217,20	5	5	1	5
SULBAKSIT	1.800,00	1,90	3.420,00	5	3	1	5
KLOVIREX	48,00	6,09	292,32	1	1	1	1
FACTIVE	240,00	56,00	13.440,00	5	1	1	5
GENTHAVER	1.440,00	0,61	878,40	5	3	1	5
KLASID	36,00	27,90	1.004,40	5	3	1	5
DECLARIT	540,00	7,00	3.780,00	5	3	1	5
MENEKLIN 300 mg	1.200,00	3,70	4.440,00	3	3	1	5
MENEKLIN 600 mg	840,00	4,58	3.847,20	3	5	1	5
POTANT	72,00	2,80	201,60	5	5	1	5
POLGYL	1.800,00	3,44	6.192,00	1	5	1	5

continued on following page

Table 11 continued

Drug	Annual Usage Amount	Unit Price (TL)	Annual Usage (TL)	Criticality	Expire Date Limitation	Limitation of Warehouse Space	Availability of the Substitute Item
MOFELOX	660,00	9,00	5.940,00	5	1	1	5
DEPOSILIN	780,00	8,00	6.240,00	5	1	5	5
PENISILIN	168,00	4,36	732,48	5	1	1	5
CEFAKS	108,00	4,10	442,80	3	3	1	5
SEFFUR	480,00	1,20	576,00	3	1	1	5
CIFLOSIN	780,00	1,30	1.014,00	5	3	1	5
EQIZOLIN	9.000,00	1,69	15.210,00	3	3	1	5

Table 12. The weighted normalized decision matrix

Drugs	Unit Cost	Criticality	Expire Date Limitation	Limitation of Warehouse Space	Availability of the Substitute Item
EQICEFT	0,144	0,317	0,150	0,009	0,004
TARGOCID	6,170	0,317	0,054	0,009	0,094
LEFOX	0,015	0,317	0,150	0,009	0,094
INVANZ	10,639	0,317	0,006	0,009	0,094
SULZON	0,021	0,317	0,150	0,009	0,004
MOPEM	1,144	0,317	0,150	0,009	0,094
ZIDIM	0,025	0,317	0,150	0,009	0,094
VANCOTEK	0,277	0,317	0,150	0,009	0,094
CANDISEPT	0,018	0,114	0,150	0,009	0,094
UNACEFIN	0,073	0,317	0,150	0,009	0,004
CEFPERAZON	0,288	0,317	0,150	0,009	0,004
CIPROPOL	0,011	0,317	0,150	0,228	0,094
PNEMOX	0,023	0,317	0,054	0,228	0,004
TEZARACIN	0,925	0,317	0,054	0,009	0,094
IESEF	0,096	0,317	0,054	0,009	0,094
POLINOKSID	0,323	0,317	0,150	0,228	0,094
TIGEJECT	0,780	0,317	0,150	0,009	0,094
ZOVIRAX	0,139	0,013	0,006	0,009	0,004
ASIRAX	0,145	0,013	0,150	0,009	0,004

continued on following page

Table 12 continued

Drugs	Unit Cost	Criticality	Expire Date Limitation	Limitation of Warehouse Space	Availability of the Substitute Item
COLISOD	0,673	0,013	0,150	0,009	0,094
MOXSACIN	0,075	0,317	0,150	0,009	0,004
AMIZECSIN	0,003	0,317	0,150	0,009	0,094
AMOKLAVIN	0,042	0,317	0,006	0,009	0,094
PENBISIN	0,031	0,317	0,150	0,009	0,094
SULBAKSIT	0,009	0,317	0,054	0,009	0,094
KLOVIREX	0,088	0,013	0,006	0,009	0,004
FACTIVE	7,410	0,317	0,006	0,009	0,094
GENTHAVER	0,001	0,317	0,054	0,009	0,094
KLASID	1,839	0,317	0,054	0,009	0,094
DECLARIT	0,116	0,317	0,054	0,009	0,094
MENEKLIN 300 mg	0,032	0,114	0,054	0,009	0,094
MENEKLIN 600 mg	0,050	0,114	0,150	0,009	0,094
POTANT	0,019	0,317	0,150	0,009	0,094
POLGYL	0,028	0,013	0,150	0,009	0,094
MOFELOX	0,191	0,317	0,006	0,009	0,094
DEPOSILIN	0,151	0,317	0,006	0,228	0,094
PENISILIN	0,045	0,317	0,006	0,009	0,094
CEFAKS	0,040	0,114	0,054	0,009	0,094
SEFFUR	0,003	0,114	0,006	0,009	0,094
CIFLOSIN	0,004	0,317	0,054	0,009	0,094
EQIZOLIN	0,007	0,114	0,054	0,009	0,094

After determining positive and negative ideal solution values, the separation measures (μ_i^+ and μ_i^-) of each drug item from the positive and negative ideal solutions were calculated using Eq. (13) and Eq. (14), respectively. Following this, the relative closeness T for each drug item to the ideal solution could be determined as shown in Table 13.

Table 13. The separation distance and Relative closeness value of each drug item

Drugs	μ_i^+	μ_i^-	T
EQICEFT	10,50	0,37	0,03
TARGOCID	4,48	6,18	0,58
LEFOX	10,63	0,35	0,03
INVANZ	0,26	10,64	0,98
SULZON	10,62	0,34	0,03
MOPEM	9,50	1,19	0,11
ZIDIM	10,62	0,35	0,03
VANCOTEK	10,36	0,44	0,04
CANDISEPT	10,63	0,20	0,02
UNACEFIN	10,57	0,34	0,03
CEFPERAZON	10,35	0,44	0,04
CIPROPOL	10,63	0,41	0,04
PNEMOX	10,62	0,38	0,03
TEZARACIN	9,72	0,98	0,09
IESEF	10,55	0,34	0,03
POLINOKSID	10,32	0,52	0,05
TIGEJECT	9,86	0,85	0,08
ZOVIRAX	10,51	0,14	0,01
ASIRAX	10,50	0,20	0,02
COLISOD	9,97	0,69	0,07
MOXSACIN	10,57	0,34	0,03
AMIZECSIN	10,64	0,35	0,03
AMOKLAVIN	10,60	0,32	0,03
PENBISIN	10,61	0,35	0,03
SULBAKSIT	10,63	0,32	0,03
KLOVIREX	10,56	0,09	0,01
FACTIVE	3,24	7,42	0,70
GENTHAVER	10,64	0,32	0,03
KLASID	8,80	1,87	0,17
DECLARIT	10,53	0,34	0,03
MENEKLIN 300 mg	10,61	0,15	0,01
MENEKLIN 600 mg	10,59	0,20	0,02

continued on following page

Table 13 continued

Drugs	μ_i^+	μ_i^-	T
POTANT	10,62	0,35	0,03
POLGYL	10,62	0,17	0,02
MOFELOX	10,45	0,37	0,03
DEPOSILIN	10,49	0,41	0,04
PENISILIN	10,60	0,32	0,03
CEFAKS	10,60	0,15	0,01
SEFFUR	10,64	0,14	0,01
CIFLOSIN	10,64	0,32	0,03
EQIZOLIN	10,64	0,14	0,01

If any drug item has a higher relative closeness value, it means that it is closer to the distance from ideal solution and it is farther from the negative ideal solution, so it is the best inside ranking. Therefore, drugs were ranked in descending order according to their closeness value and grouped into A, B, and C classes. To determine the differences between the classic ABC and the proposed method, the classic ABC analysis was also applied to the current data set. Table 14 contains the comparison results of the Fuzzy AHP-TOPSIS and classic ABC analysis.

There is no specific percentage rule to determine the boundaries between inventory classes in multi-criteria inventory classification methods. In this study, the limits for the inventory classes are obtained in the Fuzzy AHP-TOPSIS on the following basis. Out of 41 antibiotic drugs, 6 (%15) were classified as A category, 18 (%44) as B category, and the remaining as C category. Additionally, it can be seen that the Fuzzy AHP-TOPSIS provides different results when compared with the classical ABC analysis. For instance, the drug named "KLASID" is classified as class A item by the Fuzzy AHP-TOPSIS method, while it is classified as a class C item by the classic ABC analysis. These classification differences arise from the computational logic of the methods. Since the classical ABC analysis is solely based on the annual usage rate, the corresponding drug classified as a C class item in this method. However, it is classified as a class A item by the Fuzzy AHP-TOPSIS method because it is a very critical drug, it also has a short expiration date, and there are no alternative drugs available in case of absence of this drug. As can be seen here, the classic ABC method is a simple but not appropriate method for drug classification because it ignores the criteria that may be very important for drug classification.

Table 14. Comparison results of fuzzy AHP-TOPSIS and classic ABC analysis

Drug	T	Fuzzy AHP-TOPSIS	Classic ABC
INVANZ	0,98	A	A
FACTIVE	0,70	A	B
TARGOCID	0,58	A	A
KLASID	0,17	A	C
MOPEM	0,11	A	A
TEZARACIN	0,09	A	A
TIGEJECT	0,08	B	C
COLISOD	0,07	B	B
POLINOKSID	0,05	B	C
VANCOTEK	0,04	B	A
CEFPERAZON	0,04	B	A
DEPOSILIN	0,04	B	B
CIPROPOL	0,04	B	B
PNEMOX	0,03	B	C
MOFELOX	0,03	B	B
EQICEFT	0,03	B	A
PENBISIN	0,03	B	C
ZIDIM	0,03	B	C
POTANT	0,03	B	C
LEFOX	0,03	B	C
AMIZECSIN	0,03	B	C
MOXSACIN	0,03	B	B
UNACEFIN	0,03	B	A
DECLARIT	0,03	B	B
SULZON	0,03	C	B
IESEF	0,03	C	C
PENISILIN	0,03	C	C
SULBAKSIT	0,03	C	C
AMOKLAVIN	0,03	C	C
CIFLOSIN	0,03	C	C
GENTHAVER	0,03	C	C
ASIRAX	0,02	C	C

continued on following page

Table 14 continued

Drug	T	Fuzzy AHP-TOPSIS	Classic ABC
MENEKLIN 600 mg	0,02	C	B
CANDISEPT	0,02	C	B
POLGYL	0,02	C	B
CEFAKS	0,01	C	C
MENEKLIN 300 mg	0,01	C	B
EQIZOLIN	0,01	C	A
ZOVIRAX	0,01	C	C
SEFFUR	0,01	C	C
KLOVIREX	0,01	C	C

SOLUTIONS AND RECOMMENDATIONS

In this study, an integrated MCDM was proposed to solve multi-criteria inventory classification problems. The multi-criteria inventory classification methods, which take into account several important criteria simultaneously, are appropriate for healthcare inventory management. In this method, two very well-known methods (Fuzzy AHP and TOPSIS) were combined. The application results showed that the proposed method is able to yield accurate prediction of inventory classes.

FUTURE RESEARCH DIRECTIONS

As a future study, different MCDMs such as PROMETHEE, ELECTRE, and Grey relational analysis may be applied to solve multi-criteria inventory classification problems. Besides, the performance of the proposed method can be compared with other methods.

CONCLUSION

Recently, the studies focusing on healthcare operation management issues have gained more attention in the literature. Traditionally, operations management optimization problems such as distribution and inventory management are not the main concerns of the healthcare institutions. However, it has been proven that successful inventory and distribution management can provide significant cost savings and potential revenue for organizations. For this reason, healthcare organizations should have well-established inventory management systems to provide quality medical services timely and cost-effectively.

Hospitals hold a vast amount of inventory, which is composed of many different items with different importance level. Ensuring the availability of vital and essential items in the hospital is the main purpose of hospital inventory management. Especially maintaining the regular availability of drugs is crucial for ensuring sustainable medical service in hospitals. However, inventory management is a complex activity for hospitals and can be time-consuming and costly for hospitals if not handled systematically.

Inventory classification helps organizations with such complex activities to determine important and critical items to manage them appropriately. The classical ABC analysis is one of the most popular single-criterion inventory classification methods. Even though the classical ABC analysis is easy to implement, it may not be as efficient and comprehensive as the multi-criteria based inventory classification methods. The multi-criteria inventory classification methods are not only comprehensive but also reasonably easy to perform. In the literature, the multi-criteria inventory classification methods are generally studied with a general framework. However, the inventory classification problem has industry-specific character because evaluation criteria and their priorities change according to the industry. The aim of this study is to present a scientific framework about multi-criteria inventory classification for healthcare organizations. In this study, a two-stage integrated method was presented in which the Fuzzy AHP result weights are used as input weights by TOPSIS. The reason for applying the fuzzy AHP is the advantage of its ability to solve complex problems that may be a conflict of interest between multiple objectives. In the Fuzzy AHP, using linguistic terms for pairwise comparisons makes the evaluation process more preferable for decision makers. Additionally, the Fuzzy AHP is able to generate more accurate and reasonable judgements for real-life problems. The TOPSIS method is an effective method thanks to its competence of visualizing the performance of alternatives and providing a scalar value that accounts for both the best and worst alternatives simultaneously. On the other hand, the TOPSIS method is an easy, fast, and effective method. Therefore, it can be said that the Fuzzy AHP-TOPSIS method provides a simple and practical solution to healthcare organizations dealing with complex inventory management problems on a daily basis. The proposed method does not require any complex calculation knowledge as it can be easily programmed into a spreadsheet. Based on these advantages, the use of the proposed method to classify pharmaceutical items will significantly improve the efficiency of healthcare inventory management. Besides, the proposed method is able to accurately classify a large number of inventory items. For this reason, it is a suitable method for hospital inventory management. Another contribution of this method is that it extends the existing limited health inventory management literature from a new perspective.

REFERENCES

Antonoglou, D., Kastanioti, C., & Niakas, D. (2017). ABC and VED Analysis of Medical Materials of a General Military Hospital in Greece. *Journal of Health Management, 19*(1), 170–179. doi:10.1177/0972063416682643

Arora, M., & Gigras, Y. (2018). Importance of Supply Chain Management in Healthcare of Third World Countries. *International Journal of Supply and Operations Management, 5*(1), 101–106.

Begik, M., Hamurcu, M., & Eren, T. (2017). Stok kontrolde ABC analizi ve analitik ağ süreci yönteminin ısı cihazları firmasında uygulanması. *Kırıkkale Üniversitesi Sosyal Bilimler Dergisi, 7*(1), 197–216.

Behzadian, M., Otaghsara, S. K., Yazdani, M., & Ignatius, J. (2012). A state-of the-art survey of TOPSIS applications. *Expert Systems with Applications, 39*(17), 13051–13069. doi:10.1016/j.eswa.2012.05.056

Bhattacharya, A., Sarkar, B., & Mukherjee, S. K. (2007). Distance-based consensus method for ABC analysis. *International Journal of Production Research, 45*(15), 3405–3420. doi:10.1080/00207540600847145

Cakir, O., & Canbolat, M. S. (2008). A web-based decision support system for multi-criteria inventory classification using fuzzy AHP methodology. *Expert Systems with Applications, 35*(3), 1367–1378. doi:10.1016/j.eswa.2007.08.041

Chang, D. Y. (1996). Applications of the extent analysis method on fuzzy AHP. *European Journal of Operational Research, 95*(3), 649–655. doi:10.1016/0377-2217(95)00300-2

Çıtak, Ş. (2013). *Bir Elektronik Firmasında Çok Ölçütlü Stok Sınıflandırma.* Yüksek Lisans Tezi, Gazi Üniversitesi, Fen Bilimleri Enstitüsü.

Cohen, M. A., & Ernst, R. (1988). Multi-Item Classification and Generic Inventory Stock Contr. *Production and Inventory Management Journal, 29*(3), 6.

Demir, H., & Gümüşoğlu, Ş. (2003). *Üretim Yönetimi.* İstanbul, Turkey: Beta Basım Yayım Dağıtım.

Dwivedi, S., & Kothiyal, P. (2012). Inventory management: A tool of identifying items that need greater attention for control. *The Pharma Innovation, 1*(7, Part A), 125.

Ertuğrul, İ. (2013). Stok Kontrolde ABC Yöntemi ve AHP Analizlerinin İplik İşletmesine Uygulanması. *Uluslararası Alanya İşletme Fakültesi Dergisi*, *5*(1), 41–52.

Fitriana, I., Satria, R. G. D., & Setiawan, D. C. B. (2018). Medicine Inventory Management by ABC-VED Analysis in the Pharmacy Store of Veterinary Hospital, Yogyakarta, Indonesia. *Asian Journal of Animal and Veterinary Advances*, *13*, 85–90. doi:10.3923/ajava.2018.85.90

Flores, B. E., & Clay Whybark, D. J. I. J. O. O. (1986). Multiple criteria ABC analysis. *International Journal of Operations & Production Management*, *6*(3), 38–46. doi:10.1108/eb054765

Fu, Y., Lai, K. K., Miao, Y., & Leung, J. W. (2016). A distance-based decision-making method to improve multiple criteria ABC inventory classification. *International Transactions in Operational Research*, *23*(5), 969–978. doi:10.1111/itor.12193

Gupta, S., & Sunil, K. (2000). *Hospital stores management: An integrated approach* (pp. 14–1). India: Jaypee. doi:10.5005/jp/books/10360

Guvenir, H. A., & Erel, E. (1998). Multicriteria inventory classification using a genetic algorithm. *European Journal of Operational Research*, *105*(1), 29–37. doi:10.1016/S0377-2217(97)00039-8

Hadi-Vencheh, A. (2010). An improvement to multiple criteria ABC inventory classification. *European Journal of Operational Research*, *201*(3), 962–965. doi:10.1016/j.ejor.2009.04.013

Haszlinna Mustaffa, N., & Potter, A. (2009). Healthcare supply chain management in Malaysia: A case study. *Supply Chain Management*, *14*(3), 234–243. doi:10.1108/13598540910954575

Hatefi, S. M., Torabi, S. A., & Bagheri, P. (2014). Multi-criteria ABC inventory classification with mixed quantitative and qualitative criteria. *International Journal of Production Research*, *52*(3), 776–786. doi:10.1080/00207543.2013.838328

Kabir, G., & Sumi, R. S. (2014). Power substation location selection using fuzzy analytic hierarchy process and PROMETHEE: A case study from Bangladesh. *Energy*, *72*, 717–730. doi:10.1016/j.energy.2014.05.098

Kilic, A., Aygün S., Keskin, G. A., & Baynal, K. (2014). Çok kriterli ABC analizi problemine farklı birbakış açısı: bulanık analitik hiyerarşi prosesi-ideal çözüme yakınlığa göre tercih sıralama tekniği. *Pamukkale üniversitesi mühensilik bilimleri dergisi*, 20(5), 179-188.

Kobu, B. (2017). *Üretim yönetimi*. İstanbul, Turkey: Beta Basım.

Kubler, S., Robert, J., Derigent, W., Voisin, A., & Le Traon, Y. (2016). A state-of the-art survey & testbed of fuzzy AHP (FAHP) applications. *Expert Systems with Applications*, *65*, 398–422. doi:10.1016/j.eswa.2016.08.064

Kumar, S., & Chakravarty, A. (2015). ABC–VED analysis of expendable medical stores at a tertiary care hospital. *Medical Journal, Armed Forces India*, *71*(1), 24–27. doi:10.1016/j.mjafi.2014.07.002 PMID:25609859

Kwon, I. W. G., Kim, S. H., & Martin, D. G. (2016). Healthcare supply chain management; strategic areas for quality and financial improvement. *Technological Forecasting and Social Change*, *113*, 422–428. doi:10.1016/j.techfore.2016.07.014

Ladhari, T., Babai, M. Z., & Lajili, I. (2016). Multi-criteria inventory classification: New consensual procedures. *IMA Journal of Management Mathematics*, *27*(2), 335–351. doi:10.1093/imaman/dpv003

Liou, T. S., & Wang, M. J. J. (1992). Ranking fuzzy numbers with integral value. *Fuzzy Sets and Systems*, *50*(3), 247–255. doi:10.1016/0165-0114(92)90223-Q

Lolli, F., Ishizaka, A., & Gamberini, R. (2014). New AHP-based approaches for multi-criteria inventory classification. *International Journal of Production Economics*, *156*, 62–74. doi:10.1016/j.ijpe.2014.05.015

Millstein, M. A., Yang, L., & Li, H. (2014). Optimizing ABC inventory grouping decisions. *International Journal of Production Economics*, *148*, 71–80. doi:10.1016/j.ijpe.2013.11.007

Nag, K., & Helal, M. (2018, December). Multicriteria Inventory Classification of Diabetes Drugs Using a Comparison of AHP and Fuzzy AHP Models. *Proceedings 2018 IEEE International Conference on Industrial Engineering and Engineering Management (IEEM)* (pp. 1456-1460). IEEE. 10.1109/IEEM.2018.8607678

Ng, W. L. (2007). A simple classifier for multiple criteria ABC analysis. *European Journal of Operational Research*, *177*(1), 344–353. doi:10.1016/j.ejor.2005.11.018

Nigah, R., Devnani, M., & Gupta, A. K. (2010). ABC and VED analysis of the pharmacy store of a tertiary care teaching, research and referral healthcare institute of India. *Journal of Young Pharmacists, 2*(2), 201-205.

Ozdemir, A., & Zveri, O. (2004). Çok Kriterli Envanter Sınıflandırmasında Analitik Hiyerarşi Süreci Analizinin Uygulanması. *Dokuz Eylül Üniversitesi İktisadi ve İdari Bilimler Fakültesi Dergisi, 19*(2), 137-154.

Ozguven, N. (2011). Vakif üniversitesi tercihinin analitik hiyerarşi süreci ile belirlenmesi. *Dumlupınar Üniversitesi Sosyal Bilimler Dergisi*, (30), 279-290.

Park, J., Bae, H., & Bae, J. (2014). Cross-evaluation-based weighted linear optimization for multi-criteria ABC inventory classification. *Computers & Industrial Engineering*, *76*, 40–48. doi:10.1016/j.cie.2014.07.020

Partovi, F. Y., & Anandarajan, M. (2002). Classifying inventory using an artificial neural network approach. *Computers & Industrial Engineering*, *41*(4), 389–404. doi:10.1016/S0360-8352(01)00064-X

Partovi, F. Y., & Burton, J. (1993). Using the analytic hierarchy process for ABC analysis. *International Journal of Operations & Production Management*, *13*(9), 29–44. doi:10.1108/01443579310043619

Ramanathan, R. (2006). ABC Inventory Classification With Multiple- Criteria Using Weighted Linear Optimization. *Computers & Operations Research*, *33*(3), 695–700. doi:10.1016/j.cor.2004.07.014

Samuel, C., Gonapa, K., Chaudhary, P. K., & Mishra, A. (2010). Supply chain dynamics in healthcare services. *International Journal of Health Care Quality Assurance*, *23*(7), 631–642. doi:10.1108/09526861011071562 PMID:21125959

Şen, C. G., & Çınar, G. (2010). Evaluation and pre-allocation of operators with multiple skills: A combined fuzzy AHP and max-min approach. *Expert Systems with Applications*, *37*(3), 2043–2053. doi:10.1016/j.eswa.2009.06.075

Soylu, B., & Akyol, B. (2014). Multi-criteria inventory classification with reference items. *Computers & Industrial Engineering*, *69*, 12–20. doi:10.1016/j.cie.2013.12.011

Tanrıverdi, Y. (2010). *Tedarik Zinciri Ve Stok Yönetimi Üzerine Bir Uygulama*. Yüksek Lisans Tezi, Pamukkale Üniversitesi, Sosyal Bilimler Enstitüsü.

Tsai, C. Y., & Yeh, S. W. (2008). A multiple objective particle swarm optimization approach for inventory classification. *International Journal of Production Economics*, *114*(2), 656–666. doi:10.1016/j.ijpe.2008.02.017

Uthayakumar, R., & Priyan, S. (2013). Pharmaceutical supply chain and inventory management strategies: Optimization for a pharmaceutical company and a hospital. *Operations Research for Health Care*, *2*(3), 52–64. doi:10.1016/j.orhc.2013.08.001

Vahidnia, M. H., Alesheikh, A. A., & Alimohammadi, A. (2009). Hospital site selection using fuzzy AHP and its derivatives. *Journal of Environmental Management*, *90*(10), 3048–3056. doi:10.1016/j.jenvman.2009.04.010 PMID:19477577

Yeşilyurt, Ö., Sulak, H., & Bayhan, M. (2014). Sağlık Sektöründe Stok Kontrol Faaliyetlerinin ABC ve VED Analizleriyle Değerlendirilmesi: Isparta Devlet Hastanesi Örneği. *Süleyman Demirel Üniversitesi İktisadi ve İdari Bilimler Fakültesi Dergisi*, *20*(1), 365–376.

Zhou, P., & Fan, L. (2007). A note on multi-criteria ABC inventory classification using weighted linear optimization. *European Journal of Operational Research*, *182*(3), 1488–1491. doi:10.1016/j.ejor.2006.08.052

ADDITIONAL READING

Kahraman, C. (Ed.). (2008). *Fuzzy multi-criteria decision making: theory and applications with recent developments* (Vol. 16). Springer Science & Business Media. doi:10.1007/978-0-387-76813-7

Kelly, D. L. (2007). *Applying quality management in healthcare: A systems approach.* Chicago, IL: Health Administration Press.

McLaughlin, D. B., & Hays, J. M. (2008). *Healthcare operations management.* Health Administration Press.

Ozcan, Y. A. (2005). *Quantitative methods in health care management: techniques and applications* (Vol. 4). John Wiley & Sons.

Saaty, T. L. (2000). *Fundamentals of decision making and priority theory with the analytic hierarchy process* (Vol. 6). RWS publications.

Silver, E. A., Pyke, D. F., & Peterson, R. (1998). *Inventory management and production planning and scheduling* (Vol. 3, p. 30). New York: Wiley.

Srichetta, P., & Thurachon, W. (2012). Applying fuzzy analytic hierarchy process to evaluate and select product of notebook computers. *International Journal of Modeling and Optimization*, *2*(2), 168–173. doi:10.7763/IJMO.2012.V2.105

Stevenson, W. J., Hojati, M., & Cao, J. (2007). *Operations management* (Vol. 8). Boston: McGraw-Hill/Irwin.

Walshe, K., & Smith, J. (Eds.). (2011). *Healthcare management. McGraw-Hill Education.* UK: KEY.

KEY TERMS AND DEFINITIONS

Classification: It is an ordered set of related categories used to group data according to its similarities.

Fuzzy Logic: It is a form of multi-valued logic obtained from fuzzy set theory to deal with reasoning that is approximate rather than precise.

Healthcare: It is a health improvement effort via diagnosis, prevention and treatment of illnesses.

Supply Chain: It is the collection of steps that a company takes to transform raw components into final products and deliver them to customers.

Chapter 8
Interval Type II Fuzzy Number Generation From Data Set Applied to Sedation Stage Classification

Efendi Nasibov
https://orcid.org/0000-0002-7273-1473
Dokuz Eylul University, Turkey

Sinem Peker
Yaşar University, Turkey

ABSTRACT

There are several ways to summarize the data set by using measures of locations, dispersions, charts, and so on. But how can the data set be represented or shown when uncertainty exists in the environment process? Usage of the fuzzy number can be a way to handle the uncertainty in the representation of the data set. This chapter focuses on the membership function construction from the data set and introduces the formulas for the interval Type-2 generalized bell-shaped fuzzy number generation based on the data set. The bispectral index scores (BIS) are processed to see the ability of the offered methods in the construction of the interval Type -2 generalized bell-shaped membership function in the real data set. The obtained membership functions are used for a classification problem of sedation stages according to BIS data sets. Classification accuracies are calculated.

DOI: 10.4018/978-1-7998-2581-4.ch008

INTRODUCTION

The one of the way of the representing the uncertain, incomplete information in decision-making, data mining, pattern recognition is using fuzzy numbers and several fuzzy sets theories have been introduced to handle imprecise and uncertain or incomplete information (Ban and Coroianu, 2012; Torres-Blanc et al., 2018, Cheng et al., 2008).

There are various studies where classification, pattern recognition, fuzzy modelling based on the data sets are considered. For example, Shahmoradi and Shouraki (2018) introduced a novel fuzzy sequential pattern recognition tool and they applied this method in speech and handwriting recognition. Solanki and Pandey (2019) focused on predominant instrument recognition and proposed a deep convolution neural network framework where an arbitrary number of instruments from an audio signal with variable length is estimated. Sousa et al. (2019) worked on classification of potential fire outbreaks and offered a fuzzy modeling approach based on thermal images. The evaluations of membership functions from the data set is one of the topics in the classification problems, pattern recognition, fuzzy modeling (Kaufmann et al. 2015, Choi and Rhee, 2009, Bouhentala et al., 2018). For example, Kaufmann et al. (2015) proposed a method for the membership function generation from the data for inductive fuzzy classification. Choi and Rhee (2009) introduced three novel interval type-2 fuzzy membership function generation methods, focusing on heuristics, histograms, and interval type 2 fuzzy C-means. Yang and Bose (2006) mentioned about the importance of the automatic fuzzy membership generation for the pattern recognition and introduced a scheme for the generation of fuzzy membership function by using self-organizing future map. Nasibov and Peker (2011) focused on the generation of the membership function of exponential fuzzy number and evaluated the formulas of unknown parameters based on a minimization problem where the frequencies were used. The offered method was applied on a classification problem dealing with the bispectral index scores (BIS).

There are other various methods focused on the membership function generation. For example, Muhuri and Shukla (2017), underlined the advantages of semi elliptic membership function and introduced a technique for Type-2 semi elliptic membership function. Liao (2017) proposed an extended π interval type-2 membership function and a procedure of the generation of a set of them. Chen et al. (2009) introduced an approach that processes the items in a divide-and-conquer strategy to find the minimum supports, membership functions, and fuzzy association rules. Medasani et al. (1998) focused on an overview of membership function techniques for the pattern recognition and mentioned about the membership function based on the perception, heuristic methods, histogram-based methods, transformation of the probability distributions to the possibility distributions, and so on.

Although the Type I fuzzy sets are often used in the works for mapping the uncertainty in mathematical form, sometimes Type II fuzzy numbers are needed in order to be handle the uncertainty originated from many sources (Shukla and Muhuri, 2019).

In this paper, the construction of the membership function from the data set is handled and an interval Type II generalized bell shaped fuzzy number is focused on. In the foundations of the unknown parameters of this fuzzy number, the percentiles of the data set are used. For the foundation of the core of the fuzzy number, firstly, the intervals are obtained from the percentiles. The percentiles are used as the lower and upper limits of the constructed intervals. After the foundations of the intervals, the interval with narrowest width is detected. This interval is assigned as the interval that includes the core of the fuzzy number. Because the aforementioned interval may represent the peak of the distribution. To obtain unknown parameters dealing with the spreads, the minimization problem is taken into account. In the minimization problem, the sum of the squares of the distances between the limits of the intervals that corresponds to percentiles and the level cuts of fuzzy number with equal alpha-increasing level are considered. The offered method gives an interval type II generalized fuzzy number when the core of the fuzzy number does not fall in the first interval or last interval. The formulas of it are given in Theorem 1. In addition, the problem of how can be a fuzzy number obtained if the core of fuzzy number lies within the first or last interval is handled. For this problem, two additional theorems are introduced. Those theorems satisfy the mixture type of fuzzy numbers based on the data set. The fuzzy number, which has the left part that shows Type I fuzzy number characteristics and the right part that shows Type II characteristics is investigated in Theorem 2. Similarly, a fuzzy number shown Type I and Type II fuzzy number characteristics in the right and left part is searched in Theorem 3.

The proposed construction methods of fuzzy numbers based on the data set are applied on a classification problem of the bispectral index scores that correlates with the sedation stages. 21 real data sets are used in the classification problem. Each data set separated into the training and test data sets. Each training set is obtained by the drawing of a random sample of 204 rows from each data set, and the test set is formed from the remaining 102 rows. After the construction of the training set, the minimum, the maximum, the percentiles of bispectral index scores within each sedation stages are calculated and the fuzzy numbers are constructed by offered formulas in Theorem 1-3 for each sedation stage. Later, each bispectral index score in test set is taken into account, its membership degree for each sedation stage is calculated, and the sedation stage with the maximum membership degree is detected. The sedation stages are predicted with the maximum level criteria in the classification problem. After that, the number of correct predicted sedation stages and the classification accuracy are calculated for each set. Sufficient satisfactory results are obtained in the majority of the data sets.

BACKGROUND

Let $A \in F(E)$ be a fuzzy number, and $\mu_A(x)$ is membership function of A, where $F(E)$ is the space of fuzzy numbers. The fuzzy number A can be represented via α -cuts, A_α, such that:

$$A = \bigcup_{\alpha \in [0,1]} (\alpha, A_\alpha) \tag{2.1}$$

where

$$\forall a \in [0,1] : A_\alpha = [L_A(\alpha), R_A(\alpha)] \subset (-\infty, \infty)$$

and $L\_A:[0,1] \to (-\infty,\infty)$ is monotonically non-decreasing left continuous function, $R\_A:[0,1] \to (-\infty,\infty)$ is monotonically non-increasing left continuous function. Here, $L_A(\alpha)$ and $R_A(\alpha)$ are inverse functions of left-hand and right- hand sides functions of $\mu_A(x)$, respectively and they can be defined by (Nasibov and Peker, 2008; Ban and Coroianu, 2012):

$$L_A(\alpha) = \inf\{x \in \mathbb{R} : \mu_A(x) \geq \alpha\} \tag{2.2}$$

$$R_A(\alpha) = \sup\{x \in \mathbb{R} : \mu_A(x) \geq \alpha\} \tag{2.3}$$

The membership function of fuzzy number, $\mu_A(x)$, $\mu_A : \mathbb{R} \to [0,1]$ can be given by

$$\mu_A(x) = \begin{cases} 0 & , \quad x \leq a_1 \\ \mu_A^L(x) & , \quad a_1 \leq x \leq a_2 \\ 1 & , \quad a_2 \leq x \leq a_3 \\ \mu_A^R(x) & , \quad a_3 \leq x \leq a_4 \\ 0 & , \quad x \geq a_4 \end{cases} \tag{2.4}$$

where are $\mu_A^L(x)$ is non-decreasing and $\mu_A^R(x)$ is non-increasing continuous functions. In special cases, $a_1 = -\infty$ and $a_4 = +\infty$ can be taken (Chanas, 2001).

There are various fuzzy numbers such as triangular, trapezoidal, parametric trapezoidal (semi-trapezoidal), exponential, generalized bell-shaped fuzzy numbers and so on. The membership function of parametric trapezoidal fuzzy number can be defined by (Nasibov and Peker, 2008)

$$\mu_A(x) = \begin{cases} 0 & , \quad x \le a_1 \\ 1 - \left(\dfrac{a_2 - x}{a_2 - a_1} \right)^{s_L} & , \quad a_1 \le x \le a_2 \\ 1 & , \quad a_2 \le x \le a_3 \\ 1 - \left(\dfrac{x - a_3}{a_4 - a_3} \right)^{s_R} & , \quad a_3 \le x \le a_4 \\ 0 & , \quad x \ge a_4 \end{cases} \tag{2.5}$$

where

$$L_A(\alpha) = a_2 - (a_2 - a_1)(1 - \alpha)^{\frac{1}{s_L}} \tag{2.6}$$

$$R_A(\alpha) = a_3 + (a_4 - a_3)(1 - \alpha)^{\frac{1}{s_R}} \tag{2.7}$$

In the case that $s_L = s_R = 1$, the membership function in (2.5) results in the membership function of trapezoidal fuzzy number. In addition, if both $s_L = s_R = 1$ and $a_2 = a_3$, then (2.5) gives the membership function of triangular fuzzy number.

The membership function of exponential fuzzy number is as following,

$$\mu_A(x) = \begin{cases} e^{-\left(\frac{a - x}{\sigma_L} \right)^{s_L}} & , \quad x \le a \\ e^{-\left(\frac{x - a}{\sigma_R} \right)^{s_R}} & , \quad x \ge a \end{cases} \tag{2.8}$$

where

$$L_A(\alpha) = a - \sigma_L(-\ln \alpha)^{\frac{1}{s_L}} \tag{2.9}$$

$$R_A(\alpha) = a + \sigma_R(-\ln\alpha)^{\frac{1}{s_R}} \tag{2.10}$$

The membership function of generalized bell-shaped fuzzy number can be given by

$$\mu_A(x) = \begin{cases} \dfrac{1}{1+\left(\dfrac{a-x}{\sigma_L}\right)^{2s_L}} & , \quad x \leq a \\ \dfrac{1}{1+\left(\dfrac{x-a}{\sigma_R}\right)^{2s_R}} & , \quad x \geq a \end{cases} \tag{2.11}$$

where

$$L_A(\alpha) = a - \left(\frac{1-\alpha}{\alpha}\right)^{\frac{1}{2s_L}} \sigma_L \tag{2.12}$$

$$R_A(\alpha) = a + \left(\frac{1-\alpha}{\alpha}\right)^{\frac{1}{2s_R}} \sigma_R \tag{2.13}$$

For different s_L and s_R values the shapes of generalized bell-shaped membership functions are given in Figure 1.

Figure 1. Generalized bell-shaped fuzzy numbers with different s_L and s_R values.

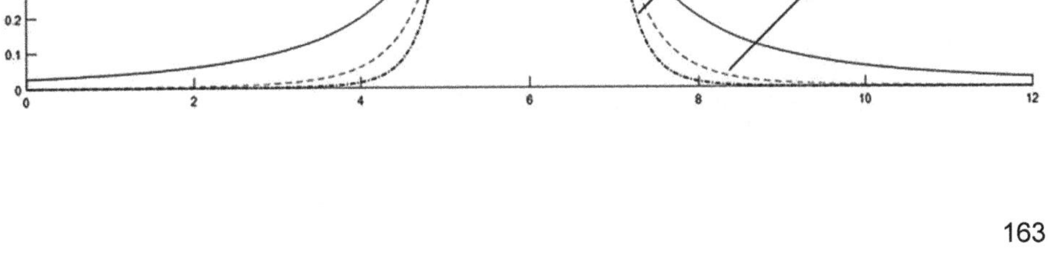

The membership functions definitions in (2.4), (2.5), (2.8), (2.11) are known as Type I membership function. They give a crisp membership degree in $[0,1]$ for an element $x \in X$, where X is the universe of discourse (Rakshit et al., 2016). Accordingly, a Type I fuzzy set can be defined by

$$A = \{(x, \mu_A(x)) | \mu_A(x) \in H, \forall x \in X\} \tag{2.14}$$

where $\mu_A : X \to H$. A type II fuzzy set $\tilde{A}$ can be defined by

$$\tilde{A} = \{(x, \mu_{\tilde{A}}(x)) | \mu_{\tilde{A}}(x) \in \tilde{P}(H), \forall x \in X\} \tag{2.15}$$

where $\tilde{P}(H)$ is the set of fuzzy sets in H (Greenfield and Chiclana, 2018). Here, the membership degree of x in $\tilde{A}$ is a Type I fuzzy value (Ngan, 2018).

The footprint of uncertainty of Type II fuzzy set can be denoted by

$$FOU(\tilde{A}) = \bigcup_{x \in X} J_x \tag{2.16}$$

and it represents "the union of all the primary membership degree". For the continuous Type II fuzzy sets lower membership function, $\mu_{A_l}(x)$, and upper membership function, $\mu_{A_u}(x)$, can be used to denote FOU such as (Mo et al., 2014)

$$FOU(\tilde{A}) = \bigcup_{x \in X} [\mu_{A_l}(x), \mu_{A_u}(x)] \tag{2.17}$$

An interval Type II generalized bell shaped fuzzy number can be defined by $\mu_{A_l}(x)$, lower membership function, $\mu_{A_u}(x)$, upper membership function such that

$$\mu_{A_l}(x) = \begin{cases} \dfrac{1}{1 + \left(\dfrac{t_{A_l} - x}{\sigma_{A_{lL}}}\right)^{2s_{lL}}}, & x \le t_{A_l} \\ \dfrac{1}{1 + \left(\dfrac{x - t_{A_l}}{\sigma_{A_{lR}}}\right)^{2s_{lR}}}, & x \ge t_{A_l} \end{cases} \tag{2.18}$$

$$\mu_{A_u}(x)=\begin{cases}\dfrac{1}{1+\left(\dfrac{t_{A_u}-x}{\sigma_{A_{uL}}}\right)^{2s_{uL}}}, & x\le t_{A_u}\\[2ex] \dfrac{1}{1+\left(\dfrac{x-t_{A_u}}{\sigma_{A_{uR}}}\right)^{2s_{uR}}}, & x\ge t_{A_u}\end{cases} \tag{2.19}$$

where $t_{A_l}=t_{A_u}$, $s_{lL}=s_{uL}$, $s_{lR}=s_{uR}$ and

$$L_{A_l}(\alpha)=t_{A_l}-\left(\frac{1-\alpha}{\alpha}\right)^{\frac{1}{2s_{lL}}}\sigma_{A_{lL}} \tag{2.20}$$

$$R_{A_l}(\alpha)=t_{A_l}+\left(\frac{1-\alpha}{\alpha}\right)^{\frac{1}{2s_{lR}}}\sigma_{A_{lR}} \tag{2.21}$$

$$L_{A_u}(\alpha)=t_{A_u}-\left(\frac{1-\alpha}{\alpha}\right)^{\frac{1}{2s_{uL}}}\sigma_{A_{uL}} \tag{2.22}$$

$$R_{A_u}(\alpha)=t_{A_u}+\left(\frac{1-\alpha}{\alpha}\right)^{\frac{1}{2s_{uR}}}\sigma_{A_{uR}} \tag{2.23}$$

In Figure 2, an interval Type II generalized bell-shaped fuzzy number is demonstrated where $s_{lL}=s_{lR}=s_{uL}=s_{uR}=1$.

Figure 2. The visual demonstration of an interval type II generalized bell shaped fuzzy number.

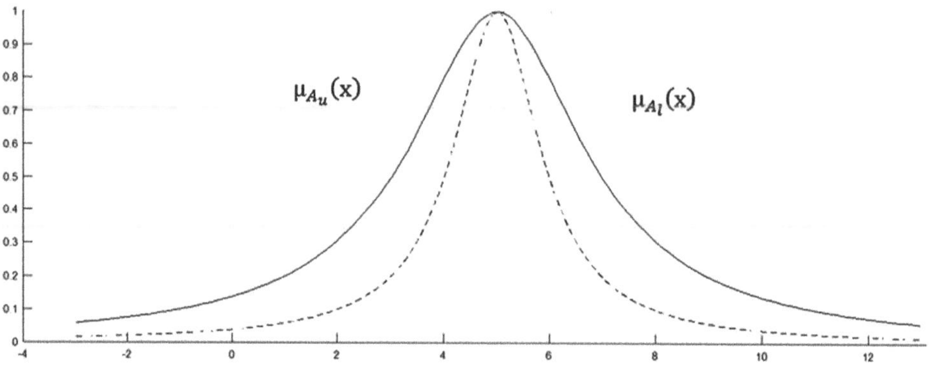

Interval Type II Generalized Bell-Shaped Fuzzy Number GENERATED FROM A Data Set

Various methods about the construction of the membership functions are proposed in the literature by considering the histograms, transformation of the probability distributions to possibility distributions and so on. In recent works, there is an increasing trend on the subject of Type II fuzzy numbers constructions. In this study, interval Type II generalized bell-shaped fuzzy number is considered and a scheme for its construction based on the data set is proposed. In the evaluations of the lower and upper membership functions of interval Type II generalized bell-shaped fuzzy number, the percentiles of the data set are used.

The steps of offered schemes are as following:

1. Obtain the intervals of which the lower and upper limits are sequential percentiles and detect the interval with the narrowest width.
2. Calculate the average value of the lower limit and upper limit of the interval with narrowest width as the core of the fuzzy number since this interval may represent the peak of the distribution.
3. Obtain the spreads of the fuzzy numbers by using formulas that are obtained via the minimization problems based on the sum of the squares of the distances between the x values that corresponds to percentiles and the alpha cuts of fuzzy number with equal increasing level.

The visual demonstration of x value that corresponds to given percentile is given in Figure 3.

Figure 3. The visual demonstration of the intervals.

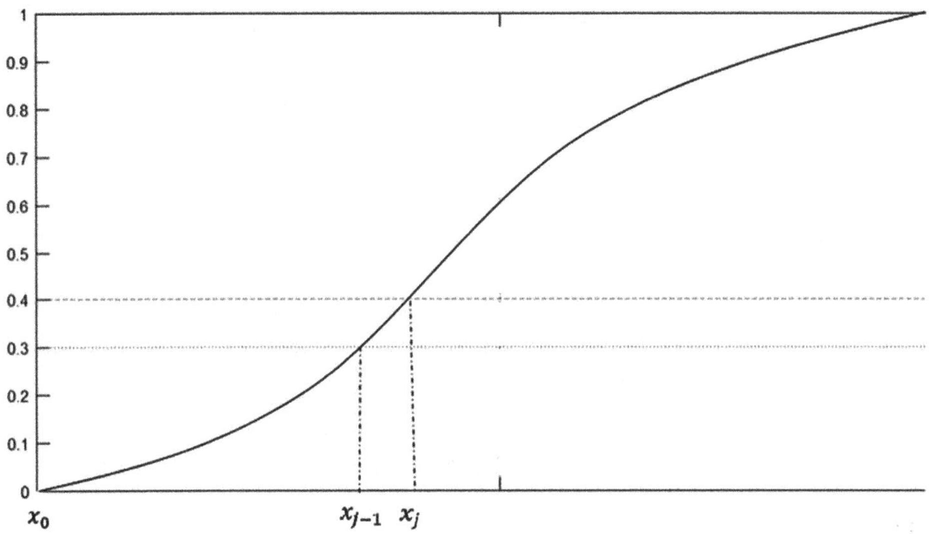

In Figure 3, the intervals where lower and upper limits correspond to sequential percentiles are as following,

$$x_1 - x_2, \ldots, x_{j-1} - x_j, \ldots, x_{n-1} - x_n$$

In the real data sets, Ogive graphs may be used to find these intervals.

Let's consider an interval Type II generalized bell-shaped fuzzy number with the lower and upper membership functions in (2.18) and (2.19), respectively. The core value of the membership function is decided to take as the average value of the lower and upper limit of interval with the narrowest width to construct the nearest interval Type II generalized bell-shaped fuzzy number based on data set in Theorem 1. Because the frequency of the number of the observations that fall the narrowest width is expected as the maximum frequency. Therefore, it is reasonable to think that this interval may represent the peak of the distribution of the data set. After the detection of the interval with the narrowest width by using percentiles of the data set, the number of the intervals up to this interval is counted for the determination of the number of alpha cuts of the pattern functions. Alpha cuts are determined with equal increasing levels where $L_{Au}(1)$ corresponds to x_1 and $L_{Al}(1)$ corresponds to x_2 in the calculation of the distances.

Let $x_{j-1}-x_j$ is the interval with narrowest width. It is expected that the number of observations that falls in this interval is greater or equal than the number observations that falls in other intervals. In the first step of scheme, this interval is detected and then the core of the interval Type II generalized bell-shaped fuzzy number is calculated by the following formula

$$t_{A_l}=t_{A_u}=\frac{x_{j-1}+x_j}{2} \tag{3.1}$$

in the second step. The values of $\sigma_{A_{uL}}$, $\sigma_{A_{lL}}$, $\sigma_{A_{uR}}$, $\sigma_{A_{lR}}$ or σ_{A_L}, σ_{A_R} are calculated by introduced Theorem 1, Theorem 2, and Theorem 3 in the third step.

Theorem 1 considers the construction of interval Type II generalized bell-shaped fuzzy number when the core of it does not fall in the first or the last raw. In addition, it is supposed that the numbers of alpha cuts are equivalent to $j-1$ in the left part of the fuzzy number, $n-j+1$ in the right part of the fuzzy number for the upper membership function, and they are equal to in order $j-2$ and $n-j$ for the lower membership function for the lower membership function. In the foundations of unknown parameters of $\sigma_{A_{uL}}$, $\sigma_{A_{lL}}$, $\sigma_{A_{uR}}$, $\sigma_{A_{lR}}$, the following objective function are taken into account in the minimization problem,

$$O_1=\left[\sum_{i=1}^{j-1}\left(x_i-t_{A_u}+\left(\frac{1-\alpha}{\alpha}\right)^{\frac{1}{2s_{uL}}}\sigma_{A_{uL}}\right)^2+\sum_{i=j}^{n}\left(x_i-t_{A_u}-\left(\frac{1-\alpha}{\alpha}\right)^{\frac{1}{2s_{uR}}}\sigma_{A_{uR}}\right)^2\right]$$

$$+\left[\sum_{i=2}^{j-1}\left(x_i-t_{A_l}+\left(\frac{1-\alpha}{\alpha}\right)^{\frac{1}{2s_{lL}}}\sigma_{A_{lL}}\right)^2+\sum_{i=j}^{n-1}\left(x_i-t_{A_l}-\left(\frac{1-\alpha}{\alpha}\right)^{\frac{1}{2s_{lR}}}\sigma_{A_{lR}}\right)^2\right] \tag{3.2}$$

In this minimization problem, the following equalities with unknown parameters $\sigma_{A_{uL}}$, and $\sigma_{A_{uR}}$ are solved for the construction of the upper membership function,

$$\frac{\delta O_1}{\delta\sigma_{A_{uL}}}=0 \tag{3.3}$$

$$\frac{\delta O_1}{\delta \sigma_{A_{uR}}} = 0 \tag{3.4}$$

Similarly, the following equalities are solved with respect to unknown parameters $\sigma_{A_{lL}}$, and $\sigma_{A_{lR}}$ for the construction of lower membership function,

$$\frac{\delta O_1}{\delta \sigma_{A_{lL}}} = 0 \tag{3.5}$$

$$\frac{\delta O_1}{\delta \sigma_{A_{lR}}} = 0 \tag{3.6}$$

Theorem 1: For the given $s_{A_{uL}}$, $s_{A_{uR}}$, $s_{A_{lL}}$, $s_{A_{lR}}$ values, the $\sigma_{A_{uL}}$, $\sigma_{A_{uR}}$, $\sigma_{A_{lL}}$, $\sigma_{A_{lR}}$ parameters of an interval Type II generalized bell shaped fuzzy number evaluated from the minimization problem of O_1 in (3.2) are as following,

$$\sigma_{A_{uL}} = \frac{-\sum_{i=1}^{j-1} x_i \left(\frac{j-1-i}{i}\right)^{\frac{1}{2s_{uL}}} + t_{A_u} \sum_{i=1}^{j-1} \left(\frac{j-1-i}{i}\right)^{\frac{1}{2s_{uL}}}}{\sum_{i=1}^{j-1} \left(\frac{j-1-i}{i}\right)^{\frac{2}{2s_{uL}}}} \tag{3.7}$$

$$\sigma_{A_{uR}} = \frac{\sum_{i=j}^{n} x_i \left(\frac{i-j}{n-i+1}\right)^{\frac{1}{2s_{uR}}} - t_{A_u} \sum_{i=j}^{n} \left(\frac{i-j}{n-i+1}\right)^{\frac{1}{2s_{uR}}}}{\sum_{i=j}^{n} \left(\frac{i-j}{n-i+1}\right)^{\frac{2}{2s_{uR}}}} \tag{3.8}$$

$$\sigma_{A_{lL}} = \frac{-\sum_{i=2}^{j-1} x_i \left(\frac{j-i}{i-1}\right)^{\frac{1}{2s_{lL}}} + t_{A_l} \sum_{i=2}^{j-1} \left(\frac{j-i}{i-1}\right)^{\frac{1}{2s_{lL}}}}{\sum_{i=2}^{j-1} \left(\frac{j-i}{i-1}\right)^{\frac{2}{2s_{lL}}}} \tag{3.9}$$

$$\sigma_{A_{lR}} = \frac{\sum_{i=j}^{n-1} x_i \left(\frac{i-j+1}{n-i}\right)^{\frac{1}{2s_{lR}}} - t_{A_l} \sum_{i=j}^{n-1} \left(\frac{i-j+1}{n-i}\right)^{\frac{1}{2s_{lR}}}}{\sum_{i=j}^{n-1} \left(\frac{i-j+1}{n-i}\right)^{\frac{2}{2s_{lR}}}} \tag{3.10}$$

where $2 < j < n-1$, and t_{A_l}, t_{A_u} are calculated by (3.1)

Proof: Let consider that the number of alpha cuts is equivalent to $j-1$ in the left part of the fuzzy number, $n-j+1$ in the right part of the fuzzy number for the upper membership function, and they are equal to in order $j-2$ and $n-j$ for the lower membership function. Accordingly, the minimization problem of O_1 holds to the following form taking into account the alpha cuts with equal increasing level,

$$\min \left\{ \begin{array}{l} \sum_{i=1}^{j-1} \left(x_i - t_{A_u} + \left(\frac{1-\frac{i}{j-1}}{\frac{i}{j-1}} \right)^{\frac{1}{2s_{uL}}} \sigma_{A_{uL}} \right)^2 + \sum_{i=j}^{n} \left(x_i - t_{A_u} - \left(\frac{1-\frac{n-i+1}{n-j+1}}{\frac{n-i+1}{n-j+1}} \right)^{\frac{1}{2s_{uR}}} \sigma_{A_{uR}} \right)^2 \\ + \sum_{i=2}^{j-1} \left(x_i - t_{A_l} + \left(\frac{1-\frac{i-1}{j-1}}{\frac{i-1}{j-1}} \right)^{\frac{1}{2s_{lL}}} \sigma_{A_{lL}} \right)^2 + \sum_{i=j}^{n-1} \left(x_i - t_{A_l} - \left(\frac{1-\frac{n-i}{n-j+1}}{\frac{n-i}{n-j+1}} \right)^{\frac{1}{2s_{lR}}} \sigma_{A_{lR}} \right)^2 \end{array} \right\}$$

By using this minimization problem, the equality dealing with $\sigma_{A_{uL}}$ is obtained by solving the following equality

$$2\sum_{i=1}^{j-1}\left(x_i - t_{A_u} + \left(\frac{1-\frac{i}{j-1}}{\frac{i}{j-1}}\right)^{\frac{1}{2s_{uL}}}\sigma_{A_{uL}}\right)\left(\frac{1-\frac{i}{j-1}}{\frac{i}{j-1}}\right)^{\frac{1}{2s_{uL}}} = 0$$

and $\sigma_{A_{uL}}$ is extracted as following,

$$\sigma_{A_{uL}} = \frac{-\sum_{i=1}^{j-1} x_i\left(\frac{j-1-i}{i}\right)^{\frac{1}{2s_{uL}}} + t_{A_u}\sum_{i=1}^{j-1}\left(\frac{j-1-i}{i}\right)^{\frac{1}{2s_{uL}}}}{\sum_{i=1}^{j-1}\left(\frac{j-1-i}{i}\right)^{\frac{2}{2s_{uL}}}}$$

In a similar way, the formulas of $\sigma_{A_{uR}}$ can be obtained by solving

$$-2\sum_{i=j}^{n}\left(x_i - t_{A_u} - \left(\frac{1-\frac{n-i+1}{n-j+1}}{\frac{n-i+1}{n-j+1}}\right)^{\frac{1}{2s_{uR}}}\sigma_{A_{uR}}\right)\left(\frac{1-\frac{n-i+1}{n-j+1}}{\frac{n-i+1}{n-j+1}}\right)^{\frac{1}{2s_{uR}}} = 0$$

and from the related equality

$$\sigma_{A_{uR}} = \frac{\sum_{i=j}^{n} x_i\left(\frac{i-j}{n-i+1}\right)^{\frac{1}{2s_{uR}}} - t_{A_u}\sum_{i=j}^{n}\left(\frac{i-j}{n-i+1}\right)^{\frac{1}{2s_{uR}}}}{\sum_{i=j}^{n}\left(\frac{i-j}{n-i+1}\right)^{\frac{2}{2s_{uR}}}}$$

is found.

For the lower membership function,

$$\min\left[\sum_{i=2}^{j-1}\left(x_i - t_{A_l} + \left(\frac{1-\frac{i-1}{j-1}}{\frac{i-1}{j-1}}\right)^{\frac{1}{2s_{lL}}}\sigma_{A_{lL}}\right)^2 + \sum_{i=j}^{n-1}\left(x_i - t_{A_l} - \left(\frac{1-\frac{n-i}{n-j+1}}{\frac{n-i}{n-j+1}}\right)^{\frac{1}{2s_{lR}}}\sigma_{A_{lR}}\right)^2\right]$$

can be taken into account. For the $\sigma_{A_{lL}}$ and $\sigma_{A_{lR}}$, the following equalities are solved, respectively.

$$2\sum_{i=2}^{j-1}\left(x_i - t_{A_l} + \left(\frac{1-\frac{i-1}{j-1}}{\frac{i-1}{j-1}}\right)^{\frac{1}{2s_{lL}}}\sigma_{A_{lL}}\right)\left(\frac{1-\frac{i-1}{j-1}}{\frac{i-1}{j-1}}\right)^{\frac{1}{2s_{lL}}} = 0$$

$$-2\sum_{i=j}^{n-1}\left(x_i - t_{A_l} - \left(\frac{1-\frac{n-i}{n-j+1}}{\frac{n-i-1}{n-j}}\right)^{\frac{1}{2s_{lR}}}\sigma_{A_{lR}}\right)\left(\frac{1-\frac{n-i}{n-j+1}}{\frac{n-i}{n-j+1}}\right)^{\frac{1}{2s_{lR}}} = 0$$

From the above equalities,

$$\sigma_{A_{lL}} = \frac{-\sum_{i=2}^{j-1} x_i\left(\frac{j-i}{i-1}\right)^{\frac{1}{2s_{lL}}} + t_{A_l}\sum_{i=2}^{j-1}\left(\frac{j-i}{i-1}\right)^{\frac{1}{2s_{lL}}}}{\sum_{i=2}^{j-1}\left(\frac{j-i}{i-1}\right)^{\frac{2}{2s_{lL}}}}$$

and

$$\sigma_{A_{lR}} = \frac{\sum_{i=j}^{n-1} x_i \left(\frac{i-j+1}{n-i}\right)^{\frac{1}{2s_{lR}}} - t_{A_l} \sum_{i=j}^{n-1} \left(\frac{i-j+1}{n-i}\right)^{\frac{1}{2s_{lR}}}}{\sum_{i=j}^{n-1} \left(\frac{i-j+1}{n-i}\right)^{\frac{2}{2s_{lR}}}}$$

are obtained, which ends the proof.

If the "$x_1 - x_2$" interval is the interval with the narrowest width, then the left part of the interval Type II generalized bell shaped fuzzy number cannot be calculated by Theorem 1. In that case, Theorem 2 can be a remedy for the construction of the mixture type of fuzzy numbers based on the data set. Theorem 2 evaluate a fuzzy number such that the left part of fuzzy number show Type I characteristic while the right part of fuzzy number show Type II characteristics. The formulas of unknown parameters are obtained by the solution of the minimization problem with the following objective function

$$O_2 = \left[\left(x_{\min} - t_{A_u} + \left(\frac{1-\alpha_{\min}}{\alpha_{\min}} \right)^{\frac{1}{2s_L}} \sigma_{A_L} \right)^2 \right] + \left[\sum_{i=j}^{n} \left(x_i - t_{A_u} - \left(\frac{1-\alpha}{\alpha} \right)^{\frac{1}{2s_{uR}}} \sigma_{A_{uR}} \right)^2 + \sum_{i=j}^{n-1} \left(x_i - t_{A_l} - \left(\frac{1-\alpha}{\alpha} \right)^{\frac{1}{2s_{lR}}} \sigma_{A_{lR}} \right)^2 \right] \quad (3.11)$$

where x_{min} is the minimum value of the data set and α_{min} is a very small membership value of fuzzy number, which is decided by decision maker.

Theorem 2: The $\sigma_{A_{uR}}$, $\sigma_{A_{lR}}$ parameters of mixture type generalized bell shaped fuzzy number evaluated from the minimization problem of O_2 in (3.11) are as in (3.8) and (3.10), respectively for the given s_{A_L}, $s_{A_{uR}}$, $s_{A_{lR}}$ values. And the parameter of σ_{A_L} is as following,

$$\sigma_{A_L} = \frac{-x_{\min} + t_{A_u}}{\left(\frac{1-\alpha_{\min}}{\alpha_{\min}} \right)^{\frac{1}{2s_L}}} \quad (3.12)$$

where $\alpha_{\min} > 0$.

Proof: The following equality is solved to find the unknown parameter σ_{A_L},

$$2\left(x_{\min} - t_{A_u} + \left(\frac{1-\alpha_{\min}}{\alpha_{\min}}\right)^{\frac{1}{2s_L}} \sigma_{A_L}\right) = 0$$

and it results that

$$\sigma_{A_L} = \frac{-x_{\min} + t_{A_u}}{\left(\frac{1-\alpha_{\min}}{\alpha_{\min}}\right)^{\frac{1}{2s_L}}}$$

which ends the proof. It is clear that the foundations of formulas $\sigma_{A_{uR}}$, $\sigma_{A_{lR}}$ gives the same results in Theorem 1.

If the " $x_{n-1} - x_n$ " interval is the interval with the narrowest width, Theorem 3 is offered to construct the mixture type of fuzzy numbers based on the data set. Because, the right part of the interval Type II fuzzy number cannot be calculated by Theorem 1. Theorem 3 satisfy a fuzzy number such that the left part of fuzzy number show Type II characteristic while right part of fuzzy number show Type I characteristics. In the foundations of $\sigma_{A_{uL}}$, $\sigma_{A_{lL}}$, σ_{A_R} unknown parameters, the following objective function in the minimization problem is used,

$$O_3 = \left[\left(x_{\max} - t_{A_u} - \left(\frac{1-\alpha_{\min}}{\alpha_{\min}}\right)^{\frac{1}{2s_R}} \sigma_{A_R}\right)^2\right] + \left[\sum_{i=2}^{j-1}\left(x_i - t_{A_l} + \left(\frac{1-\alpha}{\alpha}\right)^{\frac{1}{2s_{lL}}} \sigma_{A_{lL}}\right)^2 + \sum_{i=1}^{j-1}\left(x_i - t_{A_u} + \left(\frac{1-\alpha}{\alpha}\right)^{\frac{1}{2s_{uL}}} \sigma_{A_{uL}}\right)^2\right] \quad (3.13)$$

where $x_{\max}$ is the maximum value of the data set and α_{min} is a very small membership value of fuzzy number, which is decided by decision maker.

Theorem 3: The $\sigma_{A_{uL}}$, $\sigma_{A_{lL}}$ parameters of mixture type generalized bell shaped fuzzy number evaluated from the minimization problem of O_3 in (3.13) are as in (3.7) and (3.9), respectively for the given $s_{A_{uL}}$, $s_{A_{lL}}$, s_{A_R} values. And the parameter of σ_{A_R} is as following,

$$\sigma_{A_R} = \frac{x_{\max} - t_{A_u}}{\left(\frac{1-\alpha_{\min}}{\alpha_{\min}}\right)^{\frac{1}{2s_R}}} \tag{3.14}$$

where $\alpha_{\min} > 0$.

Proof: The unknown parameter σ_{A_R} is obtained by solving the following equality

$$-2\left(x_{\max} - t_{A_u} - \left(\frac{1-\alpha_{\min}}{\alpha_{\min}}\right)^{\frac{1}{2s_R}} \sigma_{A_R}\right) = 0$$

and

$$\sigma_{A_R} = \frac{x_{\max} - t_{A_u}}{\left(\frac{1-\alpha_{\min}}{\alpha_{\min}}\right)^{\frac{1}{2s_R}}}$$

is obtained, which ends the proof. It is clear that the foundations of formulas $\sigma_{A_{uL}}$, $\sigma_{A_{lL}}$ give the same results in Theorem 1.

A BIS Classification Application

Electroencephalography (EEG) is dealing with brain electrical activity and it is used in various cases. For example, it may be wanted to aid diagnosis of epilepsy (Zaiwalla, 2018). The Bispectral Index Score (BIS) is a monitoring instrument for depth of anesthesia and it is derived from an EEG analysis such that the depth of anesthesia is shown as a single value (Liu et al., 2019). BIS correlates the levels of sedation and it is used as a measure of sedation (Barbato et al., 2017).

The construction of the membership functions based on the data set is one of the methods used in the classification problems. In this section, the introduced technique for the construction of the interval type II generalized bell-shaped fuzzy number is processed in a classification problem to see efficiency of the membership functions. As the data sets, the same data sets used by Nasibov and Ulutagay (2010) except one are handled, 21 data sets dealing with bispectral index scores obtained using the electroencephalograph signals are processed.

In order to be apply a classification procedure and to obtain a classification accuracy for each data set, firstly, a random sample of 204 rows is selected from each data set to construct the training sets. The test sets are extracted from the remaining rows after the selection of the training sets from the data set that involves 306 rows. Hence, each data set separate into the training set with 204 rows and the test set with 102 rows. The training sets are used for the construction of fuzzy numbers, and the test sets are used for the calculation of the classification accuracy.

After the extraction of the training sets, the minimum, the maximum values and the percentiles of the BIS are found for each sedation stage. By using these values, the $\sigma_{A_{uL}}$, $\sigma_{A_{lL}}$, $\sigma_{A_{uR}}$, $\sigma_{A_{lR}}$ or σ_{A_L}, σ_{A_R} are calculated by formulas introduced Theorems 1-3 and the obtained results are given in Table 1-11. As shown in tables, 67 sedation stages are handled and for each sedation stages generalized bell shaped fuzzy numbers are calculated. Among 67 fuzzy numbers, 52 of them are constructed via Theorem 1 and the interval Type II generalized bell shaped fuzzy numbers are obtained. 7 of them evaluated by Theorem 2 and the mixture type fuzzy numbers which includes Type I characteristic on the left parts and Type II characteristic on the right parts of them are found. 8 of them are evaluated by Theorem 3 and the fuzzy numbers which show Type II characteristic on the left parts of them and Type I characteristics on the right part of them are constructed. After the foundation of fuzzy numbers, the average value of $\mu_{A_l}(x)$ and $\mu_{A_u}(x)$ is calculated for each interval Type II generalized bell shaped fuzzy numbers and mixture type fuzzy numbers.

The membership degree of each bispectral index score for each sedation stage is calculated in the handled test set and the maximum membership degree is detected. This maximum membership degree is taken into account for the prediction of the sedation stage in BIS classifying. After the classification, the number of correct predictions that are the same with expert decisions are count for each test set. The number of correct points divide the number of points in the test set to calculate the classification accuracy. Table 12 gives the classification accuracies with the parameters obtained by using Theorems 1-3 and maximum level criteria in the membership degrees. It is observed that majority of the 21 data set give sufficient satisfactory results.

Table 1. Percentiles of training sets 1-2 and calculated parameters via theorems 1-3

		Training Set of Set 1					Training Set of Set 2	
		S. Stage 1	S. Stage 2	S. Stage 3	S. Stage 4	S. Stage 5	S. Stage 2	S. Stage 3
Min		,2520	,2050	,5650	,819	,872	,2640	,5280
Max		,5820	,7980	,8160	,899	,977	,8260	,9650
Percentile	10	,310200	,337100	,601500	,82250	,87200	,300000	,564500
	20	,332200	,373600	,627600	,83220	,87320	,324000	,605000
	30	,356100	,396200	,681100	,83930	,87610	,352700	,628500
	40	,368200	,407600	,697600	,84440	,88380	,376400	,645000
	50	,375500	,429000	,704500	,84500	,92850	,389000	,672500
	60	,388000	,461800	,791200	,84940	,97220	,400200	,720000
	70	,393900	,498700	,805000	,87150	,97640	,491200	,755000
	80	,405600	,547200	,808600	,88260	,97700	,577200	,821000
	90	,564100	,600100	,811900	,89410	.	,655900	,848000
t		,39095	,4019	,81025	,8447	,9767	,3946	,63675
$\sigma_{A_{UL}}$		,036953	,044661	,090442	,012478	,058211	,049711	,049851
$\sigma_{A_{UR}}$		,102092	,091948	-	,026408	-	,159452	,106442
$\sigma_{A_{IL}}$		,024787	,017621	,071057	,006282	,050634	,032755	,020294
$\sigma_{A_{IR}}$		,009122	,062461	-	,01755	-	,096024	,079476
σ_{A_R}		-	-	,006608	-	3,02E-05	-	-

Table 2. Percentiles of training sets 3-4 and calculated parameters via theorem 1-3

		Training Set of Set 3			Training Set of Set 4		
		S. Stage 2	**S. Stage 3**	**S. Stage 4**	**S. Stage 1**	**S. Stage 2**	**S. Stage 3**
Min		,3080	,4780	,8330	,2110	,2840	,7080
Max		,7870	,8760	,9610	,3790	,7920	,9120
Percentile	10	,402800	,672000	,840200	,264000	,333900	,755000
	20	,444400	,738000	,852600	,275600	,353000	,792000
	30	,478500	,764800	,881400	,282000	,368000	,807000
	40	,499000	,783600	,893200	,291600	,378600	,819000
	50	,530000	,804000	,898000	,302500	,407500	,829500
	60	,565600	,813400	,910600	,316000	,431400	,846000
	70	,602400	,828800	,934400	,323000	,462800	,872000
	80	,635400	,834600	,940000	,331800	,517400	,873000
	90	,667900	,838800	,953800	,342000	,559700	,891500
t		,48875	,8367	,8956	,2788	0,3733	,8725
$\sigma_{A_{UL}}$		,061165	,057804	,033959	,0148	0,02803	,051576
$\sigma_{A_{UR}}$		,091313	-	,032721	,03068	0,0881	,019
$\sigma_{A_{lL}}$		,027987	,037134	,020784	,0032	0,012982	,037375
$\sigma_{A_{lR}}$		,068879	-	,02334	,024448	0,061315	,0005
σ_{A_R}		-	,00395	-	-	-	-

Table 3. Percentiles of training sets 5-6 and calculated parameters via theorem 1-3

		Training Set of Set 5				Training Set of Set 6	
		S. Stage 1	S. Stage 2	S. Stage 3	S. Stage 4	S. Stage 2	S. Stage 3
Min		,1790	,3430	,6080	,8150	,2740	,5140
Max		,3570	,8020	,8910	,8760	,6560	,7110
Percentile	10	,193300	,415200	,640100	,815000	,333600	,538200
	20	,211800	,481800	,655800	,815000	,362000	,565600
	30	,232400	,526400	,670100	,826200	,374000	,623600
	40	,248600	,570400	,704000	,848600	,397000	,636000
	50	,258500	,605000	,742500	,871000	,411000	,645000
	60	,265600	,622000	,770200	,873000	,423800	,654600
	70	,280800	,645000	,803700	,875000	,437000	,662000
	80	,308600	,700400	,819000	.	,474000	,673600
	90	,339500	,747800	,834000	.	,510200	,696200
t		,26205	,6135	,66295	,815	,368	,6583
$\sigma_{A_{UL}}$		,035841	,101387	,02285	-	,0344	,052421
$\sigma_{A_{UR}}$		,044198	,077931	,088628	,034593	,061251	,025767
$\sigma_{A_{lL}}$		,02331	,063821	,00715	-	,006	,033301
$\sigma_{A_{lR}}$		,023406	,043136	,074117	,028782	,044054	,009702
σ_{A_L}		-	-	-	0	-	-

Table 4. Percentiles of training sets 7-8 and calculated parameters via theorem 1-3

		Training Set of Set 7			Training Set of Set 8		
		S. Stage 2	**S. Stage 3**	**S. Stage 4**	**S. Stage 3**	**S. Stage 4**	**S. Stage 5**
Min		,2440	,2850	,8100	,4680	,7040	,7300
Max		,7460	,8320	,9100	,9130	,9100	,9200
Percentile	10	,305400	,592000	,810000	,538600	,748600	,815400
	20	,347600	,648000	,829200	,597600	,799800	,828800
	30	,385200	,681000	,848000	,642000	,817700	,840100
	40	,430000	,697000	,861200	,697000	,825000	,848600
	50	,465000	,717000	,868500	,729000	,828000	,860000
	60	,488600	,744000	,884600	,768200	,839000	,863200
	70	,526200	,769000	,905000	,800300	,852300	,871000
	80	,591800	,792000	,906000	,826000	,868000	,877800
	90	,650600	,813000	.	,846000	,883000	,897000
t		,4768	,689	,9055	,836	,8265	,8616
$\sigma_{A_{UL}}$		,093386	,066468	,044059	,125501	,038471	,024409
$\sigma_{A_{UR}}$		,102589	,063718	-	-	,029788	,01914
$\sigma_{A_{IL}}$		,064628	,025456	,033581	,096786	,012903	,016106
$\sigma_{A_{IR}}$		,058938	,048486	-	-	,019567	,008858
σ_{A_R}		-	-	,000452	,007739	-	-

Table 5. Percentiles of training sets 9-10 and calculated parameters via theorem 1-3

		Training Set of Set 9			Training Set of Set 10			
		S. Stage 3	**S. Stage 4**	**S. Stage 5**	**S. Stage 1**	**S. Stage 2**	**S. Stage 3**	**S. Stage 4**
Min		,4720	,7640	,8430	,2360	,4040	,5030	,7400
Max		,8560	,9110	,9420	,4150	,6470	,8430	,8910
Percentile	10	,620000	,809500	,874800	,269000	,433300	,607100	,740000
	20	,645600	,824000	,886000	,281600	,456000	,646600	,741600
	30	,693400	,832000	,892000	,288700	,486300	,726500	,749100
	40	,709000	,841000	,895000	,302400	,505200	,748200	,784800
	50	,744000	,846500	,900000	,311500	,540500	,756500	,809500
	60	,755600	,855000	,906000	,320400	,571600	,785000	,835800
	70	,776000	,871000	,911000	,332600	,583000	,820700	,877100
	80	,790400	,887000	,915200	,349200	,609200	,826800	,887800
	90	,816000	,900000	,921600	,370000	,617900	,833900	.
t		0,7498	,84375	,8935	,28515	,61355	,82375	,7408
$\sigma_{A_{UL}}$		,070702	,019813	,0127	,01615	,081116	,093888	-
$\sigma_{A_{UR}}$		,03932	,030132	,014111	,037501	-	,01015	,069596
$\sigma_{A_{lL}}$		,048887	,010972	,004667	,00355	,06563	,068065	-
$\sigma_{A_{lR}}$		,023047	,020328	,010464	,027605	-	,00305	,054447
σ_{A_R}, σ_{A_L}						,003362		8,04E-05

Table 6. Percentiles of training sets 11 and calculated parameters via theorem 1-3

		Training Set of Set 11				
		S. Stage 1	S. Stage 2	S. Stage 3	S.Stage 4	S. Stage 5
Min		,2840	,3320	,3980	,7760	,3950
Max		,6940	,5940	,8910	,9710	,8210
Percentile	10	,306800	,358200	,446500	,812000	,399500
	20	,322800	,388400	,510000	,865000	,435400
	30	,333800	,397600	,568500	,904500	,457100
	40	,349600	,427000	,623000	,926000	,499200
	50	,357000	,432000	,672000	,938500	,509500
	60	,369800	,460600	,724000	,946000	,542200
	70	,378800	,489200	,781000	,950500	,621900
	80	,393200	,516600	,837000	,953000	,718600
	90	,426200	,558600	,862000	,960500	,800300
t		,3533	,4295	,8495	,95175	,50435
$\sigma_{A_{UL}}$		,028223	,042234	,180412	,050858	,064116
$\sigma_{A_{UR}}$		,034868	,066884	-	,00875	,151045
$\sigma_{A_{lL}}$		,017184	,024122	,145263	,029826	,03915
$\sigma_{A_{lR}}$		,019691	,042695	-	,00125	,094433
σ_{A_R}				,004171	-	-

Table 7. Percentiles of training sets 12-13 and calculated parameters via theorem 1-3

		Training Set of Set 12				Training Set of Set 13		
		S. Stage 1	**S. Stage 2**	**S. Stage 3**	**S. Stage 4**	**S. Stage 3**	**S. Stage 4**	**S. Stage 5**
Min		,2760	,3740	,4110	,4340	,5560	,8210	,8440
Max		,3860	,9630	,9750	,9740	,9160	,9720	,9720
Percentile	10	,284000	,374000	,491800	,534800	,582000	,868100	,879600
	20	,287000	,462000	,566000	,575600	,609000	,878400	,892000
	30	,293000	,708000	,612800	,613400	,621000	,896000	,899000
	40	,295000	,775000	,639000	,642600	,730000	,909400	,905400
	50	,298000	,788000	,683000	,733000	,749000	,917000	,911000
	60	,316000	,789000	,718400	,802800	,772000	,925200	,916600
	70	,342000	,888000	,760200	,844000	,797000	,935000	,923000
	80	,353000	,955000	,825000	,887400	,840000	,944200	,932800
	90	,366000	.	,872000	,954200	,879000	,961000	,948800
t		0,294	,7885	,6259	,628	,615	,9132	,9082
$\sigma_{A_{UL}}$		,007637	,202809	,092801	,067543	,033	,028349	,016396
$\sigma_{A_{UR}}$		,035607	,122329	,121507	,170438	,132757	,024525	,019888
$\sigma_{A_{lL}}$		,004243	,118888	,03759	,033771	,006	,018385	,008971
$\sigma_{A_{lR}}$		,025872	,056427	,08895	,131159	,108648	,015646	,011779
σ_{A_R}		-	-	-	-	-	-	-

Table 8. Percentiles of training sets 14-15 and calculated parameters via theorem 1-3

		Training Set of Set 14			Training Set of Set 15		
		S. Stage 3	**S. Stage 4**	**S. Stage 5**	**S. Stage 3**	**S. Stage 4**	**S. Stage 5**
Min		,3510	,8580	,8230	,4730	,7050	,5290
Max		,9720	,9310	,9720	,8960	,8970	,9500
Percentile	10	,409000	,858000	,823000	,514000	,705000	,673200
	20	,426000	,858000	,828000	,524400	,723000	,830600
	30	,440000	,858000	,836000	,539000	,740000	,862600
	40	,454000	,858000	,866000	,560400	,740000	,867400
	50	,480000	,871000	,895000	,588000	,742000	,878500
	60	,526400	,884000	,904000	,640000	,743000	,887600
	70	,600000	,907500	,920000	,697000	,868000	,895700
	80	,688400	.	,947000	,782600	,889000	,916600
	90	,836800	.	.	,843400	.	,926700
t		,433	,858	0,8255	,5955	,74	,865
$\sigma_{A_{UL}}$		,024	0	-	-	,024607	,118228
$\sigma_{A_{UR}}$		,15291	,027517	,056302	,132169	,07141	,030305
$\sigma_{A_{lL}}$		,007	0	-	-	,009617	,020138
$\sigma_{A_{lR}}$		,09456	,013392	,042922	,10924	,040723	,022071
σ_{A_L}		-	-	,000251	,012312	-	-

Table 9. Percentiles of training sets 16-17 and calculated parameters via theorem 1-3

		Training Set of Set 16			Training Set of Set 17	
		S. Stage 3	S. Stage 4	S. Stage 5	S. Stage 2	S. Stage 3
Min		,5360	,7450	,7870	,3340	,4310
Max		,8870	,9070	,9770	,5810	,8200
Percentile	10	,582000	,797800	,871500	,368200	,505000
	20	,616000	,832800	,896000	,384000	,582000
	30	,647000	,846800	,905500	,396800	,618000
	40	,673000	,855000	,910000	,406000	,628000
	50	,682000	,863000	,919000	,415000	,637000
	60	,714000	,870400	,927000	,421600	,673000
	70	,745000	,881800	,938000	,435400	,699000
	80	,786000	,892400	,953000	,451800	,725000
	90	,818000	,896800	,964000	,488000	,770000
t		,6775	,8946	,90775	,4183	,6325
$\sigma_{A_{UL}}$		,056428	,036946	,023829	,025857	,064548
$\sigma_{A_{UR}}$		,075935	-	,027433	,037868	,07213
$\sigma_{A_{IL}}$		,03222	,025904	,007283	,016617	,024131
$\sigma_{A_{IR}}$		,051697	-	,01979	,017776	,047028
σ_{A_R}		-	,001246	-	-	-

Table 10. Percentiles of training sets 18-19 and calculated parameters via theorem 1-3

		Training Set of Set 18			Training Set of Set 19		
		S. Stage 2	S. Stage 3	S. Stage 4	S. Stage 2	S. Stage 3	S. Stage 4
Min		,4560	,5890	,7930	,5700	,6160	,8420
Max		,7680	,9020	,9680	,7900	,8410	,9340
Percentile	10	,565800	,698400	,793000	,592600	,691000	,842000
	20	,577000	,734000	,800200	,610000	,727200	,845200
	30	,600400	,753000	,815300	,620600	,773600	,859300
	40	,616400	,766400	,824000	,635200	,796800	,867400
	50	,653000	,777000	,857000	,661000	,806000	,869500
	60	,665600	,797600	,906800	,678600	,813200	,876000
	70	,681200	,810200	,944000	,697400	,818000	,897000
	80	,699600	,822800	,965600	,709800	,820600	,926800
	90	,732600	,834400	.	,737200	,828000	.
t		,5714	,7717	,7966	,6153	,8193	,7717
$\sigma_{A_{UL}}$		-	,04049	-	,0227	,048704	,04049
$\sigma_{A_{UR}}$		,071648	,036213	,076372	,05692	,0087	,03276
$\sigma_{A_{lL}}$		-	,02009	-	,0053	,03047	,02009
$\sigma_{A_{lR}}$		,057215	,026984	,057584	,04383	,0013	,022072
$\sigma_{A_{L}}$		,011598	-	,000362	-	-	-

Table 11. Percentiles of training sets 20-21 and calculated parameters via theorem 1-3

		Training Set of Set 20			Training Set of Set 21		
		Stage 2	**Stage 3**	**Stage 4**	**Stage 2**	**Stage 3**	**Stage 4**
Min		,3350	,6240	,5370	,3850	,4120	,8850
Max		,5150	,8540	,9720	,8220	,8790	,9280
Percentile	10	,350400	,657200	,694000	,417000	,461600	,885000
	20	,360600	,692000	,728000	,436400	,508200	,885000
	30	,367200	,714000	,770500	,452100	,525800	,891600
	40	,379400	,750200	,803000	,468800	,545400	,904800
	50	,389000	,769000	,827000	,489000	,577000	,918000
	60	,403800	,784200	,845000	,504000	,624600	,922000
	70	,419400	,794400	,875500	,519900	,657400	,926000
	80	,481000	,830800	,890000	,546600	,708800	.
	90	,510400	,841400	,934000	,643200	,757400	.
t		,3639	,7893	,88275	,4965	,517	,885
$\sigma_{A_{UL}}$		,0135	,062645	,085773	,044059	,0554	-
$\sigma_{A_{UR}}$		,059627	,04121	,05125	,073316	,107351	,022294
$\sigma_{A_{lL}}$		,0033	,043655	,06491	,031316	,0088	-
$\sigma_{A_{lR}}$		,040677	,024918	,00725	,026424	,079782	,017686
σ_{A_L}		-	-	-	-	-	0

Table 12. Classification accuracies using offered parameters

Data Set	n_{test}	Correct Estimation	Classification Accuracy	Data Set	n_{test}	Correct Estimation	Classification Accuracy
1	102	68	,666667	12	102	24	,235294
2	102	86	,843137	13	102	39	,382353
3	102	83	,813725	14	102	87	,852941
4	102	88	,862745	15	102	74	,72549
5	102	78	,764706	16	102	78	,764706
6	102	93	,911765	17	102	96	,941176
7	102	79	,77451	18	102	55	,539216
8	102	39	,382353	19	102	69	,676471
9	102	83	,813725	20	102	63	,617647
10	102	79	,77451	21	102	69	,676471
11	102	64	,627451				

SOLUTIONS AND RECOMMENDATIONS

In this chapter, one of the methods dealing with the construction of the interval Type II generalized bell-shaped fuzzy number based on the data set introduced. The percentiles are used in the offered method and the core of the fuzzy numbers is obtained by considering narrowest interval of which the lower and upper boundaries consist of percentiles. However, it is unable to find the lower and upper membership functions by this method when the core of the fuzzy numbers lies between the 1st and 2nd percentiles, and between the (n-1)th and nnd percentiles. In those cases, the lower and upper membership functions cannot be calculated with offered Theorem 1 for the left or right part. As a remedy for this situation, the additional Theorems are offered as Theorem 2-3 in the chapter. These theorems satisfy mixture type fuzzy numbers where one part of it shows the characteristics of Type I fuzzy number while the other part of shows Type II characteristics. In other words, the methods which combines Type II fuzzy number characteristics and Type I fuzzy number characteristics are offered.

FUTURE RESEARCH DIRECTIONS

In future researches, the effects of $s_{A_{uL}}$, $s_{A_{uR}}$, $s_{A_{lL}}$, $s_{A_{lR}}$ values that are decided by decision makers can be investigated on the construction of the interval Type II generalized bell shaped membership function based on the data set. Alternative methods may be introduced for selection of the optimal values of the parameters $s_{A_{uL}}$, $s_{A_{uR}}$, $s_{A_{lL}}$, $s_{A_{lR}}$ according to different criteria.

CONCLUSION

In this study, the construction of an interval Type II generalized membership function based on the data set is studied. The percentiles of the data set are used for the forming of the intervals, and the limits of these intervals are processed in the calculation of the core and the spreads of the related fuzzy numbers. The interval with the narrowest width is taken as the interval that involves the core of the fuzzy number because the number of observations that falls in this interval may be equal or greater than the number observations that falls in the other intervals and this interval may represent the peak of the distribution. The average value of the lower and upper limits of this interval is taken as the core of the fuzzy number. For the foundation of the left and the right spreads of the related fuzzy number, a minimization problem that is based on the sum of the squares of the distances between percentiles and alpha cuts of the fuzzy number with equal increasing levels is solved. In Theorem 1, the formulas of the left and right spreads of the lower and upper membership functions of the interval Type II generalized bell shaped fuzzy number are found if the core of the fuzzy number does not take any value in the first or last interval. When the core of fuzzy number falls in the first interval, Theorem 1 is inapplicable for the foundation of the left spreads of the lower and upper membership functions of the fuzzy number. For this case, Theorem 2 can be used for the foundation of fuzzy number that reflects the characteristics of Type I fuzzy number on the left part and the characteristics of Type II fuzzy number on the right part of the fuzzy number. If the core of fuzzy number falls in the last interval, Theorem 3 can be applied to obtain a fuzzy number that reflects the characteristics of Type I fuzzy number on its right part and the characteristics of Type II fuzzy number on its left part. Similarly, both Theorem 2 and Theorem 3 are based on the minimization problems where the sum of the squares of the distances between the percentiles and the alpha cuts of the fuzzy number with equal increasing levels are used.

The offered methods for the fuzzy number construction based on the data set are applied on a classification problem to see their efficiency. 21 real data set dealing with bispectral index scores and sedation stages are used in the classification problem and the observations are aimed to assign the correct sedation stages. Each data set separated into the training and the test sets. The minimum, the maximum values and the percentiles of the bispectral index scores are found for each sedation stage in the training sets for the construction of the fuzzy numbers. The offered theorems are applied to construct fuzzy numbers for each sedation stage in each training set. The test sets are used to obtain the classification accuracies. For classification, firstly, the average values of $\mu_{A_l}(x)$ and $\mu_{A_u}(x)$ are calculated for each interval Type II generalized bell shaped fuzzy numbers and mixture type fuzzy numbers. After that, the membership degree of each bispectral index score for each sedation stage is calculated and the maximum membership degree is used for the prediction of the sedation stage in BIS classifying. After the classification, the number of correct predictions for each test set is counted and the classification accuracy is calculated. In the majority of the related data set, the sufficient satisfactory results are observed.

ACKNOWLEDGMENT

The data sets used in the experiment dealing with bispectral index series were provided by Professor M. Özgören.

REFERENCES

Ban, A. I., & Coroianu, L. (2012). Nearest interval, triangular and trapezoidal approximation of a fuzzy number preserving ambiguity. *International Journal of Approximate Reasoning*, *53*(5), 805–836. doi:10.1016/j.ijar.2012.02.001

Bang, Y. K., & Lee, C. H. (2011). Fuzzy time series prediction using hierarchical clustering algorithms. *Expert Systems with Applications*, *38*(4), 4312–4325. doi:10.1016/j.eswa.2010.09.100

Barbato, M., Barclay, G., Potter, J., Yeo, W., & Chung, J. (2017). Correlation Between Observational Scales of Sedation and Comfort and Bispectral Index Scores. *Journal of Pain and Symptom Management*, *54*(2), 186–193. doi:10.1016/j.jpainsymman.2016.12.335 PMID:28063863

Bouhentala, M., Mouna G., & Kheireddine, C. (2018). Interval-valued membership function estimation for fuzzy modeling, *Fuzzy Sets and Systems*, Available online July 4, 2018.

Chanas, S. (2001). On the interval approximation of a fuzzy number. *Fuzzy Sets and Systems*, *122*(2), 353–356. doi:10.1016/S0165-0114(00)00080-4

Chen, C. H., Hong, T.-P., & Tseng, V. S. (2009). An improved approach to find membership functions and multiple minimum supports in fuzzy data mining. *Expert Systems with Applications*, *36*(6). doi:10.1016/j.eswa.2009.01.067

Cheng, C. H., Cheng, G. V., & Wang, J. W. (2008). Multi-attribute fuzzy time series method based on fuzzy clustering. *Expert Systems with Applications*, *3*(2), 1235–1242. doi:10.1016/j.eswa.2006.12.013

Choi, B. I., & Rhee, F. C. H. (2009). Interval Type-2 fuzzy membership function generation methods for pattern recognition. *Information Sciences*, *179*(13), 2102–2122. doi:10.1016/j.ins.2008.04.009

Greenfield, S., & Chiclana, F. (2018). Type-Reduced Set structure and the truncated type-2 fuzzy set. *Fuzzy Sets and Systems*, *352*, 119–141. doi:10.1016/j.fss.2018.02.012

Kaufmann, M., Meier, A., & Stoffel, K. (2015). IFC-Filter: Membership function generation for inductive fuzzy classification. *Expert Systems with Applications*, *42*(21), 8369–8379. doi:10.1016/j.eswa.2015.06.034

Liao, T. W. (2017). A Procedure for the generation of type-2 membership functions from data. *Applied Soft Computing*, *52*, 925–936. doi:10.1016/j.asoc.2016.09.034

Liu, Y. H., Qiu, D. J., Jia, L., Tan, J. T., Kang, J. M., Xie, T., & Xu, H. M. (2019). Depth of anesthesia measured by bispectral index and postoperative mortality: A meta-analysis of observational studies. *Journal of Clinical Anesthesia*, *56*, 119–125. doi:10.1016/j.jclinane.2019.01.046 PMID:30771713

Medasani, S., Kim, J., & Krishnapuram, R. (1998). An overview of membership function generation techniques for pattern recognition. *International Journal of Approximate Reasoning*, *19*(3-4), 391–417. doi:10.1016/S0888-613X(98)10017-8

Moa, H., Wang, F.-Y., Zhou, M., Li, R., & Xiao, Z. (2014). Footprint of uncertainty for type-2 fuzzy sets. *Information Sciences*, *272*, 96–110. doi:10.1016/j.ins.2014.02.092

Muhuri, P. K., & Shukla, A. K. (2017). Semi-elliptic membership function: Representation, generation, operations, deffuzification, ranking and its application to the real-time task scheduling problem. *Engineering Applications of Artificial Intelligence*, *60*, 71–82. doi:10.1016/j.engappai.2016.12.020

Nasibov, E., & Peker, S. (2011). Exponential Membership Function Based on Frequency. *Asian Journal of Mathematics and Statistics*, *4*(1), 8–20. doi:10.3923/ajms.2011.8.20

Nasibov, E. N., & Ulutagay, G. (2010). Comparative clustering analysis of bispectral index series of brain activity. *Expert Systems with Applications*, *37*(3), 2495–2504. doi:10.1016/j.eswa.2009.07.071

Ngan, S.-C. (2018). Revisiting fuzzy set operations: A rational approach for designing set operators for type-2 fuzzy sets and type-2 like fuzzy sets. *Expert Systems with Applications*, *107*, 255–284. doi:10.1016/j.eswa.2018.03.061

Rakshita, P., Saha, S., Konar, A., & Saha, S. (2016). A type-2 fuzzy classifier for gesture induced pathological disorder recognition. *Fuzzy Sets and Systems*, *305*, 95–130. doi:10.1016/j.fss.2016.05.001

Shahmoradi, S., & Shouraki, S. B. (2018). Evaluation of a novel fuzzy sequential pattern recognition tool (fuzzy elastic matching machine) and its applications in speech and handwriting recognition. *Applied Soft Computing*, *62*, 315–327. doi:10.1016/j.asoc.2017.10.036

Shukla, A. K., & Muhuri, P. K. (2019). Big-data clustering with interval type-2 fuzzy uncertainty modeling in gene expression datasets. *Engineering Applications of Artificial Intelligence*, *77*, 268–282. doi:10.1016/j.engappai.2018.09.002

Solanki, A., & Pandey, S. (2019). Music instrument recognition using deep convolutional neural networks, *International Journal of Information Technology*, 1-10.

Sousa, M. J., Moutinho, A., & Almeida, M. (2019). Classification of potential fire outbreaks: A fuzzy modeling approach based on thermal images. *Expert Systems with Applications*, *129*, 216–232. doi:10.1016/j.eswa.2019.03.030

Torres-Blanc, C., Hernández-Varela, P., & Cubillo, S. (2018). Self-contradiction for type-2 fuzzy sets whose membership degrees are normal and convex functions. *Fuzzy Sets and Systems*, *352*, 73–91. doi:10.1016/j.fss.2017.12.015

Yang, C. C., & Bose, N. K. (2006). Generating fuzzy membership function with self-organizing feature map. *Pattern Recognition Letters*, *27*(5), 356–365. doi:10.1016/j.patrec.2005.08.026

Zaiwalla, Z. (2018). To EEG or not EEG. *Paediatrics & Child Health*, *28*(6), 289–292. doi:10.1016/j.paed.2018.04.013

ADDITIONAL READING

Bigand, A., & Colot, O. (2016). Membership function construction for interval-valued fuzzy sets with application to Gaussian noise reduction. *Fuzzy Sets and Systems*, *286*, 66–85. doi:10.1016/j.fss.2015.07.001

Hong, T. P., & Chen, J. B. (1999). Finding relevant attributes and membership functions. *Fuzzy Sets and Systems*, *103*(3), 389–404. doi:10.1016/S0165-0114(97)00187-5

Hu, B. Q., & Wang, C. Y. (2014). On type-2 fuzzy relations and interval-valued type-2 fuzzy sets. *Fuzzy Sets and Systems*, *236*, 1–32. doi:10.1016/j.fss.2013.07.011

Mizumoto, M., & Tanaka, K. (1976). Some properties of fuzzy sets of type-2. *Information and Control*, *31*(4), 312–340. doi:10.1016/S0019-9958(76)80011-3

Mizumoto, M., & Tanaka, K. (1981). Fuzzy sets of type-2 under algebraic product and algebraic sum. *Fuzzy Sets and Systems*, *5*(3), 277–290. doi:10.1016/0165-0114(81)90056-7

Sanchez, M. A., Castillo, O., & Castro, J. R. (2015). Information granule formation via the concept of uncertainty-based information with Interval Type-2 Fuzzy Sets representation and Takagi–Sugeno–Kang consequents optimized with Cuckoo search. *Applied Soft Computing*, *27*, 602–609. doi:10.1016/j.asoc.2014.05.036

Torres-Blanc, C., Cubillo, S., & Hernández, P. (2017). Aggregation operators on type-2 fuzzy sets. *Fuzzy Sets and Systems*, *324*, 74–90. doi:10.1016/j.fss.2017.03.015

Zadeh, L. A. (1965). Fuzzy sets. *Information and Control*, *8*(3), 338–353. doi:10.1016/S0019-9958(65)90241-X

KEY TERMS AND DEFINITIONS

Bell-Shaped Membership Function: A special type of membership function.

Bispectral Index Score: An index reflecting the stage of brain activity.

Classification: A problem that identifies the class of the sample according to data set.

Electroencephalogram Data: Electrical signals of brain activity collected via special equipment.

Fuzzy Number: A Fuzzy set that consists of the set of real numbers with crisp membership degrees.

Fuzzy Set: A set that can have elements with different crisp membership degrees between 0 and 1 interval.

Interval Membership Function: A membership function with values as intervals.

Membership Function Generation: Construction of the parameters of the membership function retrieved from data set.

Type II Fuzzy Number: A Fuzzy Number that consists of the set of real numbers with membership degrees as Fuzzy Numbers.

Chapter 9
Detection of Chronic Disease in Primary Care Using Artificial Intelligence Techniques

Hakan Gulmez
https://orcid.org/0000-0001-5467-3743
Department of Family Medicine, İzmir Demokrasi University, Turkey

ABSTRACT

Chronic diseases are the leading causes of death and disability worldwide. By 2020, it is expected to increase to 73% of all deaths and 60% of global burden of disease associated with chronic diseases. For all these reasons, early diagnosis and treatment of chronic diseases is very important. Machine learning is an application of artificial intelligence that provides systems the ability to automatically learn and improve from experience without being explicitly programmed. Machine learning is the development of computer programs that can access data and use it to learn for themselves. The learning process starts by searching for patterns in the examples, experiences, or observations. It will make faster and better decisions in the future based on all these. The primary purpose in machine learning is to allow computers to learn automatically without human help and affect. Considering all the reasons above, this chapter finds the most appropriate artificial intelligence technique for the early detection of chronic diseases.

DOI: 10.4018/978-1-7998-2581-4.ch009

INTRODUCTION

We all know that the world population and average life expectancy are increasing. As a result of the increasing population and increasing life expectancy, the annual applications to the health sector are increasing rapidly. With these increasing applications, the examination times of physicians are shortened. Malpractice (medical malpractice) is defined as the harm caused by the physician's failure to perform standard practice, lack of skills or failure to treat the patient (Koc, 2014). Reduced examination times bring the risk of malpractice. For all these reasons, physicians should diagnose patients who come to their clinic in a short time.

Healthcare is defined as studies for health protection, treatment and rehabilitation of diseases. The aim of the health service is to increase, improve and maintain the health level of society and individuals. Healthcare services are divided into 3 classes: preventive health services, therapeutic health services and rehabilitative health services (Rakel & Rakel, n.d.). Also, therapeutic health services are divided into three groups: primary health care services, secondary health care services and tertiary health care services (AYGN et al., 2016). Health institutions provide all of the preventive, therapeutic and rehabilitative health services to the individual or families. However, the distribution of all these health services varies. Preventive health services come to the fore in primary health care services. In addition, the primary healthcare, which is first step of healthcare services, is great importance in the early diagnosis and follow-up of the diseases. Because primary healthcare cares about people rather than treatment certain diseases (Rakel & Rakel, n.d.).

Chronic diseases are affecting more and more people with increasing life span. Chronic diseases are the leading causes of death and disability worldwide. Chronic disease rates accelerate globally, progress in each region and affect all socioeconomic classes("WHO | Projections of mortality and causes of death, 2016 to 2060," 2018). Early diagnosis and treatment of chronic diseases is very important. Family physicians in primary care examine their patients regularly and keep all information digitally thanks to the patient follow-up programs they use today. In fact, these regularly recorded data provide an unprecedented opportunity for people to be diagnosed early (Rakel & Rakel, n.d.).

Machine learning is an application of artificial intelligence that provides systems the ability to automatically learn and improve from experience without being explicitly programmed. Using the machine learning technique, we can conduct research across chronic diseases and healthy individuals based on the currently selected medical data sets. Using some machine learning techniques, the prediction of chronic disease can be simplified using a variety of features to determine whether a person is at risk for chronic disease. It also takes less time for early diagnosis and treatment of diseases ("What is artificial intelligence?," n.d.).

Considering all the reasons above, the aim of this chapter is to find the most appropriate artificial intelligence technique for the early detection of chronic diseases by using the data set, which was used in a study conducted on the staff working on a university campus.

DEFINITIONS

Chronic Disease

Chronic diseases are generally defined as conditions that last for 1 year or more and require ongoing medical assistance or limit activities in daily life or both. Chronic diseases such as heart disease, cancer and diabetes are the most important causes of death and disability worldwide ("About Chronic Diseases I CDC," n.d.; "WHO I Integrated chronic disease prevention and control," 2010). These disease rates are accelerating globally, progressing in every region and affecting all socioeconomic classes. According to the World Health Organization (WHO) World Health Report 2002, death, morbidity and disability currently attributed to major chronic diseases currently account for almost 60% of all deaths and 43% of the global burden of disease. By 2020, chronic diseases are expected to rise to 73% of all deaths and 60% of global disease burden. Furthermore, in developing countries, the mortality rate from these diseases reaches 79%. Four of the most common chronic diseases are;

- Cardiovascular diseases (CVD),
- Cancer,
- Chronic obstructive pulmonary disease (COPD)
- Type 2 diabetes

These diseases are associated with common and preventable biological risk factors, particularly behavioral risk factors associated with high blood pressure, high blood cholesterol and overweight, as well as unhealthy nutrition, physical inactivity and tobacco use. Action to prevent these major chronic diseases is to try to control them and other important risk factors in a very well-integrated way and to diagnose them as early as possible. Developing an integrated approach to address all major risk factors of chronic diseases is the most cost-effective way to prevent and control them.

Family Medicine

Family medicine is a medical specialty that provides continuous and comprehensive health care for the individual and the family. It is the most comprehensive specialty combining biological, clinical and behavioral sciences (Rakel & Rakel, n.d., p. 5).

Family Physician

The family physician is a physician trained in the discipline of family medicine. Family physicians have different attitudes, skills, and knowledge (e.g. biological, behavioral, or social) that are characterized by providing continuous and comprehensive medical care, health care and preventive services to each member of a family, regardless of gender, age, or type of problem.

Primary Care

Primary health care is a community-wide approach to health and well-being that focuses on the needs and preferences of the individual, family and community. It deals with health in a broader context and focuses on the comprehensive and interrelated aspects of physical, mental and social health and well-being ("Primary health care," n.d.). In 1978 the Declaration of Alma- Ata identified primary health care as the most cost- effective way to deliver essential health services (*Declaration of Alma-Ata*, 1978). In addition to the diagnosis and treatment of acute and chronic diseases, primary health care includes disease prevention, health care, counseling and patient education in various health care settings. (e.g., office, inpatient, critical care, long-term care, home care). WHO emphasizes that primary care is the best way to cope with 21st century diseases and that better use of existing preventive measures can reduce the global burden of disease by as much as 70%.

METHODS

Artificial Intelligence

According to Encyclopedia Britannica, artificial intelligence (AI) is defined as *"The ability of a digital computer or computer-controlled robot to perform tasks commonly associated with intelligent beings. The term is frequently applied to the project of developing systems endowed with the intellectual processes characteristic of humans, such as the ability to reason, discover meaning, generalize, or learn from past experience.*"("Artificial intelligence I Definition, Examples, and Applications I Britannica.com," n.d.).

AI algorithms are designed to make decisions using real-time data. They are not like passive machines that can only respond to mechanical or predetermined responses. It combines information from various sources, analyzes the material instantly, and acts according to predictions derived from this data ("What is artificial intelligence?," n.d.).

Artificial neural networks (ANNs) use a similar pattern to the way the human brain processes information. ANN includes several neuron-like processing units that work together. They contain a large number of synapses. The network has an input layer, an output layer, and any number of hidden layers. A neuron bound to all neurons in the next layer, as shown in Figure 1 (S. H. Chen, Jakeman, & Norton, 2008).

Figure 1. Overview of artificial neural networks
(Adapted from (S. H. Chen et al., 2008)).

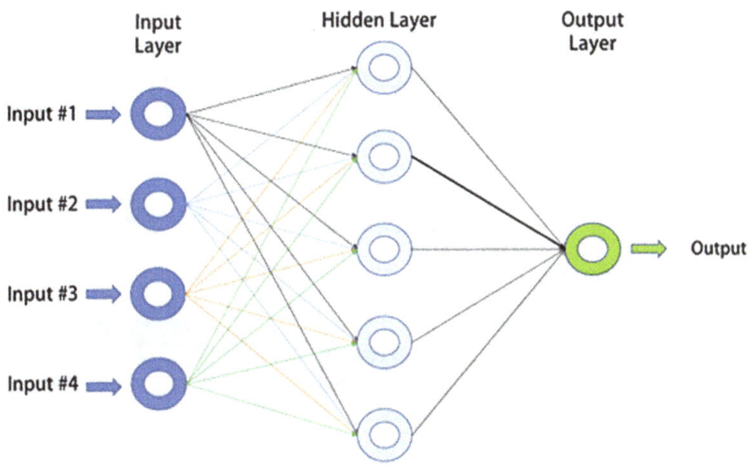

AI makes our lives easier in many different fields including industry, aerospace engineering, finance, computer science, health, aviation, weather forecasting, toys and computer games. In the field of medicine, AI systems can be used to regulate inpatient treatment services, establish staff work plan and follow up and edit patient files (Anyanwu, 2011).

Machine Learning

Machine learning is a data analysis technique that teaches computers to learn from the natural experience like humans and animals. Machine learning algorithms learn information directly from data using computational methods without relying on a predetermined equation as a model. As the number of samples available for learning increases, so does the performance of machine learning algorithms. Deep learning is a special form of machine learning ("What Is Machine Learning? | How It Works, Techniques & Applications - MATLAB & Simulink," n.d.).

Machine learning allows computers to automatically learn and predict processes to accomplish challenging tasks that cannot simply be described by humans, for example, self-driving cars, film recommendations on digital platforms, online recommendations, diagnosis in medical imaging, autonomous robotic surgery (Kannan & Vasanthi, 2019).

There are two different main models of machine learning which are supervised and unsupervised learning models (Figure 2).

Figure 2. Machine learning techniques: unsupervised and supervised learning *(Adapted from ("What Is Machine Learning? | How It Works, Techniques & Applications - MATLAB & Simulink," n.d.)).*

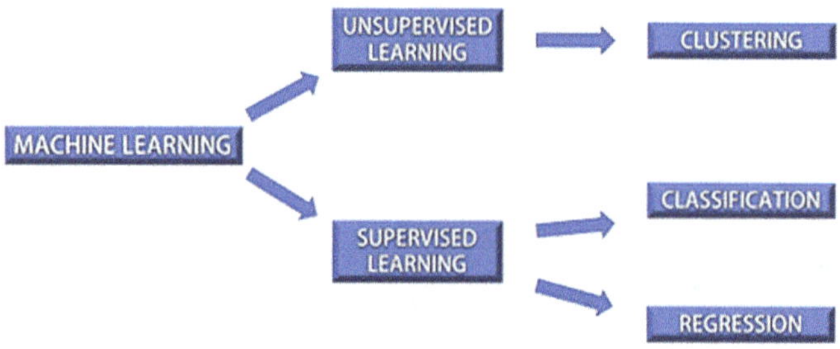

Supervised Learning

A supervised learning model receives known responses from a known set of input data. Using this knowledge develops a model to produce reasonable estimates for responding to new data. Supervised learning models are evaluated under two headings as "classification" and "regression".

Classification techniques predict different responses, such as whether an email is original or spam, or whether a tumor is malign or benign. Classification models classify input data by category. Typical application areas are medical imaging, speech recognition, credit scoring and so on. There are so many algorithms for performing classification -for example; support vector machine (SVM), semi-supervised support vector machine (S3VM), k-nearest neighbor (KNN), linear classifiers, logistic regression, naïve bayes classifier, perceptron, quadratic classifiers, k-means clustering, boosting and bagging decision tree, random forest (rf), neural networks, bayesian networks and so on (Jet & O, 2017; "What Is Machine Learning? I How It Works, Techniques & Applications - MATLAB & Simulink," n.d.).

Support Vector Machine

SVMs are among the most popular techniques of machine learning. If the data is sufficiently labeled, it usually gives excellent results. In summary, SVM is to solve the quadratic programming problem for a given training data set (Figure 3). We should remember that SVM is only available when training sets are marked. While there is a large amount of unmarked data in real life, the scope of application of SVM is limited. To solve this problem in processing large amounts of data, the semi-supervised support vector machine appeared in machine learning tasks (Nawel, Nabiha, Nilanjan, & Mokhtar, 2016).

Figure 3. An example of a problem that can be divided into two different groups. The support vectors are marked with colored squares to identify the largest margin of separation between the two groups
Source: (Adapted from (Cortes, Corinna, 1995)).

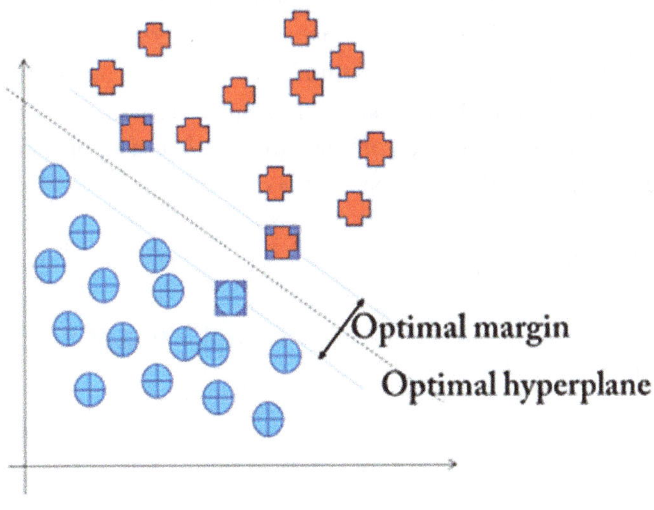

Semi-Supervised Learning Method

The semi-supervised learning method is a combination of non-supervised learning and supervised learning. In recent years, semi-supervised learning has focused on machine learning. The purpose of this method is to help improve the impact of the supervised learning method by using a large number of unlabeled data. Semi-supervised learning is recommended because unlabeled data can indeed help theoretically improve the performance of an algorithm. Semi-supervised learning algorithms are mostly based on two assumptions. These assumptions are cluster assumption and manifold assumption. The cluster assumption is used where samples in the same batch are more likely to have the same label. The manifold assumption assumes that proximal points along the manifold plane have a similar structure or similar label. Of these two assumptions, the cluster assumption reflects the global characteristics of the models, while the manifold assumption reflects local characteristics (Ding, Zhu, & Zhang, 2017).

Semi-Supervised Support Vector Machine

S3VM method first introduced by Bennet and Demiriz. S3VM is a semi-supervised learning method and is mainly based on the cluster assumption. If the training set is larger than the working set, S3VM may be considered as a method to solve the transduction risk according to the overall risk minimization principle (Bennett & Demiriz, 1998).

K-Nearest Neighbor

The KNN method is an instance-based learning method. This method stores all existing data points and classifies new data points according to the measure of similarity. The main idea of the KNN method is to give new unclassified samples to the class to which most of its K nearest neighbors belong. KNN is very effective in reducing the wrong classification error when the number of samples in the training data set is high (Saini, Singh, & Khosla, 2013).

Linear Classifiers

Linear classifiers are very successful in the field of text classification (Zhang & Iyengar, 2002).

Regression

The other supervised learning technique is regression. Regression techniques estimate continuous responses such as changes in temperature or changes in water consumption of a region. Typical applications include accurate quantitative estimation of energy performance of residential buildings using, medical situations such as cardiovascular risk prediction, big data evaluation in econometry and so on (Akay, 2018; Goldstein et al., 2016; Jihad & Tahiri, 2018).

Naïve Bayes Classifier

Naïve Bayes is popular in text classification because of its computational efficiency and relatively good predictability (J. Chen, Huang, Tian, & Qu, 2009).

Perceptron

The Perceptron algorithm was introduced by Rosenblatt in the late 1950s (Rosenblatt, 2005). The perceptron, a simple computing engine, is best related to supervised classification. Since 1950s, neural networks have been used to improve classification decision boundaries or to evaluate the assignment of new cases (Murtagh, 1991).

Quadratic Classifiers

Quadratic classifiers are very popular in pattern recognition (Fukunaga & Hayes, 1989). In addition, handwriting recognition is another area where quadratic classifiers are used (Liu, Sako, & Fujisawa, 2004).

K-Means Clustering

The most commonly used criterion for clustering is the clustering error criterion that calculates the square distance from the corresponding cluster center for each point and then receives the sum of these distances for all points in the data set. The K-mean clustering algorithm has become a popular clustering method because it minimizes clustering error (Likas, Vlassis, & J. Verbeek, 2003).

Boosting and Bagging Decision Tree

Bagging is a bootstrap community method that creates a community for individuals by training each classifier on the random distribution of the training set. Boosting classifiers are a family of methods that have focus to produce a series of classifiers.

In the boosting process, samples that are incorrectly estimated by previous classifiers in the series are selected more often than those that are correctly predicted (Maclin & Opitz, 1997).

Random Forest

Random forests add an additional layer of randomness to the bagging. In addition to set up each tree data using a different bootstrap, random forests change the way the classification or regression trees are built (Liaw & Wiener, 2002).

Neural Networks

See artificial intelligence.

Bayesian Networks

To explain the Bayesian network simply, it is an annotated oriented graph. It encodes probabilistic relationships between distinctions of interest in an uncertain reasoning problem (Heckerman, Geiger, & Chickering, 1995).

Unsupervised Learning

Unsupervised learning process should be used, when there is a set of variables and no corresponding output variables (i.e., the data are unlabeled). Because of there is no correct answer for the training data to learn from, the learning algorithm must figure out the connections in the datasets. Clustering techniques is one of the most important unsupervised learning techniques. This technique is the process of segmenting data from some breakpoints according to some similarity criteria (e.g. weight) (Alashwal, El Halaby, Crouse, Abdalla, & Moustafa, 2019).

Data Set

Machine learning models require a large amount of data to accurately predict. We can collect the necessary data sets from the data sources of health institutions. AI algorithms can be added to the data management systems used by family medicine, and many predictions can be made by using the data that physicians have already entered into the system.

In this chapter, we have introduced the dataset which was used in a study conducted on the staff working on a university campus and explained the machine learning models with ROC curve for the chronic disease predictions (Gülmez, 2013). The data were collected by face to face survey data collection technique.

Data set used in our study consists of 83 staff working on the university campus between January and February 2012. The data set has 19 features (Table 1) with 83 samples and 2 classes. The classification of a data set is achieved by utilizing a model whose parameters tuned by an appropriate technique.

We obtained 19 variables and divided the data into two groups. We formed the AI training group with 70% of the data. We used the remaining 30% for the test group. The percentage of chronic disease should not be the same in training and testing of data. We have listed 19 variables in Table 1.

Table 1. Variables used in the study

Variable
Age
Sex
Height
Weight
BMI
Education
Marital status
Number of children
Household status
How many people live at home
Year of work
Satisfaction at work
Quality of life
Satisfaction of health
Physical satisfaction
Psychological satisfaction
Social satisfaction
Environmental satisfaction
Chronic disease status

Experiment

Chronic disease is a general definition. Therefore, there is no single method for chronic disease detection. For the diagnosis of chronic disease, the question of which chronic disease should be answered first. Afterwards, examinations should be performed for the pre-diagnosed chronic disease. The number of these examinations varies according to the diseases. Of course, as the number of examinations performed increases rapidly in costs.

The time from the occurrence of chronic diseases to diagnosis is very important. Because the damage to the body increases as the diagnosis of chronic disease is delayed. This makes treatment difficult and increases the dose and number of drugs used. Thus, the cost of treatment increases, and the life expectancy is shortened. For all these reasons, early diagnosis is very important in chronic diseases. Early diagnosis improves the quality of life of patients, prevents chronic disease-related damage. In addition, treatment costs are reduced.

People apply to hospitals only when they are sick. But in the practice of family medicine this situation is different. Because family physicians should call for regular visits even if they are not sick. These control periods vary depending on the age, sex, pregnancy, occupation, illness or chronic illness of people. Many different parameters are entered into the patient follow-up systems during these checks performed by the family physician.

In this study, we used parameters similar to those recorded in patient follow-up systems in family practice. When evaluated individually, none is used for the diagnosis of chronic disease. However, when we evaluated all of them by using different machine learning techniques, we found that we could put significant results in terms of chronic disease risk.

To evaluate our data, we used different Machine learning techniques such as SVM, S3VM, KNN, linear classifiers, logistic regression, naïve bayes classifier, perceptron, quadratic classifiers, k-means clustering, boosting and bagging decision tree, random forest... In this section, we present the results of the four highest accuracy of machine learning techniques that we apply. These methods were RUSBoosted trees method of ensemble classifiers, linear SVM technique, fine KNN and weighted KNN methods. Matlab R2018a (9.4) program was used to evaluate the data and calculate the results.

Experimental Results

The results obtained from our data set with machine learning methods are as follows. The highest accuracy rate was 72.3% which obtained from the Ensemble Classifiers, RUSBoosted Trees Method. Confusion Matrix of this method is given in Table 2. Furthermore, the ROC curve and the area under curve (AUC) value (0.73) are shown in figure 4.

Table 2. Confusion matrix of ensemble classifiers, RUSBoosted trees method

	True	False
True	55%	17%
False	45%	83%
Positive Predictive Value	55%	83%
False Discovery Rate	45%	17%

Figure 4. ROC curve of ensemble classifiers, RUSBoosted trees method

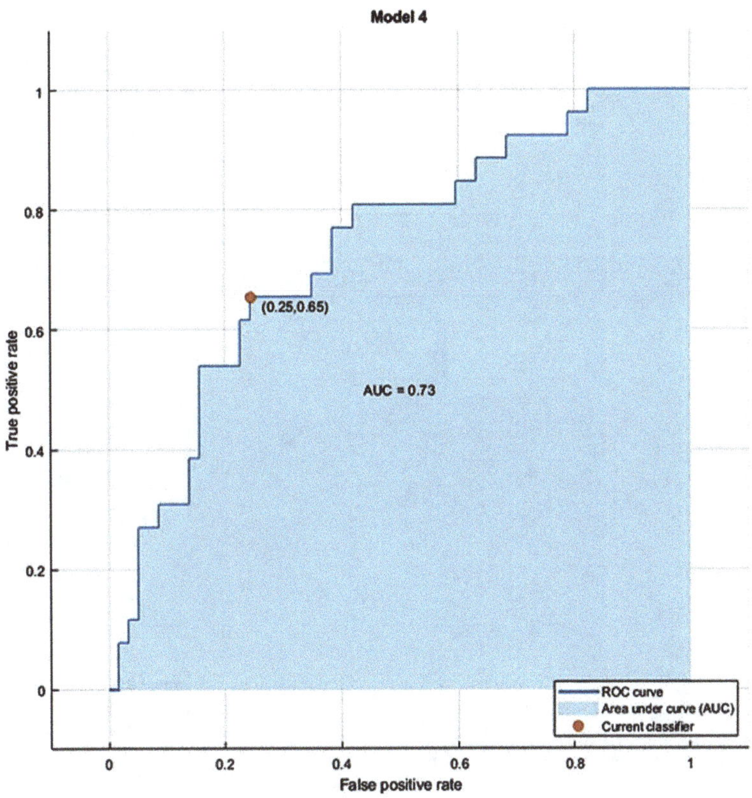

Table 3. Confusion matrix of SVM, linear SVM technique

	True	False
True	63%	28%
False	37%	72%
Positive Predictive Value	63%	72%
False Discovery Rate	37%	28%

The second highest accuracy rate was 71.1%. We obtained this result with linear SVM technique. In Table 3, Confusion Matrix of Linear SVM Technique is given. In addition, the AUC value of the ROC curve shown in figure 5 was 0.60.

Figure 5. ROC curve of SVM, linear SVM technique

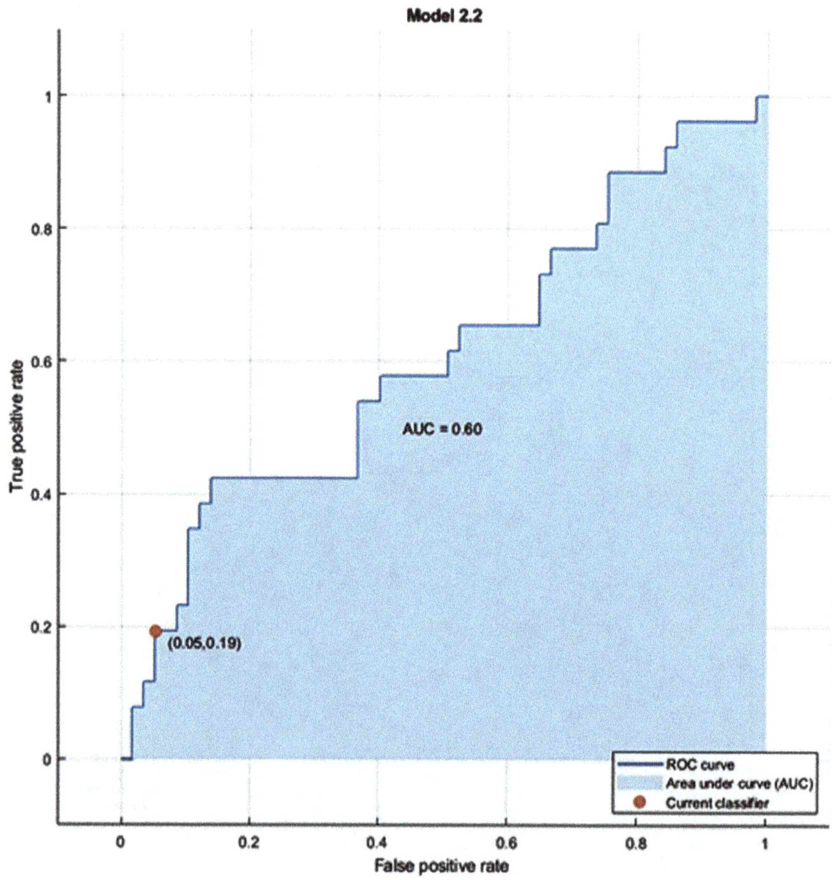

The third highest accuracy rate was obtained from fine KNN method which was one of the nearest neighbor classifiers. This accuracy rate was 69.9%. Positive predictive value and false discovery rate can be seen in Table 4. The AUC value of the ROC curve obtained by the fine KNN method was 0.67 (Figure 6).

Table 4. Confusion matrix of nearest neighbor classifiers, fine KNN method

	True	False
True	52%	20%
False	48%	80%
Positive Predictive Value	52%	80%
False Discovery Rate	48%	20%

Figure 6. ROC Curve of Nearest Neighbor Classifiers, Fine KNN method.

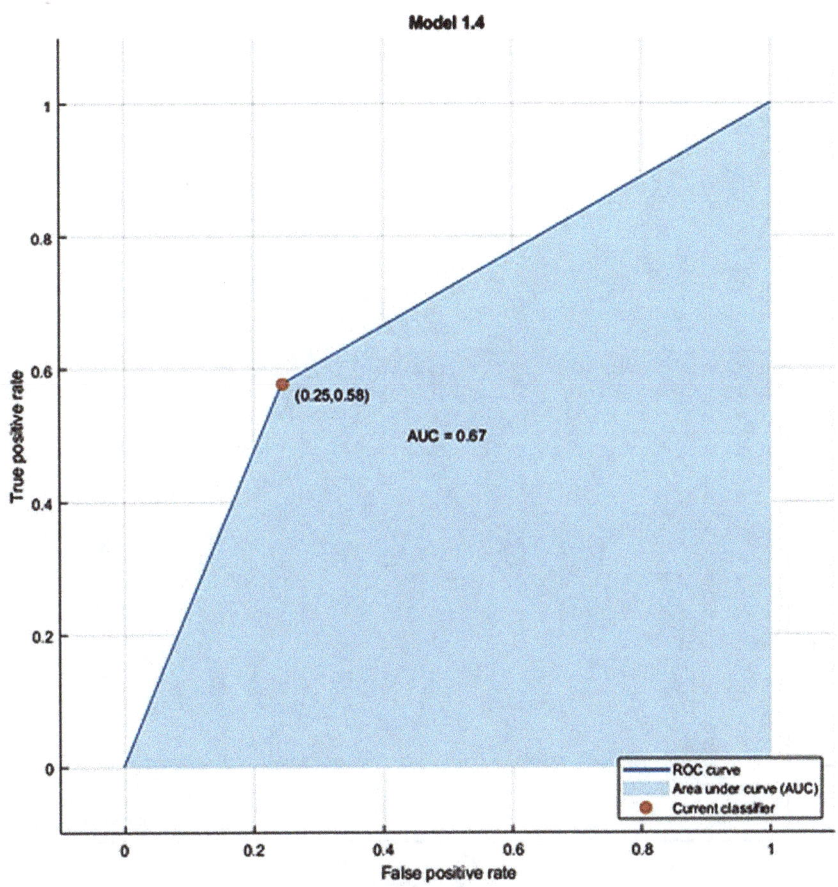

The fourth high accuracy rate of our study was 68.7%. This result was obtained by weighted KNN method which is another nearest neighbor classifier method. Positive predictive value obtained by weighted KNN method was found to be 50% and negative predictive value was 69% (Table 5). We found that the AUC value of the ROC curve formed by the weighted KNN method was 0.61 (Figure 7).

Table 5. Confusion matrix of nearest neighbor classifiers, weighted KNN method

	True	False
True	50%	31%
False	50%	69%
Positive Predictive Value	50%	69%
False Discovery Rate	50%	31%

Figure 7. ROC curve of nearest neighbor classifiers, weighted KNN method

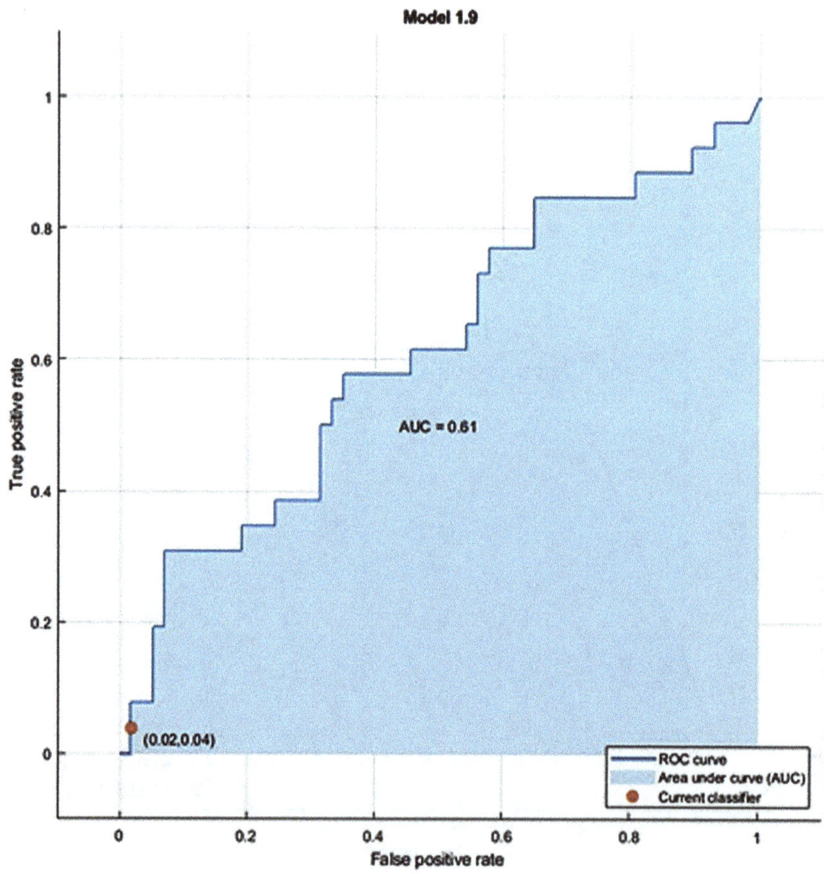

The AUC and accuracy values of these four methods with the highest accuracy rate in our study are given in Table 6. Moreover, graphical representation of AUC and accuracy values can be seen in Figure 8.

Table 6. Comparison for AUC and accuracy values between methods

	AUC	Accuracy
RUSBoosted Trees	0.73	72.3%
Linear SVM	0.60	71.1%
Fine KNN	0.67	69.9%
Weighted KNN	0.61	68.7%

Figure 8. Graphical representation of AUC and accuracy values

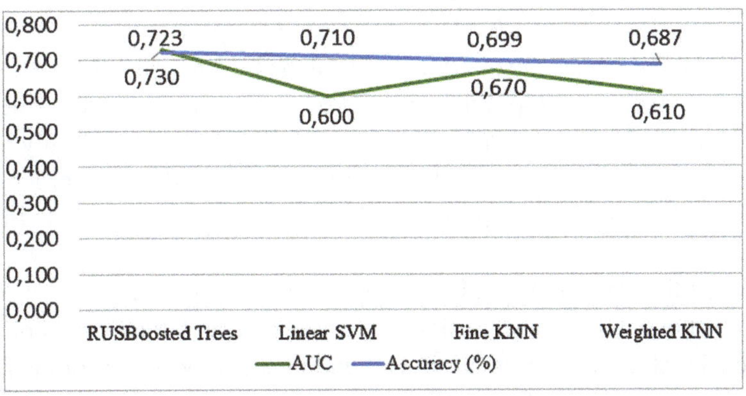

DISCUSSION

The use of AI in the field of medicine is the development of AI-equipped programs that can diagnose and decide treatment (Demirhan et al., 2010). In addition, AI systems can be used in areas such as arranging inpatient treatment services, making personnel work plans, and monitoring and editing patient files(Anyanwu, 2011). In 2007, the Artificial Intelligence in Medicine Europe (AIME) conference in Amsterdam, the Netherlands, emphasized that AI will open a new era in medicine and take place as a separate discipline in this new age (Patel et al., 2009).

The increasing population and average life expectancy in the world increase the number of applications in the field of health rapidly. As the elderly population increases, especially in chronic diseases, the duration of examination of physicians decreases with these increasing practices. Reduced examination times bring the risk of malpractice. For this reason, AI applications in the field of medicine are designed to support the daily work of healthcare workers and to assist them in the management of data and information (Jet & O, 2017; Ramesh et al., 2004).

In our study, we used 19 markers in the data set to estimate the diagnosis of chronic disease (Gülmez, 2013). We made this prediction using four different machine learning algorithms: RUSBoosted trees method of ensemble classifiers, linear SVM method, fine KNN and weighted KNN methods. We compared the performance of these algorithms with the accuracy obtained from them, as well as with ROC curves and confusion matrixes.

Seventy percent of the data was used for the training phase of machine learning. The remaining thirty percent was used to evaluate the prediction of the algorithm. When we compared the results of the AUCs and the accuracy of the models, their accuracy ranged between 68.7% and 72.3%, and the AUCs ranged between 0.61 and 0.73 (Table 6). RUS Boosted trees method was the best performing method for predicting chronic disease with 72.3% accuracy (Figure 8).

The importance and usage of AI methods in the health system is increasing day by day. As AI systems develop and use increases, it will bring many conveniences for both patients and physicians. We would like to briefly mention the family medicine system and patient registration and follow-up in family medicine in order to better explain why AI methods are important in the primary care, especially in the family medicine system.

Family medicine follows people from birth to death. They monitor, evaluate and train them not only when they are sick, but at every stage of their development. Let us first consider the situation of an adult attending a family doctor for the first time (Rakel & Rakel, n.d.). In the first application, the person's identification information, as well as general socio-demographic data and health history are recorded in detail. It is possible to make many predictions even by using only this data. It should be noted as a very detailed medical history. Vaccines that have been given so far, previous diseases, previous surgeries, food or drug allergy, current or chronic disease status, continuously used drugs and so on. After a detailed personal history, a detailed family history should also be obtained. Chronic diseases and cancers frequently seen in the family are questioned in the family history. If so, the causes of death at an early age are examined. After all this detailed assessment, the physical examination is done. In addition to these data, vital signs should be recorded. If there are other members of the family, such as parents, spouses and children, all these procedures are applied to them as well. All data are recorded in the family medicine monitoring system. The systems used today store daily recorded data on the main health care systems.

Figure 9. A. Classical treatment approach, B. Estimated treatment approach in the future

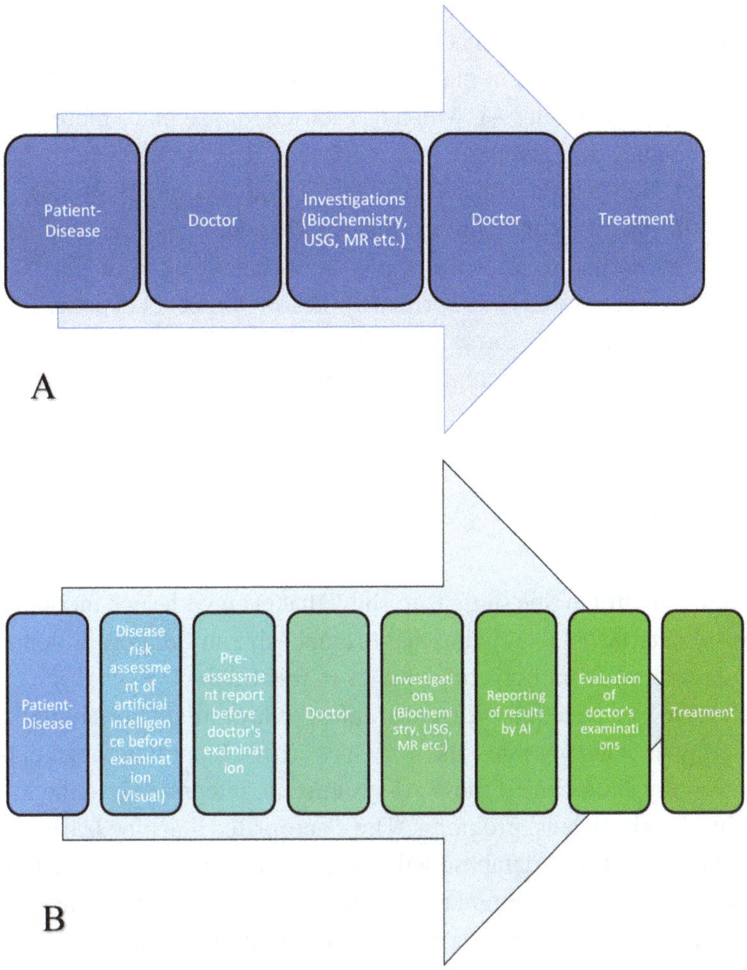

Thus, even if people change family physicians, the recorded data is transferred from the hosts to the system of the newly registered physician.

Periodic examination schedules are formed for everyone according to the health records, age, and gender of the individuals after the first registration. This planning, which was done manually from the patient follow-up files, is now created in seconds and without error thanks to the patient follow-up programs. When the physician opens the program, he sees the patients who need to follow-up for that day. The physician can easily plan the next day, week and month.

During recordings and subsequent follow-ups, an incredible data set is created. AI systems to be integrated into patient monitoring programs can use this data. In this way, the number of early diagnoses may increase with the warnings of the program, while the diseases have not yet presented symptoms. In the 9th figure, the current diagnosis and treatment plan applied to the present day and the predictive treatment approach including AI, which has started to take place more and more in the field of medicine, are given.

The data set that we used in this experimental study was not a specially prepared data set for the diagnosis of chronic disease. However, it was able to achieve predictability in chronic disease with a very high accuracy rate of 72.3%.

The limitations of our study were primarily the low number of patients. In addition, the data were obtained with forms prepared for a different study. In addition, the data were obtained with forms prepared for a different study. Therefore, the validity of the data is low.

CONCLUSION

In conclusion, our aim in this study is to show that even with such incomplete data, valuable results can be obtained. Thus, it is to emphasize how important contributions can be made with wide participation studies in this field.

AI systems to be developed with multicenter, wide participation studies can work with much higher accuracy rates and very low errors. Incredibly large data can be accessed in a very short time if these AI systems are integrated into the ministries' hosts, not just by physicians' programs. Thus, automated machine learning systems to be added to the national database will increase their success by self-training.

In this paper, we tried to summarize the possible methods for predicting chronic disease with innovative machine learning algorithms. In doing so, our aim was to draw attention to new horizons waiting for us in this field. Thanks to the developments in this field, both individuals' healthy life span will increase and the budgets that the societies should allocate for health will be reduced.

Dear editor, I would like to thank the referees for their valuable contributions and criticism. Necessary arrangements and corrections were made in accordance with the suggestions and criticisms of the referees. Current literature has been added to improve the bibliography.

Best regards.

List of changes made;

- Required references have been added to the introduction.
- The contribution of the study to the literature was emphasized.

- A graphical summary was added to the study.
- Tables reviewed.
- Applications used were announced.
- The long AUC form was added to the first place in the text.
- The figures in Figure 8 have been corrected.
- Information about the program used in calculations was given.
- Additions were made to the conclusion part of the study.
- Current literature was added to the bibliography.
- Figures were reviewed and added.
- The last section was rewritten considering the effect of the model on the current state of knowledge and practical use.
- The limitations of the study were clearly defined.
- The methods used and the discussion were reviewed.
- Data collection was explained in detail.
- The validity / reliability of the data was discussed.
- It was clearly stated that this amount of data was insufficient to generalize the result.

It was emphasized that the variables of the study were arranged for a different study.

REFERENCES

About Chronic Diseases I CDC. (n.d.). Retrieved August 31, 2019, from https://www.cdc.gov/chronicdisease/about/index.htm

Akay, E. Ç. (2018). A New Horizon in Econometrics: Big Data and Machine Learning. *Social Sciences Research Journal*, *7*(2), 41–53.

Alashwal, H., El Halaby, M., Crouse, J. J., Abdalla, A., & Moustafa, A. A. (2019). The application of unsupervised clustering methods to Alzheimer's disease. *Frontiers in Computational Neuroscience*, *13*(May), 1–9. doi:10.3389/fncom.2019.00031 PMID:31178711

Anyanwu, K. (2011). Overview and Applications of Artificial Intelligence, (June).

Artificial intelligence I Definition, Examples, and Applications I Britannica.com. (n.d.). Retrieved August 31, 2019 from https://www.britannica.com/technology/artificial-intelligence/Reasoning

Aygn, O., Gokdemir, O., Bulut, L., Yaprak, S., & Gldal, D. (2016). Evaluation of Primary Health Care Services Which Is Provided To Refugees Within a Public Health Center. *Turkish Journal of Family Medicine & Primary Care*, *10*(1), 6. doi:10.5455/tjfmpc.199143

Bennett, K. P., & Demiriz, A. (1998). Semi-Supervised Support Vector Machines. In M. S. Kearns, S. A. Solla, & D. A. Cohn (Eds.), Vol. 11). Advances in Neural Information Processing Systems Cambridge, MA: MIT Press; Retrieved from http://books.nips.cc/papers/files/nips11/0368.pdf

Bilge, U. (2007). Tıpta Yapay Zeka ve Uzman Sistemler. In *IV* (pp. 113–118). Antalya: Ulusal Tıp Bilişimi Kongresi.

Chen, J., Huang, H., Tian, S., & Qu, Y. (2009). Feature selection for text classification with Naïve Bayes. *Expert Systems with Applications*, *36*(3 PART 1), 5432–5435. doi:10.1016/j.eswa.2008.06.054

Chen, S. H., Jakeman, A. J., & Norton, J. P. (2008). Artificial Intelligence techniques: An introduction to their use for modelling environmental systems. *Mathematics and Computers in Simulation*, *78*(2–3), 379–400. doi:10.1016/j.matcom.2008.01.028

Cortes, Corinna, and V. V. (1995). Photonic neural networks and learning machines. *IEEE Expert*, *7*(5), 63–72. doi:10.1109/64.163674

Demírhan, A., Alper Kilic, Y., Güler, İ., Üniversitesi Teknoloji Fakültesi, G., & Mühendisliği Bölümü, B. (2010). *Tıpta Yapay Zeka Uygulamaları* Artificial Intelligence Applications in Medicine. Yoğun Bakım Dergisi, 9.*

Ding, S., Zhu, Z., & Zhang, X. (2017). An overview on semi-supervised support vector machine. *Neural Computing & Applications*, *28*(5), 969–978. doi:10.100700521-015-2113-7

Fukunaga, K., & Hayes, R. R. (1989). The Reduced Parzen Classifier. *IEEE Transactions on Pattern Analysis and Machine Intelligence*, *11*(4), 423–425. doi:10.1109/34.19040

Goldstein, B. A., Navar, A. M., & Carter, R. E. (2016). Moving beyond regression techniques in cardiovascular risk prediction: Applying machine learning to address analytic challenges. *European Heart Journal*, *38*(23). doi:10.1093/eurheartj/ehw302 PMID:27436868

Gülmez, H. (2013). Factors that Affecting Quality of Life of Employees. *Turkish Journal of Family Medicine & Primary Care*, *7*(4), 1. doi:10.5455/tjfmpc.38192

Heckerman, D., Geiger, D., & Chickering, D. M. (1995). Learning Bayesian Networks: The Combination of Knowledge and Statistical Data. *Machine Learning*, *20*(3), 197–243. doi:10.1007/BF00994016

Jihad, A. S., & Tahiri, M. (2018). Forecasting the heating and cooling load of residential buildings by using a learning algorithm "gradient descent", Morocco. *Case Studies in Thermal Engineering*, *12*, 85–93. doi:10.1016/j.csite.2018.03.006

Kannan, R., & Vasanthi, V. (2019). Machine Learning Algorithms with ROC Curve for Predicting and Diagnosing the Heart Disease. In Springer Briefs in Applied Sciences and Technology (pp. 63–72). doi:10.1007/978-981-13-0059-2_8

Koc, S. (2014). Forensic Medicine Related Physician Liability and Malpractice. *Toraks Cerrahisi Bulteni*, *5*(1), 14–22. doi:10.5152/tcb.2014.002

Liaw, A., & Wiener, M. (2002). *Classification and Regression by RandomForest*. Retrieved from https://www.researchgate.net/publication/228451484

Likas, A., Vlassis, N., & Verbeek, J. (2003). The global k-means clustering algorithm. *Pattern Recognition*, *36*(2), 451–461. doi:10.1016/S0031-3203(02)00060-2

Liu, C. L., Sako, H., & Fujisawa, H. (2004). Discriminative learning quadratic discriminant function for handwriting recognition. *IEEE Transactions on Neural Networks*, *15*(2), 430–444. doi:10.1109/TNN.2004.824263 PMID:15384535

Maclin, R., & Opitz, D. (1997). *An Empirical Evaluation of Bagging and Boosting Advice Refinement in Knowledge-Based SVMs View project An Empirical Evaluation of Bagging and Boosting*. AAAI Press. Retrieved from https://www.researchgate.net/publication/2262068

Murtagh, F. (1991). Multilayer perceptrons for classification and regression. *Neurocomputing*, *2*(5–6), 183–197. doi:10.1016/0925-2312(91)90023-5

Nawel, Z., Nabiha, A., Nilanjan, D., & Mokhtar, S. (2016). Adaptive semi supervised support vector machine semi supervised learning with features cooperation for breast cancer classification. *Journal of Medical Imaging and Health Informatics*, *6*(1), 53–62. doi:10.1166/jmihi.2016.1591

Osisanwo, F. Y., Akinsola, J. E. T., Awodele, O., Hinmikaiye, J. O., Olakanmi, O., & Akinjobi, J. (2017). Supervised machine learning algorithms: classification and comparison. *International Journal of Computer Trends and Technology, 48*(3), 128-138.

Patel, V. L., Shortliffe, E. H., Stefanelli, M., Szolovits, P., Berthold, M. R., Bellazzi, R., & Abu-Hanna, A. (2009). The coming of age of artificial intelligence in medicine. *Artificial Intelligence in Medicine*, *46*(1), 5–17. doi:10.1016/j.artmed.2008.07.017 PMID:18790621

Peek, N., Combi, C., Marin, R., & Bellazzi, R. (2015). Thirty years of artificial intelligence in medicine (AIME) conferences: A review of research themes. *Artificial Intelligence in Medicine*, *65*(1), 61–73. doi:10.1016/j.artmed.2015.07.003 PMID:26265491

Primary health care. (n.d.). Retrieved August 31, 2019, from https://www.who.int/news-room/fact-sheets/detail/primary-health-care

Rakel, R. E., & Rakel, D. (n.d.). *Textbook of family medicine*.

Ramesh, A. N., Kambhampati, C., Monson, J., & Drew, P. J. (2004). Artificial intelligence in medicine. *Annals of the Royal College of Surgeons of England*, *86*(5), 334–338. doi:10.1308/147870804290 PMID:15333167

Saini, I., Singh, D., & Khosla, A. (2013). QRS detection using K-Nearest Neighbor algorithm (KNN) and evaluation on standard ECG databases. *Journal of Advanced Research*, *4*(4), 331–344. doi:10.1016/j.jare.2012.05.007 PMID:25685438

Topol, E. J. (2019). High-performance medicine: The convergence of human and artificial intelligence. *Nature Medicine*, *25*(1), 44–56. doi:10.103841591-018-0300-7 PMID:30617339

What, Is. Machine Learning? | How It Works, Techniques & Applications - MATLAB & Simulink. (n.d.). Retrieved September 2, 2019, from https://www.mathworks.com/discovery/machine-learning.html

What is artificial intelligence? (n.d.). Retrieved September 1, 2019, from https://www.brookings.edu/research/what-is-artificial-intelligence/

WHO. | Integrated chronic disease prevention and control. (2010). *WHO*. Retrieved from https://www.who.int/chp/about/integrated_cd/en/

WHO. (2018). *Projections of mortality and causes of death, 2016 to 2060*. WHO.

World Health Organization. (1978). Declaration of Alma-Ata: International Conference on Primary Health Care, Alma-Ata, USSR, September 6-12, 1978. Retrieved February, 14, 2006.

Zhang, T., & Iyengar, V. S. (2002). Recommender Systems Using Linear Classifiers. *Journal of Machine Learning Research*, *2*(3), 313–334. doi:10.1162/153244302760200641

Chapter 10
Deep Learning in the Healthcare Industry:
Theory and Applications

Zahra A. Shirazi
Department of Statistical and Actuarial Sciences, The University of Western Ontario, Canada

Camila P. E. de Souza
Department of Statistical and Actuarial Sciences, The Univeristy of Western Ontario, Canada

Rasha Kashef
Electrical, Computer, and Biomedical Engineering Department, Ryerson University, Canada

Felipe F. Rodrigues
School of Management, Economics and Mathematics, King's University College at Western University, Canada

ABSTRACT

Artificial Neural networks (ANN) are composed of nodes that are joint to each other through weighted connections. Deep learning, as an extension of ANN, is a neural network model, but composed of different categories of layers: input layer, hidden layers, and output layers. Input data is fed into the first (input) layer. But the main process of the neural network models is done within the hidden layers, ranging from a single hidden layer to multiple ones. Depending on the type of model, the structure of the hidden layers is different. Depending on the type of input data, different models are applied. For example, for image data, convolutional neural networks are the most appropriate. On the other hand, for text or sequential and time series data,

DOI: 10.4018/978-1-7998-2581-4.ch010

recurrent neural networks or long short-term memory models are the better choices. This chapter summarizes the state-of-the-art deep learning methods applied to the healthcare industry.

INTRODUCTION

The healthcare industry is facing challenges as demand increases. The goal of the industry in the coming years is to manage this increasing demand while decreasing costs, adhering to mandatory legal requirements, and improving overall quality. This problem requires precise and well-managed solutions that work with the current industry while avoiding compromises to critical factors such as quality and legalities. Improvements in patient wellbeing, treatment planning, insurance risk information, and public health initiatives have already proven beneficial to the healthcare industry. Primarily, techniques such as cluster analysis, neural networks, text mining, and survival analysis have shown the potential to improve patient diagnosis in the future. For example, Survival analysis has been proven as a practical approach in determining life expectancies and hazard rates, which have been incorporated in the way insurance companies create health plans.

Deep Learning models can provide a doctor with insights into a case that can help improve the diagnosis and treatment decision making. Advances in computational technology have allowed researchers to develop and apply different Deep Learning methods to ever larger and more complex data. The application of Deep Learning in healthcare provides users the ability to create a high-level abstraction of raw data or images and develop an overall feature set. This feature set can then be utilized to understand new data quickly and draw sophisticated insights which may benefit the user. Neural networks and deep learning allow for public health users to better capture and understand structures and trends in society.

By leveraging machine learning tools, health managers and practitioners would be able to better direct resources and test new programs. While such applications can provide immense value-based healthcare, the current use of health data is exceptionally controlled, which provides a challenge to meet the full potential of such tools. This chapter samples the state-of-art neural networks and deep learning methods that have been currently utilized in the healthcare industry with a focus on classification-based, prediction-based, and clustering-based methods.

The rest of this chapter is organized as follows: Section 2 summarized the deep learning models addressed in this chapter, Section 3 discusses the current application of deep learning in health care systems and its various performance measures; finally, conclusions and future directions are presented in Section 4.

DEEP LEARNING MODELS

In this section, five of the leading deep learning analytical models are discussed. For each model, we define the basic learning fundamentals, usage, and summarize its architecture. Each model aims at either predicting, classifying, or clustering subjects based on a training set of responses/labels and features.

In general, Artificial Neural Networks (ANN) models consist of three primary layers, namely input, hidden, and output; with differences in each layer giving rise to each specific model. To pave the way of discussions in the next sections, the list of abbreviations used in this chapter is summarized in Table 1.

Table 1. List of abbreviations and symbols

Abbreviation	Description
ANN	Artificial Neural Network
AUC	Area under the ROC curve
BMU	Best Matching Unit
BPA	Back-Propagation Algorithm
CNN	Convolutional Neural Network
CPNN	Competitive Neural Network
CRF	Conditional Random Field
DDI	Drug-Drug Interaction
EHR	Electronic Health Records
FF-BP NN	Feedforward-Back Propagation Neural Network
GRU	Gated Recurrent Units
IoMT	Internet of Medical Things
KSOM	Kohonen Self-Organizing Map
LR	Logistic Regression
LSTM	Long Short-Term Memory
LVQ	Learning Vector Quantization
MLP	Multilayer Perceptron
MSE	Mean squared error
RBF	Radial Basis Function
RF	Random Forest
RMSE	Root Mean Squared Error
RNN	Recurrent Neural Network
ROC	Receiver Operating Curve
SMAPE	Symmetric Mean Absolute Percentage Error
SOM	Self-Organizing Map

Feedforward-Back Propagation Neural Networks

The Feedforward-Back Propagation Neural Network (FF-BP NN) or multilayer perceptron (MLP) neural network models are the simplest ANN models (Du, 2014). They include three main layers: input, hidden (single or multiple) and output layers. These are considered as the acyclic ANN models in which there is only one direction in the hidden layers. The Back-propagation algorithm used to fit FF-BP NN models has two phases: in the first phase called Feed Forward, the input neurons are propagated to the whole model to compute the output; in the backward phase the connection weights are adjusted based on the difference between the computed and observed information in the output layer to finally reach the best result. Moreover, in this model, all neurons from one layer are connected to all neurons of the next layer through the weights (Du, 2014; Graves, 2012). The main architecture of the FF-BP NN network is illustrated in Fig.1.

Figure 1. The Architecture of the FF-BP NN

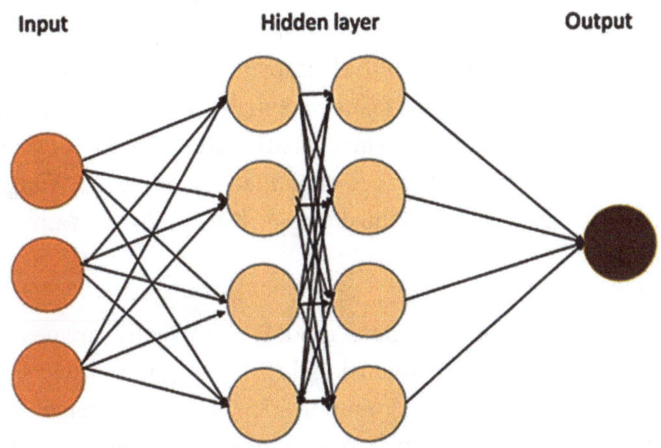

- **Input Layer:** Input data are propagated to the FF-BB NN model through this first layer. Each observation (also called neuron, unit or node) is connected to the next layer (in the MLP hidden layer) through the weights and using a pre-activation function, which is a product of the input and weights plus some bias.
- **Hidden Layer(s):** These are the deep layers in these models and could be one, two or more. All neurons from one layer are connected to all nodes of the next layer. The activation function (e.g., the sigmoid function) is fed to the

network through the inputs and then used for all hidden layers. Also, it should be noted that within each hidden layer, the weights and biases are different from each other.

- **Output Layer:** The information from the last hidden layer are fed to the output layer for classification or prediction purposes by applying the *softmax* activation function.

Convolutional Neural Network (CNN)

The CNN models are deep learning models that are mostly used for image processing and computer vision jobs. The image processing tasks can used for lots of purposes including the recognition of: faces and individuals (Lawrence, Giles, Tsoi, & Back, 1997), street signs (Luo, Yang, Tong, Wu, & Fan, 2018; Zhu et al., 2016), tumors (Cruz-Roa et al., 2014) and other applications (Howard et al., 2017; Ji, Xu, Yang, & Yu, 2013; Kim, 2014). As the general structure of ANN models, these models consist of an input layer, hidden layers, and the output layer. However, for CNN models, the hidden layers are further split into a convolution layer, a pooling layer, and a fully connected layer, as shown in Fig. 2. For the CNN models, the convolution layers extract the most important features of the images (from the input layer). The pooling layers shrink the dimension of the feature maps (the output of the convolution layers) by retaining their important features. Finally, the shrunken images are the inputs for the fully connected layer. The classification process is done in the fully connected layer. Each of these layers is explained next (Duan, Wang, Cui, Sang, & Sun, 2019; Karan, Bayraktar, Gümüşkaya, & Karlık, 2012; Yamashita, Nishio, Do, & Togashi, 2018).

- **Input Layer:** The input for these models are usually images. The images should be in the form of 2-dimensional (2-D; height and width) matrices or arrays of pixels often ranging from 0 to 255. However, images from a digital camera have three dimensions, including height, weight, and depth. The third dimension or depth consists of channels, and for the colored images, there exist three channels: Red, Green, and Blue (RGB). For the gray-scaled images the number of channels is one. So, it could be imagined that the 2-D matrices for each channel are stacked over each other.
- **Convolution Layer:** The core part of these models is this layer. The convolution operations (layers) have several kernels or filter matrices, which extract the features of the input image. These filters slide on the 2-D input matrices to extract their features, and the output of this layer are feature maps. The number of filters and their size are two important factors (arguments) for this layer. Adding more filters enables more features to be extracted from the

image, which improves the ability of the network to recognize the pattern for the test set.

- **Pooling Layer:** The dimensionality of each feature map is reduced in this layer, though their most important features and information are retained. There are different types of pooling operations: average, maximum, sum, etc. The output of this layer is the input for the fully connected layer.
- **Fully Connected Layer:** This layer is the traditional MLP in which every node from the previous layer is connected to every node in the next layer. For this layer, the activation function that is mostly used is the *softmax* activation
- **Output Layer:** The output consists of the probabilities of the images belonging to each class.

Figure 2. The schematic Architecture of the CNN network

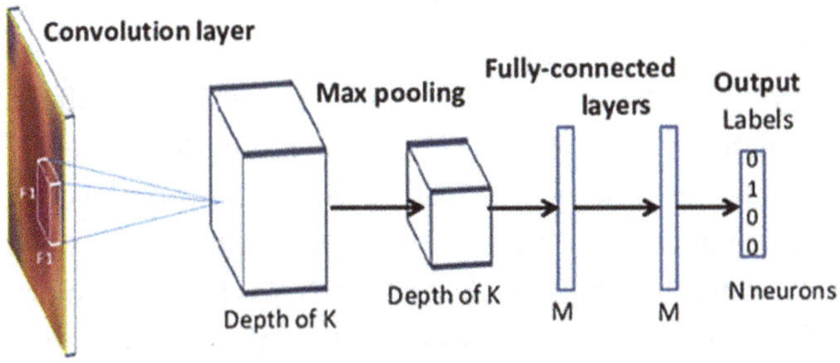

Recurrent Neural Network (RNN)

RNNs are the ANN models with cyclic connections, this means that the same task is done for each element of a sequence (e.g., each time step in the case of time series data or each word when the sequence is a sentence). In RNNs, the entire history of the previous inputs maps to each output and the activation from previous time steps are stored in the internal state of the network and then fed to the network as inputs to make decisions for the current time input (Du, 2014; Graves, 2012; Lipton, Berkowitz, & Elkan, 2015; Lipton, Kale, Elkan, & Wetzel, 2017; Singaravel, Suykens, & Geyer, 2018). Fig. 3 shows the unfolded RNN.

Figure 3. The unfolded RNN network

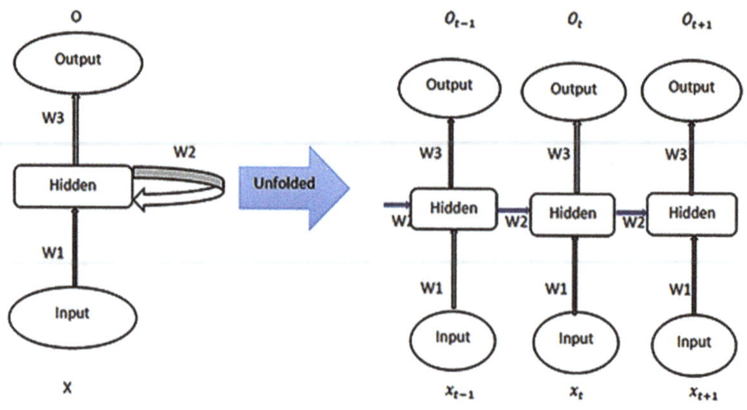

- **Input Layer:** The input data are sequential data, that is, interdependent data such as time-series data or pieces of strings, etc.
- **Hidden Layer:** Hidden layers in RNN models are slightly different than in the other ANN models. Since the data are sequential, the input from the hidden layer from previous time step as well as the input from the current time step are fed to the hidden layer related to the current time step via the activation function. Therefore, the hidden layer in an RNN is like a "memory" that retains the input from the current time as well as the information from previous time steps. Figure 3 shows the folded RNN and its unfolded shape. As can be seen from the figure, at each time, there is one input for the current time *t* and the previous information that merge and fed to the current time hidden layer by an activation function. In the folded shape, the recurrent task for the hidden layers for each element is shown, and the unrolled figure demonstrates the dependence between the current time and the previous information. As seen, in the unfolded figure, the weights are the same, which shows the same task for every element in the sequential data, so the same parameters are used rather than different parameters for each element. Indeed, the folded shape is a merge of the unfolded one.
- **Output:** The output layer gives the output, which varies according to the problem, it could be the prediction for the next time steps or next word, and so on.

Due to this cyclic structure of RNN models, the influence of the input on the hidden layers and therefore on the output layer is increases exponentially, which is called the vanishing gradient problem of RNNs. Because of the vanishing gradient property of the RNNs, these models only access 5-10 discrete time steps, which means the "memory" in the hidden layers are limited. To address this issue in the RNNs, Long Short-Term Memory (LSTM) models are designed, of which structure will be described in the next section. In general, they are widely applied for language modeling and generating text, machine translation, speech recognition, generating image description, and others.

Long Short-Term Memory (LSTM)

These LSTM models are designed to address the previously stated problem of vanishing gradient in the RNNs. Therefore, they have an input layer, hidden layers, and an output layer similar to those of the RNN. The only difference is in the structure of hidden layers wherein the summation units in recurrent hidden layers in RNNs are replaced with memory blocks in LSTM. The memory blocks consist of one or more self-connected memory cells and three multiplicative units: input, forget, and output gates. In the memory blocks, the input gate controls the flow of cell activation into the memory cell, and the outputs control the flow of cell activation from the network. The forget gate, resetting cell's memory which means it scales the internal state of the memory cell before adding it as input through self-recurrent connections of the cell (Du, 2014; Graves, 2012; Gridach, 2017; Lipton et al., 2015, 2017; Lipton, Kale, & Wetzel, 2016; Pham, Tran, Phung, & Venkatesh, 2016; Singaravel et al., 2018).

Self-Organizing Map (SOM)

The SOM models are unsupervised, competitive learning ANN models that are usually applied for clustering, visualization of patterns in high-dimensional data or classification for detecting the pattern or membership in a group. This method maps the high-dimensional data into a discretized low dimensional (i.e., one or two dimensions) feature map that preserves the most important patterns and topological relationships of the original data (Beale, 1990; Miljkovic, 2017). The SOM was first introduced by Teuvo Kohonen in the 1980s and sometimes called Kohonen feature map or Kohonen Self-Organizing Map (KSOM). As mentioned, they are unsupervised learning methods in which no prior knowledge is needed for grouping the data and the network itself learn from the relationships of the input data to categorize them. In fact, in SOM, we are dealing with unlabeled data. There are four steps in the SOM algorithm, including initialization, competition, cooperation, and synaptic adaptation (Fekihal & Yousif, 2012; Patole, Kulkarni, & Pachghare, 2010; Solano & Ghany, 2012).

- **Initialization:** The neuron weights are initialized with small random values.

- **Competition:** For each input vector and the synaptic weight, the value of the discrimination function is computed to find the similarities between the input and the neuron. The most popular discriminant functions are euclidean distance, correlation, direct cosine, and block distance. The neuron that provides the smallest measure of distance is the winner, and usually, the winning node is called the Best Matching Unit (BMU).
- **Cooperation:** The winning neuron (BMU) finds the spatial location of the topological neighborhood of the excited neurons, and hence, the neighboring neurons can cooperate.
- **Synaptic Adaptation:** The excited neurons decrease their values of the discriminant function related to the input pattern vector by using a suitable weight adjustment process.

Advantages and Disadvantages of the Deep Learning Models

Table 2 summarizes the advantages and disadvantages of the previously mentioned deep learning models.

Table 2. A Summary of the advantages and disadvantages of the deep learning models

	CNN	RNN	LSTM	SOM
Advantages	Since the CNN models are parallelized, they are faster in speed compared to other models such as RNNs. Also, they have enough capacity to extract features from the input matrix.	RNNs are good choices for sequence labelling data and they can take different types of data and representations and find the sequential patterns in them. These models are designed for one-dimensional sequences, although, they are flexible in the use of contexts which makes them a desirable choice even for image and video processing that are multidimensional.	LSTMs can store, and have access to information for long time spans. Because of their long-range memory, they perform well (compared to RNNs) on learning context-free and context-sensitive languages. They have applications in very different types of real-world data including: Music generation, reinforcement learning, speech recognition, handwritten recognition, language modeling and so on.	SOMs are very good data mining tool for data visualization, particularly for non-linear data and exploratory data analysis, it is an easy and simple algorithm to understand, and finally, they represent the topological clustering of data.
Disadvantages	Modeling long word relationships by using CNNs is difficult. Another drawback is that these models do not keep track of the position of the words in the sentences because they do not have the recurrence of the RNN models which leads to loss of information in doing the word order tasks.	One of the biggest disadvantages of RNNs is that they have difficulty for storing information for long periods of time, due to that difficulty, they have access to a limited range of context which is an issue when dealing with sequence labelling data. Another problem of RNNs is their one direction access to the contextual information, however, for time series data that does not matter, but for the sequence labelling data, it is better to have bidirectional access.	Because of its structure, LSTM requires more time, and memory to train and these models are sensitive to different random weights initializations.	It should be mentioned that it is a time-consuming algorithm due to the increasing number of computations, which leads to the slow training process. Moreover, there does not exist a rule-of-thumb for various parameters in the algorithm.

Performance Measures

Validation is the process of estimating how well the model output fits the underlying structure of the real output/data. A good validation should be invariant to the changes in data size, features, and types. Validation methods can be categorized into two classes, external validation, and internal validation. External measures evaluate the results based on some supervised information available while internal ones evaluate the result based on the information intrinsic to the data alone. To assess the performance of the ANN models, different validation metrics are used depending on the objective of the analysis: binary classification, multi-class classification, and prediction of a continuous quantity. Table 3 provides a summary of the most commonly used validation metrics, along with references.

Table 3. Validation metrics used in deep learning

Binary Classification	
Area under the receiver operating characteristic (ROC) curve analysis (sensitivity, specificity, accuracy, precision, F1-score, AUC)	(Fawcett, 2006)
C-statistics	(Caetano, Sonpavde, & Pond, 2018)
Rand index	(Yeh & Yang, 2017)
Multi-class Classification	
Jaccard index	(Levandowsky & Winter, 1971)
V-measure	(Rosenberg & Hirschberg, 2007)
F-measure	(Rezaei & Franti, 2016)
hF-measure	(Draszawka & Szymański, 2011)
L-measure	(Dalli, 2003)
Cross-entropy	(Goodfellow lan, Bengio Yoshua, 2016)
Purity	(Deepa & Revathy, 2012)
Normalized mutual information	(Rendón, Abundez, Arizmendi, & Quiroz, 2011)
Davis Bolden index	(Petrovic, 2006)
Prediction	
MSE, RMSE, SMAPE	(Armstrong, n.d.)
R^2	(Faraway, 2016)

APPLICATION IN HEALTHCARE: VISION AND DIRECTIONS

The CNNs are widely used in healthcare for different purposes including, but not limited to, diagnosis/detection of diseases, prediction of future risks, analysis of neuropathologies, lesion detection, image segmentation, classification, drug-drug interactions, etc. The RNN models are widely used in the healthcare for prediction, classification, and diagnosis purposes. Beyond those, because in EHR and sequential data, there are lots of missing values, another use of RNNs is to find the pattern of those missing data to improve the classification and prediction. The LSTMs are used for prediction, diagnosis, detection, classification, progression, and intervention of diseases as well as drug name recognition and clustering the patients.

FF-BP NN Healthcare Applications

In Shayea, Refae, & Yaseen (2013), a neural network for medical diagnosis was proposed by using FF-BP NN with tan-sigmoid transfer functions. Diagnosis data on acute nephritis, heart disease, and spondylolisthesis disease were used, and the results showed an accuracy (percent of cases correctly classified) of 100%, 88% and 82% on the diagnosis of acute nephritis, heart disease, and spondylolisthesis, respectively, based on the simulation sample. In Al-Shayea & Bahia (2010), the research objective was to evaluate ANNs in urinary disease diagnosis. For that purpose, an FF-BP NN was used for disease diagnosis and applied to data generated by a medical expert as a test set. The results showed the properties of the FF-BP NN to learn the patterns corresponding to disease symptoms, and an accuracy of 99% when it was applied to the simulation sample. Shukla et al. (2009) presented the results of applying an FF-BP NN on the diagnosis of thyroid gland disorders. The FF-BP NN was trained using three ANN algorithms: BPA, RBF, and the LVQ. The authors concluded that ANNs could be effectively used for the diagnosis of thyroid disorders. When comparing the performance of three neural network architectures, the LVQ-based network was found to have the best accuracy of diagnosis, which was 98%. More recently, Kar and Majumder (2017) present a Levenberg–Marquardt (LM) FF-BP NN, achieving 100% accuracy in brain cancer detection.

CNN Applications in Medical Classification and Diagnosis

The CNN model is considered by several authors including but not limited to the following examples. Feng et al. (2017) applied LR, RF and MG-CNN to the Hospital Quality Monitoring (HSQM) data to primarily predict the length of stay in the hospital. Experimental results show that the MG-CNN has better performance when compared to LR and RF models. In Cheng, Wang, Zhang, & Hu (2016), different

CNN-based models including: BP CNN (Basic CNN), EF CNN (Temporal Early Fusion CNN), LF CNN (Temporal Late Fusion CNN) and SF CNN (Temporal Slow Fusion CNN) are introduced and applied to EHR data used for diagnosis, medication, lab tests and procedures. A comparison study using ten-fold cross-validation showed that SF CNN performed better than the other CNN-based models.

In Nguyen, Tran, Wickramasinghe, & Venkatesh (2017), a new CNN-based algorithm called DEEPR was proposed and applied to EHR data for predicting future risks such as readmission after discharge, the onset of a specific disease and worsening from a condition. It was concluded that the proposed DEEPR achieves superior accuracy (around 81%) compared to traditional techniques such as Regularized LR.

In Esteva et al. (2017), CNN was used on clinical image data for diagnosis of skin cancer and the final results match with the performance of dermatologists. Yasaka et al. (2018) applied CNN on CT images of liver masses for differentiating them, the results showed a median AUC of 84% for the test data, which demonstrates a high diagnosis performance of CNN in the differentiation of liver masses. Liu et al. (2016) have applied CNN on DDI corpus data of the 2013 DDI Extraction challenge and their findings showed that CNN-based DDI extraction method achieves an F-score of 69.75% that outperforms the existing best performing method by 2.75%. Also, Zou et al. (2019) have applied CNN to different datasets for mammographic breast cancer diagnosis (MBCD). They found out that based on how to use CNN techniques, MBCD could be broadly categorized into three groups. A CNN was proposed by Lakhani & Sundaram (2017) and applied to four datasets to classify the images of chest radiographs. They concluded that their proposed CNN could accurately classify tuberculosis at chest radiography with an AUC of 0.99.

A computationally efficient dual pathway model with 11-layers, 3-D CNN, and 3-D fully connected CRF was recommended by (Kamnitsas et al., 2017). The model was applied to MRI data of 66 patients with moderate to severe traumatic brain injury for the planning of treatment strategies, monitoring of disease progression, prediction of patient outcome.

In Yamashita et al. (2018), a 3D-CNN was applied to three different datasets: CT images of lung nodules, medical images of a segmentation system of the uterus, and a dataset of chest radiographs. Their goal was to study the application of 3D-CNN in radiology, including classification, segmentation, detection, and others. They concluded that using CNN is useful for improving radiological results and patient care. In Murata et al. (2019), the authors developed a CNN to detect maxillary sinusitis from panoramic radiographs. Their model performs equivalently to a panel of experienced radiologists and far outperformed inexperienced residents. They conclude by proposing that their model be used as a diagnosis support tool for inexperienced dentists.

In Abiyev & Ma'aitah (2018), the three models, including CNN, FF-BP NN, and CPNN, were compared to each other. They considered a simulated dataset of chest diseases for diagnosis purposes using medical X-Rays. Their findings showed that CNN had achieved the highest recognition rate and the lowest MSE for both training and test data.

In Tajbakhsh et al. (2016), a pre-trained fine-tuned deep CNN and fully-trained deep CNN were compared. Their goal was to apply those models for medical image analysis including lesion detection, image classification, and image segmentation. Among their conclusions, they found that in most cases, a pre-trained CNN with adequate fine-tuning dominates a CNN that is trained from scratch.

RNN Applications in Prediction and Diagnosis

In Choi et al. (2016), RNN models are used for predicting diagnosis and medication categories. A longitudinal time-stamped EHR data of 260,000 patients and 2,128 physicians over eight years was used, and they concluded that their model not only can outperform several baseline models, but it is also very robust, being generalizable to other platforms. The RNN models using GRU is another common type of RNN. This model was used in many studies such as (Che & Liu, 2017; Che, Purushotham, Cho, Sontag, & Liu, 2018; Choi et al., 2016).

An RRN-based human activity recognition model was used in (Park et al., 2016) for applications in health monitoring and home care, the model used twelve datasets of human activities sequences containing twelve activities for activity recognition tasks. Results showed that their RRN model was able to reliably recognize human activity with an average AUC of 99.55% for all activities, outperforming previous hidden Markov-based models.

In Choi et al. (2017), the authors applied a GRU model to EHR data for detecting relationships among time-stamp events (eg., disease diagnosis, medication orders, procedure orders, etc.) and heart failure. They concluded that the GRU model improved the detection performance of heart failure incidents within shorter observation windows, compared to previous models that disregarded temporality. (Che & Liu, 2017; Che et al., 2018) have applied GRU models on various sets of EHR data aiming to address, among other things, issues of missing/incomplete data in disease prediction models. Their results showed that their GRU model outperformed the existing baselines, particularly concerning missing data in EHR. In other work related to missing values in health-related data, Turabieh, Abu Salem, & Abu-El-Rub (2018) proposed a Dynamic Layered RNN to predict any missing value in IoMT data. They applied their model to a mammographic mass dataset and a hepatocellular carcinoma dataset. They concluded that the proposed model was able to replace missing data for IoMT applications with high accuracy.

In Ma et al. and Suo et al. (2017; 2017) the authors had applied Attention-based Bidirectional RNN model on temporal time-series EHR data for the goal of diagnosis prediction (e.g., diabetes and osteopenia, respectively). Their models have shown valid and effective results with better accuracy for diagnosis prediction when applied to these data.

More recently, Ghanvatkar & Rajan (2019) developed a multi-time scale RNN to predict mortality in intensive care units using both dense and sparse clinical time series data. The proposed method outperforms other state-of-the-art mortality models (e.g., KNN and LSTM) in predictive accuracy (measured by F1-score).

LSTM Applications in Diagnosis Classification and Predictions

In Lipton et al. (2016), the authors directly modeled the missing data extracted from EHR data using LSTM for diagnosis classifications. In Liu et al. (2017), an LSTM was applied to a large Chinese doctor-patient communication dataset. Their goal was to use LTSM models to study a medical self-diagnosis android (namely Relevant Symptom Generation). Their results showed an improvement in performance by over 30% when comparing LSTM to alternative methods.

An LSTM-based algorithm called DeepCare was proposed by Pham et al. (2016) to study disease progression and predict future outcomes. The authors applied DeepCare to data from a cohort of patients with diabetes. Results showed that DeepCare (F-score = 79.1%) improved risk prediction of future hospital readmission by 7.7% when compared to a RF baseline method (F-score = 71.4%).

LSTM was also applied on MIT-BIH arrhythmia dataset in Van der Westhuizen & Lasenby (2017) for classification purposes, which results in the average score reduction for the method.

A Bidirectional LSTM-CRF applied to drug name recognition was modelled by Jauregi Unanue, Zare Borzeshi, & Piccardi (2017). The model was applied to three different data sets and showed better performance compared to a CRF-only baseline model.

A Time-aware LSTM (T-LSTM) was proposed by Baytas et al. (2017) and applied to data from the Parkinson's Progression Markers Initiative to cluster patients into clinical subtypes. An acceptable representation of temporal patient data was obtained using the proposed model.

In Ballinger et al. (2018), a multi-task LSTM was built and applied to a dataset consisting of 57,675 data records from wearable heart rate sensors to detect multiple medical conditions. Results showed that the proposed model has high detection accuracy (80% - 85%). In Maragatham & Devi (2019) a LSTM was applied to EHR data for diagnosis and prediction of heart failure. It was concluded that the model improved accuracy in heart failure.

An LSTM was proposed by Radha et al (2019) for modeling long-term sleep architectural patterns using heart rate variability. The model was validated on a dataset comprising 292 participants with a wide range of ages and pathological profiles and attained an accuracy of 77.00±8.90% across the entire database.

The SOM Applications for Categorization Problem in Healthcare Systems

In Chou, Cheng, & Chang (2007), the authors evaluated drug utilization and laboratory test on two levels of SOM and Rough Set theory (RST) or SOM-SOM-RST model to a clinical database containing 3083 records. They concluded that the proposed SOM-SOM-RST model successfully and effectively detected patients whose diagnosis codes have been changed during the period of investigation. It attains an accuracy of approximately 98%.

Simiarly, Zheng, Wang, & Black (2008) first presented a new computational approach for clustering analysis of daily-living human activities within a smart home environment, which may lead to significant applications in healthcare. They applied Growing SOM to a dataset generated by a 30-year-old woman who spent free time at a one-bedroom apartment for about two weeks. Their findings showed that relevant patterns in the data and data collection errors, as well as unusual, abnormal behaviors, were better detected and understood by using their proposed method.

In Gil et al. (2009) the authors studied the development of medical decision support systems of diseases. They wanted to aid medical specialists in obtaining reliable diagnosis while decreasing the number of tests. Unsupervised ANN models like KSOM, Growing Cell-Structures and supervised ANNs of multilayer perceptron were applied to data of 300 patients with dysfunctions of lower urinary tract. Results showed the proposed models were able to distinguish and classify between ill and healthy patients with average accuracy above 80%.

In Lloyd et al. (2009), the authors described a SOM-based procedure, namely SOM Discrimination Index, for identifying candidate marker compounds and compared it to a more traditional approach using partial least squares regression coefficients. As an application, the authors considered data arising from nuclear magnetic resonance spectroscopy of 96 human saliva samples from two groups (control and treatment) with 49 explanatory variables consisting of bucketed intensities. They concluded that SOMs could be employed to determine which variables are most significant in discriminating among groups. Also, their implementation showed a number of safeguards and advantages over partial least squares regression.

On the other hand, Tuckova et al. (2011) focused on the analysis of disordered children's speech with the diagnosis of Specific Language Impairment (SLI), also named as Developmental Dysphasia (DD), and the analysis of the expressive speech by using KSOM and supervised SOM. The results demonstrated the ability of the models to classify emotions and the SLI patients successfully.

In Fekihal & Yousif (2012), the SOM neural network is used as a clustering technique for classifying mental illness. They proposed using a novel Self Organizing Feature Map (SOFM) model to classify transcribed speech samples and determine mental disorders. The SOFM has been applied on 200 text files comprising the original message plus their replies. They concluded that SOFM is a reliable method and achieved a high accuracy of 97% in the classification of the input text and predicting mental illness or not.

In Solano & Ghany (2012), the authors used the SOM neural network to produce a tool named SOM-Visualize to enable the visualization of the Philippine Regional Health Data to uncover several patterns that may exist within the dataset.

In Tirunagari et al. (2015), the aimed to explore survey data regarding self-care behaviors in Type-1 diabetic patients. They performed the analysis of the self-care factors using SOMs on data from 611 patients' responses for 15 self-care behavior questions. The results obtained using SOMs corresponded well to the expectations of the clinicians in identifying similar patient profiles that are in need of adjusting their lifestyles.

In Jha et al. (2018) they proposed a modified visual KSOM-based clustering approach to monitor patient flow to diagnostic units. Results showed a group efficiency of 93.8% and 88.34% for binary data and sequential datasets, respectively. More recently, Pourkia et al. (2019) demonstrated how different types of SOMs can be effectively used to provide visual interpretation of healthcare data to hospital administration.

Hybrid Deep Learning Methods

In Muhammad et al. (2017), the authors showed that a hybrid deep learning method outperforms standard optical coherence tomographic (OCT) and visual field clinical metrics in distinguishing eyes previously classified as either healthy or with mild glaucoma. The proposed hybrid approach consists of using a CNN to extract features from OCT scans followed by a random forest classifier based on these features to predict the existence of glaucomatous damage.

In Zhang & An (2017), they proposed a hybrid deep CNN architecture for medical image reconstruction that contains three layers: one bicubic interpolation layer predetermined by mathematics deduction and two convolutional layers which learn from training images.

Finally, Almubarak (2018) explored a hybrid method to classify different types of cervical cancer. Their proposed framework consists of combining handcrafted features along with CNN features from digitized histology images and using those as input to a classifier.

Taxonomy of the deep learning methods based on the learning strategy is presented in table 4.

Table 4. Taxonomy of the deep learning methods in healthcare industry

Classification-Based Methods	Prediction-Based Methods	Clustering-Based Methods
CNN, CPNN, SSOM, DCNN, DEEPER	RNN, LSTM, LSTM-CRF,RBF, Dynamin L-RNN	KSOM, GCS, SOM-SOM-RST, T-LSTM

CONCLUSION

The goal of the healthcare industry in the coming years is to manage this increasing demand while decreasing costs, adhering to mandatory legal requirements and improving overall quality. This large problem requires precise and well managed solutions that work with the current industry while avoiding compromises to key factors such as quality and legalities. Deep Learning presents potential towards this goal. Improvements in patient well-being, treatment planning, insurance risk information and public health initiatives have already proven beneficial to the healthcare industry. As such, techniques such as deep learning have shown potential to go beyond improving patient diagnosis in the future. Overall the impact of using deep learning big data can have on healthcare systems is limitless. In this chapter, the state-of-art deep learning models are discussed along with their architecture, impact, and applications in various healthcare systems.

REFERENCES

Abiyev, R. H., & Ma'aitah, M. K. S. (2018). Deep Convolutional Neural Networks for Chest Diseases Detection. *Journal of Healthcare Engineering*, 1–11. doi:10.1155/2018/4168538 PMID:30154989

Al-Shayea, Q., & Bahia, I. (2010). Urinary system diseases diagnosis using artificial neural networks. *IJCSNS, 10*(7). Retrieved from https://resolver.1science.com/proquest/?id=f586b4f2b6fce265b0bd04f39031ff86e6e16dfd

Al Shayea, Q., El Refae, G., & Yaseen, S. (2013). Artificial neural networks for medical diagnosis using biomedical dataset. *International Journal of Behavioural & Healthcare Research*, *4*(1), 45–63. doi:10.1504/IJBHR.2013.054519

Almubarak, H. (2018). *Deep Learning and Localized Features Fusion for Medical Image Classification*. Retrieved from http://search.proquest.com/docview/2068551083/

Armstrong, J. S. (n.d.). Long-range forecasting: from crystal ball to computer / J. Scott Armstrong. In *Long-range forecasting : from crystal ball to computer* (2nd ed.). New York: Wiley.

Ballinger, B., Hsieh, J., Singh, A., Sohoni, N., Wang, J., & Tison, G. H., … Pletcher, M. J. (2018). Deepheart: Semi-supervised sequence learning for cardiovascular risk prediction. *32nd AAAI Conference on Artificial Intelligence, AAAI 2018*, 2079–2086. AAAI press.

Baytas, I. M., Xiao, C., Zhang, X., Wang, F., Jain, A. K., & Zhou, J. (2017). Patient subtyping via time-aware LSTM networks. *Proceedings of the ACM SIGKDD International Conference on Knowledge Discovery and Data Mining, Part F129685*, 65–74. 10.1145/3097983.3097997

Beale, R. (1990). Neural computing: an introduction / R. Beale and T. Jackson. In Neural computing: an introduction. Bristol, UK: Hilger.

Caetano, S. J., Sonpavde, G., & Pond, G. R. (2018). C-statistic: A brief explanation of its construction, interpretation and limitations. *European Journal of Cancer, 90*, 130, 132.

Che, Z., & Liu, Y. (2017). Deep learning solutions to computational phenotyping in health care. *IEEE International Conference on Data Mining Workshops, ICDMW, 2017-November*, 1100–1109. 10.1109/ICDMW.2017.156

Che, Z., Purushotham, S., Cho, K., Sontag, D., & Liu, Y. (2018). Recurrent Neural Networks for Multivariate Time Series with Missing Values. *Scientific Reports*, *8*(1), 6085. doi:10.103841598-018-24271-9 PMID:29666385

Cheng, Y., Wang, F., Zhang, P., & Hu, J. (2016). Risk prediction with electronic health records: A deep learning approach. *Proceedings 16th SIAM International Conference on Data Mining 2016, SDM 2016*, 432–440. 10.1137/1.9781611974348.49

Choi, E., Bahadori, M. T., Schuetz, A., Stewart, W. F., & Sun, J. (2016). Doctor AI: Predicting Clinical Events via Recurrent Neural Networks. *JMLR Workshop and Conference Proceedings*, *56*, 301–318. Retrieved from http://www.ncbi.nlm.nih.gov/pubmed/28286600 PMID:28286600

Choi, E., Schuetz, A., Stewart, W. F., & Sun, J. (2017). Using recurrent neural network models for early detection of heart failure onset. *Journal of the American Medical Informatics Association*, *24*(2), 361–370. doi:10.1093/jamia/ocw112 PMID:27521897

Chou, H. C., Cheng, C. H., & Chang, J. R. (2007). Extracting drug utilization knowledge using self-organizing map and rough set theory. *Expert Systems with Applications*, *33*(2), 499–508. doi:10.1016/j.eswa.2006.05.020

Cruz-Roa, A., Basavanhally, A., González, F., Gilmore, H., Feldman, M., & Ganesan, S. … Madabhushi, A. (2014). Automatic detection of invasive ductal carcinoma in whole slide images with convolutional neural networks. In M. N. Gurcan, & A. Madabhushi (Eds.), Medical Imaging 2014: Digital Pathology (Vol. 9041, pp. 1–15). doi:10.1117/12.2043872

Dalli, A. (2003). *Adaptation of the F-measure to cluster-based lexicon quality evaluation*. doi:10.3115/1641396.1641404

Deepa, M., & Revathy, P. (2012). Validation of Document Clustering based on Purity and Entropy measures. *International Journal of Advanced Research in Computer and Communication Engineering*, *1*(3), 147–152.

Draszawka, K., & Szymański, J. (2011). External validation measures for nested clustering of text documents. *Studies in Computational Intelligence, 369*, 207, 225.

Du, K.-L. (2014). Neural Networks and Statistical Learning [electronic resource] / In K.-L. Du, & M. N. S. Swamy (Eds.), Neural Networks and Statistical Learning (1st ed. 20). London, UK: Springer London.

Duan, P., Wang, T., Cui, M., Sang, H., & Sun, Q. (2019). Multi-person pose estimation based on a deep convolutional neural network. *Journal of Visual Communication and Image Representation, 62*, 245, 252.

Esteva, A., Kuprel, B., Novoa, R. A., Ko, J., Swetter, S. M., Blau, H. M., & Thrun, S. (2017). Dermatologist-level classification of skin cancer with deep neural networks. *Nature*, *542*(7639), 115–118. doi:10.1038/nature21056 PMID:28117445

Faraway, J. J. (2016). Extending the linear model with R : generalized linear, mixed effects and nonparametric regression models / Julian J. Faraway, University of Bath, UK. In *Extending the linear model with R : generalized linear, mixed effects and nonparametric regression models (2nd ed.)*. Boca Raton, FL: CRC Press. doi:10.1201/b21296

Fawcett, T. (2006). An introduction to ROC analysis. *Pattern Recognition Letters, 27*(8), 861, 874.

Fekihal, M. A., & Yousif, J. H. (2012). Self-Organizing Map Approach for Identifying Mental Disorders. *International Journal of Computer Applications, 45*(7), 25, 30. Retrieved from https://resolver.1science.com/proquest/?id=9d8b94ada26ae94ece6c6ec6524c845f5e289ee5

Feng, Y., Min, X., Chen, N., Chen, H., Xie, X., Wang, H., & Chen, T. (2017). Patient outcome prediction via convolutional neural networks based on multi-granularity medical concept embedding. *Proceedings - 2017 IEEE International Conference on Bioinformatics and Biomedicine, BIBM 2017, 2017-January*, 770–777. 10.1109/BIBM.2017.8217753

Ghanvatkar, S., & Rajan, V. (2019). Deep recurrent neural networks for mortality prediction in intensive care using clinical time series at multiple resolutions. *Proceedings of ICIS*. Munich, Germany. Academic Press.

Gil, D., Johnsson, M., Garcia Chamizo, J. M., Paya, A. S., & Fernandez, D. R. (2009). Application of artificial neural networks in the diagnosis of urological dysfunctions. *Expert Systems with Applications*, *36*(3), 5754–5760. doi:10.1016/j.eswa.2008.06.065

Goodfellow, I., Bengio, Y., & Courville, A. (2016). Deep learning. MIT press. Retrieved from MIT Press website: https://books.google.com.mx/books?hl=en&lr=&id=omivDQAAQBAJ&oi=fnd&pg=PR5&dq=deep+learning+ian+goodfellow&ots=MMT-hrrBQQ&sig=Ue-yavSqPS_vg2AQFhGKKaBY-5U&redir_esc=y#v=onepage&q=deep learning ian goodfellow&f=false

Graves, A. (2012). Supervised sequence labelling. In Supervised sequence labelling with recurrent neural networks (pp. 5-13). Berlin, Germany: Springer.

Gridach, M. (2017). Character-level neural network for biomedical named entity recognition. *Journal of Biomedical Informatics, 70*, 85, 91.

Howard, A. G., Zhu, M., Chen, B., Kalenichenko, D., Wang, W., Weyand, T., … Adam, H. (2017). *MobileNets: Efficient Convolutional Neural Networks for Mobile Vision Applications*.

Jauregi Unanue, I., Zare Borzeshi, E., & Piccardi, M. (2017). Recurrent neural networks with specialized word embeddings for health-domain named-entity recognition. *Journal of Biomedical Informatics, 76*, 102–109. doi:10.1016/j.jbi.2017.11.007 PMID:29146561

Jha, R. K., Sahay, B. S., Chattopadhyay, M., & Gajpal, Y. (2018). A visual approach to enhance coordination among diagnostic units using self-organizing map. *Decision (Washington, D.C.), 45*(1), 27–41. doi:10.100740622-017-0170-8

Ji, S., Xu, W., Yang, M., & Yu, K. (2013). 3D Convolutional Neural Networks for Human Action Recognition. *IEEE Transactions on Pattern Analysis and Machine Intelligence, 35*(1), 221, 231.

Kamnitsas, K., Ledig, C., Newcombe, V. F. J., Simpson, J. P., Kane, A. D., Menon, D. K., ... Glocker, B. (2017). Efficient multi-scale 3D CNN with fully connected CRF for accurate brain lesion segmentation. *Medical Image Analysis, 36*, 61–78. doi:10.1016/j.media.2016.10.004 PMID:27865153

Kar, S., & Majumder, D. (2017). A mathematical theory of shape and neuro-fuzzy methodology-based diagnostic analysis: a comparative study on early detection and treatment planning of brain cancer. *International Journal of Clinical Oncology, 22*(4), 667, 681.

Karan, O., Bayraktar, C., Gümüşkaya, H., & Karlık, B. (2012). Diagnosing diabetes using neural networks on small mobile devices. *Expert Systems With Applications, 39*(1), 54, 60.

Kim, Y. (2014). *Convolutional Neural Networks for Sentence Classification*. Retrieved from https://arxiv.org/abs/1408.5882

Lakhani, P., & Sundaram, B. (2017). Deep learning at chest radiography: Automated classification of pulmonary tuberculosis by using convolutional neural networks. *Radiology, 284*(2), 574–582. doi:10.1148/radiol.2017162326 PMID:28436741

Lawrence, S., Giles, C. L., Tsoi, A. C., & Back, A. D. (1997). Face recognition: A convolutional neural-network approach. *IEEE Transactions on Neural Networks, 8*(1), 98, 113. doi:10.1109/72.554195 PMID:18255614

Levandowsky, M., & Winter, D. (1971). Distance between sets [5]. *Nature, 234*(5323), 34,35.

Lipton, Z. C., Berkowitz, J., & Elkan, C. (2015). *A Critical Review of Recurrent Neural Networks for Sequence Learning*. Academic Press.

Lipton, Z. C., Kale, D. C., Elkan, C., & Wetzel, R. (2017). Learning to Diagnose with LSTM Recurrent *Neural Networks*. Academic Press.

Lipton, Z. C., Kale, D. C., & Wetzel, R. (2016). *Modeling Missing Data in Clinical Time Series with RNNs*. Academic Press.

Liu, C., Sun, H., Du, N., Tan, S., Fei, H., & Fan, W. … Zhang, C. (2017). Augmented LSTM framework to construct medical self-diagnosis android. *Proceedings - IEEE International Conference on Data Mining, ICDM*, 251–260. 10.1109/ICDM.2016.157

Liu, S., Tang, B., Chen, Q., & Wang, X. (2016). Drug-Drug Interaction Extraction via Convolutional Neural Networks. *Computational and Mathematical Methods in Medicine, 2016*, 1–8. doi:10.1155/2016/6918381 PMID:26941831

Lloyd, G. R., Wongravee, K., Silwood, C. J. L., Grootveld, M., & Brereton, R. G. (2009). Self Organising Maps for variable selection: Application to human saliva analysed by nuclear magnetic resonance spectroscopy to investigate the effect of an oral healthcare product. *Chemometrics and Intelligent Laboratory Systems, 98*(2), 149–161. doi:10.1016/j.chemolab.2009.06.002

Luo, H., Yang, Y., Tong, B., Wu, F., & Fan, B. (2018). Traffic Sign Recognition Using a Multi-Task Convolutional Neural Network. *IEEE Transactions on Intelligent Transportation Systems, 19*(4), 1100,1111.

Ma, F., Chitta, R., Zhou, J., You, Q., Sun, T., & Gao, J. (2017). Dipole: Diagnosis prediction in healthcare via attention-based bidirectional recurrent neural networks. *Proceedings of the ACM SIGKDD International Conference on Knowledge Discovery and Data Mining, Part F129685*, 1903–1911. 10.1145/3097983.3098088

Maragatham, G., & Devi, S. (2019). LSTM Model for Prediction of Heart Failure in Big Data. *Journal of Medical Systems, 43*(5), 1, 13.

Miljkovic, D. (2017). Brief review of self-organizing maps. *Proceedings 2017 40th International Convention on Information and Communication Technology, Electronics and Microelectronics (MIPRO)*, 1061–1066. 10.23919/MIPRO.2017.7973581

Muhammad, H., Fuchs, T. J., De Cuir, N., De Moraes, C. G., Blumberg, D. M., Liebmann, J. M., ... Hood, D. C. (2017). Hybrid Deep Learning on Single Wide-field Optical Coherence tomography Scans Accurately Classifies Glaucoma Suspects. *Journal of Glaucoma, 26*(12), 1086–1094. doi:10.1097/IJG.0000000000000765 PMID:29045329

Murata, M., Ariji, Y., Ohashi, Y., Kawai, T., Fukuda, M., Funakoshi, T., ... Ariji, E. (2019). Deep-learning classification using convolutional neural network for evaluation of maxillary sinusitis on panoramic radiography. *Oral Radiology*, *35*(3), 301–307. doi:10.100711282-018-0363-7 PMID:30539342

Nguyen, P., Tran, T., Wickramasinghe, N., & Venkatesh, S. (2017). Deepr: A Convolutional Net for Medical Records. *IEEE Journal of Biomedical and Health Informatics*, *21*(1), 22–30. doi:10.1109/JBHI.2016.2633963 PMID:27913366

Park, S. U., Park, J. H., Al-Masni, M. A., Al-Antari, M. A., Uddin, M. ., & Kim, T.-S. (2016). A Depth Camera-based Human Activity Recognition via Deep Learning Recurrent Neural Network for Health and Social Care Services. *Procedia Computer Science, 100*, 78, 84.

Patole, V., Kulkarni, D., & Pachghare, V. K. (2010). Self-Organizing Maps to Build Intrusion Detection System. *International Journal of Computer Applications, 1*(8), 1, 4. Retrieved from https://resolver.1science.com/proquest/?id=3ffd17e15fc7228301415445ba5972a3a06ab95a

Petrovic, S. (2006). A Comparison Between the Silhouette Index and the Davies-Bouldin Index in Labelling IDS Clusters. *11th Nordic Workshop on Secure IT-Systems*, 53–64. Retrieved from https://xp-dev.com/svn/b_frydrych.../silhuetteIndexRegulaStopu.pdf

Pham, T., Tran, T., Phung, D., & Venkatesh, S. (2016). DeepCare: A deep dynamic memory model for predictive medicine. Lecture Notes in Computer Science (Including Subseries Lecture Notes in Artificial Intelligence and Lecture Notes in Bioinformatics), 9652, 30, 41. Springer Verlag.

Pourkia, J., Rahimi, S., & Baghaei, K. T. (2019). Hospital Data Interpretation: A Self-Organizing Map Approach. In R. B. Kearfott, I. Batyrshin, M. Reformat, M. Ceberio, & V. Kreinovich (Eds.), *Fuzzy Techniques: Theory and Applications* (pp. 493–504). Cham, Switzerland: Springer International Publishing. doi:10.1007/978-3-030-21920-8_44

Radha, M., Fonseca, P., Moreau, A., Ross, M., Cerny, A., Anderer, P., ... Aarts, R. M. (2019). Sleep stage classification from heart-rate variability using long short-term memory neural networks. *Scientific Reports*, *9*(1), 1–11. doi:10.103841598-019-49703-y PMID:31578345

Rendón, E., Abundez, I., Arizmendi, A., & Quiroz, E. (2011). Internal versus external cluster validation indexes. *International Journal of Computers and Communications, 5*(1), 27, 34. Retrieved from https://resolver.1science.com/proquest/?id=bf2a5cfbebe590efcee9d581287c290126a44cc7

Rezaei, M., & Franti, P. (2016). Set Matching Measures for External Cluster Validity. *IEEE Transactions on Knowledge and Data Engineering, 28*(8), 2173,2186.

Rosenberg, A., & Hirschberg, J. (2007). V-Measure: A Conditional Entropy-Based External Cluster Evaluation Measure. *Proceedings of the 2007 Joint Conference on Empirical Methods in Natural Language Processing and Computational Natural Language Learning*, 410-420. Prague, Czech Republic: Association for Computational Linguistics.

Shukla, A., Tiwari, R., Kaur, P., & Janghel, R. R. (2009). Diagnosis of thyroid Disorders using Artificial Neural Networks. *Proceedings 2009 IEEE International Advance Computing Conference, IACC 2009*, 1016, 1020. 10.1109/IADCC.2009.4809154

Singaravel, S., Suykens, J., & Geyer, P. (2018). Deep-learning neural-network architectures and methods: Using component-based models in building-design energy prediction. *Advanced Engineering Informatics, 38*, 81, 90.

Solano, G., & Ghany, M. (2012). *Visualization of Multivariate Health Data using Self-Organizing Maps*. Porto, Portugal: Mathematical Models and Methods in Modern Science.

Suo, Q., Ma, F., Canino, G., Gao, J., Zhang, A., Veltri, P., & Agostino, G. (2017). A Multi-Task Framework for Monitoring Health Conditions via Attention-based Recurrent Neural Networks. *AMIA ... Annual Symposium Proceedings. AMIA Symposium, 2017*, 1665–1674.

Tajbakhsh, N., Shin, J. Y., Gurudu, S. R., Hurst, R. T., Kendall, C. B., Gotway, M. B., & Liang, J. (2016). Convolutional Neural Networks for Medical Image Analysis: Full Training or Fine Tuning? *IEEE Transactions on Medical Imaging, 35*(5), 1299–1312. doi:10.1109/TMI.2016.2535302 PMID:26978662

Tirunagari, S., Poh, N., Hu, G., & Windridge, D. (2015). *Identifying Similar Patients Using Self-Organising Maps: A Case Study on Type-1 Diabetes Self-care Survey Responses*. Retrieved from http://arxiv.org/abs/1503.06316

Tuckova, J., Bartu, M., Zetocha, P., & Grill, P. (2011). Self-organizing maps as data classifiers in medical applications. *NCTA 2011 - Proceedings of the International Conference on Neural Computation Theory and Applications*. 10.5220/0003722604220429

Turabieh, H., Abu Salem, A., & Abu-El-Rub, N. (2018). Dynamic L-RNN recovery of missing data in IoMT applications. *Future Generation Computer Systems, 89*, 575–583. doi:10.1016/j.future.2018.07.006

van der Westhuizen, J., & Lasenby, J. (2017). *Techniques for visualizing LSTMs applied to electrocardiograms.* Retrieved from http://arxiv.org/abs/1705.08153

Yamashita, R., Nishio, M., Do, R., & Togashi, K. (2018). Convolutional neural networks: an overview and application in radiology. *Insights into Imaging, 9*(4), 611, 629.

Yasaka, K., Akai, H., Abe, O., & Kiryu, S. (2018). Deep learning with convolutional neural network for differentiation of liver masses at dynamic contrast-enhanced CT: A preliminary study. *Radiology, 286*(3), 887–896. doi:10.1148/radiol.2017170706 PMID:29059036

Yeh, C.-C., & Yang, M.-S. (2017). Evaluation measures for cluster ensembles based on a fuzzy generalized Rand index. *Applied Soft Computing, 57*, 225, 234.

Zhang, Y., & An, M. (2017). Deep Learning- and Transfer Learning-Based Super Resolution Reconstruction from Single Medical Image. *Journal of Healthcare Engineering, 2017*, 20. doi:10.1155/2017/5859727 PMID:29065625

Zheng, H., Wang, H., & Black, N. (2008). Human activity detection in smart home environment with self-adaptive neural networks. *Proceedings of 2008 IEEE International Conference on Networking, Sensing and Control, ICNSC*, 1505–1510. 10.1109/ICNSC.2008.4525459

Zhu, Z., Liang, D., Zhang, S., Huang, X., Li, B., & Hu, S. (2016). Traffic-Sign Detection and Classification in the Wild. *Proceedings of the IEEE Computer Society Conference on Computer Vision and Pattern Recognition, 2016*, 2110, 2118. IEEE Computer Society. 10.1109/CVPR.2016.232

Zou, L., Yu, S., Meng, T., Zhang, Z., Liang, X., & Xie, Y. (2019). A Technical Review of Convolutional Neural Network-Based Mammographic Breast Cancer Diagnosis. *Computational and Mathematical Methods in Medicine, 2019*, 1–16. doi:10.1155/2019/6509357 PMID:31019547

Chapter 11
Smart Cataract Detector:
An Image Processing-Based Mobile Application for Cataract Detection

M. Manikandakumar
https://orcid.org/0000-0003-2648-7139
Thiagarajar College of Engineering, India

ABSTRACT

Eyes react to light. Cataract, a common eye disease, clouds the lens of the eye, which decreases vision and can cause blindness. It can be in one or both eyes. The most major cause of cataract is ageing. Cataract also can be found in children and can occur due to eye injuries and inflammation. As mobile technology emerges to a greater extent, designing an application would help people perform a self check-up without meeting the doctors in person, thus saving time and cost. The pre-diagnosis of cataracts is costly for poor people. Time taken by the machine to detect cataract is greater, so the doctor can't attend as many patients. A cheap, reliable mobile application that helps diagnose cataract would cut cost and simplify diagnosis. This chapter proposes the development of smart phone application to detect the presence of cataract using image processing techniques.

IINTRODUCTION

A cataract is a type of eye disease that causes blindness. Ophthalmologists who perform Cataract detection take a lot of time to take the right decision. Smartphones popularity has helped in the development of mobile applications. Smartphones are considered to be the platforms that offer cost-effective solutions for many

DOI: 10.4018/978-1-7998-2581-4.ch011

problems in various domains like healthcare, agriculture, IoT, etc., Hence, a medical practitioner is no longer required to appear in person to monitor the patients. The short version of cataract is myopia and the long-term version is called blindness. A cataract is found to occur in the eye lens. The lens is made up of proteins and they are arranged in an organized manner. So cataract occurs due to the accumulation of proteins in the lens. The symptoms of cataract include cloudy or blurred vision, increasing difficulty with vision at night, yellowing of colors that would eventually lead to blindness. A congenital cataract is one of the types of cataracts which affects children. It can also occur due to eye injuries that have affected the lens. Cataracts can also be a genetic disorder.

A cataract is classified into three types based on the area of protein deposition. They are named as nuclear cataracts, cortical cataract, and posterior sub-capsular cataracts. Nuclear cataract as the name suggests develops a cloudy layer of proteins on the nucleus of the lens. The type of cataract normally affects the elderly. A cortical cataract develops in the cortex of the lens which surrounds the lens. A posterior sub-capsular cataract develops at the back of the lens. People suffering from diabetes and those taking steroids are also at the risk of having such cataracts.

Figure 1. Normal eye vs. cataract eye

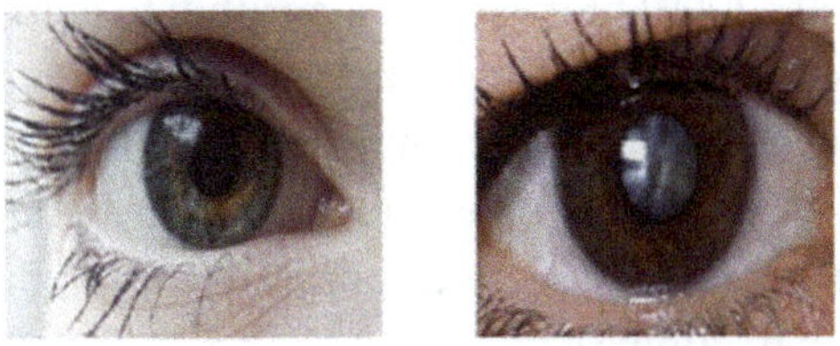

The software has developed during 2011 (Md. Anayet U. Patwari, Muammar D. Arif, Md. N. A. Chowdhury, A. Arefin and Md. I. Imam, 2011) that uses the digital images of healthy and cataract affected eyes for detection, classification, and evaluation of cataracts. Digital images of a few patients with different degrees of nuclear cataract, few patients with different cortical cataracts along with few samples of normal and healthy people were considered for the research. The healthy eyes were given as a reference to the developed system. The presence of the cataract is then detected by comparing the cataract affected with the mean grey intensity of the healthy eyes obtained and hence the cataract could be decided. The technique has 94.96% of accuracy and 95.14% reliability. The algorithms of the developed software are sensitive to grey-level variations which leads to the error measured in several cases. In this scenario, developing more complex algorithms for the detection of cataract leads to reduce the error rate at the expected level. The algorithm, proposed by (Shashwat Pathak and Basant Kumar, 2016) automatically detects the presence of cataract using diagnostic opinion from color images. To develop an inexpensive, convenient algorithm for cataract detection was considered as the goal. The simulations were performed with a simulation tool. The proposed algorithm was applied by creating a simple graphical user interface (GUI) in the simulation tool. The GUI gets a true-color image as input and it undergoes the conversion of true-color images into grayscale followed by performing the contrast enhancement by applying the Gaussian filter. The software will calculate texture parameter i.e. standard deviation and have decided the presence of cataract. The proposed method gave 98% accuracy. The computer-aided detection (CAD) of cataract proposed (Albab Ahmad Khan, M. Usman Akram, Ahmad Tariq, Faraz Tahir, and Kamran Wazir, 2017 & Wong et al., 2007) aims to detect the cataract automatically. The proposed system uses the techniques of image processing and classification algorithms. For the detection of cataract through the CAD system, the picture of the patient with retina in focus is accessed and then it localizes the iris and pupil of the eye. To isolate the lens, a localization algorithm is used and cropping is done for feature extraction. Texture analysis of the obtained image is analyzed to find out whether the eye is affected by cataract. The classifier used in this system is the Support Vector Machine (SVM). The system is developed and tested on a locally gathered cataract dataset. (Abraham et al., 2009) proposed an algorithm to help the review person in evaluating result images for finding the presence of illness. Precise feature detection and extraction is considered primary for cataract detection. (Xu, Zhifei, and Pengfei Shi, 2006) developed an algorithm for accurate identification and estimation of eye pupil features. The center and radius calculations of the pupil need to be extracted as part of the feature extraction.

PROPOSED SYSTEM

The chapter proposes a simple, low-cost mobile application. The proposed application has five functions which include the pre-assessment test, cataract test, vision ability test, generation of test results and finally advice prescribed. Users must attend the pre-assessment test, the cataract test and the vision ability test to get greater accuracy of results for their eye-examination. Each module is provided with instructions on how to attend the test. The proposed application has been created in two languages i.e. English and Tamil. Language-based cataract detection will aid people in rural areas worldwide. The user can provide his or her choice of language based on the need. For information gathering, case studies were done at three hospitals in Madurai, to know more about cataracts, their causes, symptoms and the treatment involved to cure cataracts. The experts shared their knowledge and provided valuable guidance to develop the application. The application was designed using the Android Studio developer kit. The user interface section of the application i.e., the user input will gather the basic information about the user like name, age, gender. This page will then navigate to the Pre-assessment test than to the cataract test and finally to the vision test to generate the test results.

DATA COLLECTION

The input for the cataract test is a color image of the eye which is captured through a mobile camera or that can be loaded from the locally created dataset. The eye images are collected from various sources like the healthy eye, old aged and those working in sectors like glass cutting, people who are working in welding workshops, people working under sunlight for a long period and people wearing glasses due to myopia. The images collected were stored in a repository to create a dataset for future purposes. Privacy and security aspects of the created datasets are also an important point of concern. Challenges related to privacy and security of big data (Manikandakumar, M., and E. Ramanujam, 2018) have to be addressed and properly maintained for any kind of datasets including the collected and locally stored cataract image data set. Image data collection, Pre Processing of collected images, Enhancement or improvements of the images, applying Feature Extraction methodologies and Classification of normal eye and affected eye are the important fundamental activities of this proposed work. Steps for performing the transformation and scaling of RGB and Grayscale images are to be carefully designed. The height factors of the images will be between 900 and 200 pixels (Kumar, S., Pathak, S., & Kumar, B., 2019).

Pre-Assessment Test

A cataract is caused due to some specific reasons. The reasons are identified and based on the identified reasons this phase has been designed. This phase has a few questions that are major physical reasons for causing cataracts. The users have to attend the test and answer the questions. Some of the questions include genetic reasons, age factor, and eye injuries; working under sunlight, etc., the pre-assessment phase was designed based on the input gathered from the hospitals where the interactions were conducted. The probabilities for causing cataracts have been identified. This phase is designed as the ophthalmologists were unable to discuss all the major questions that are reasons for cataract with the patient at the time of checkup. This phase will be provided as a report to the users which can be taken to their eye doctor at the time of the visit to the hospitals.

Cataract Test

In this phase, the image collected will be taken as the input. The image of the lens is first extracted from the patient's photo by cropping them with a specific region of interest. The RGB image is then converted to a resized greyscale for reducing the calculation load. The presence of the cataract is then detected by comparison with the mean grey intensity of healthy eyes which will be provided as threshold values. Cataract detection is achieved by performing the proposed steps. Sometimes, examining the gradient vectors with radial constraint and two-way image gradients to perform the removal of errors are challenging issues in radial mapping as well as in center localization of eye. To overcome this kind of issue appropriate mechanisms such as preprocessing, setting up of adaptive skin color threshold and Gradients of the Inward Direction need to be followed properly. Need to give proper Weightages to the features of iris. Specific features of these iris would be applied based on the geometric approaches (Ahuja, K., Banerjee, R., Nagar, S., Dey, K., & Barbhuiya, F., 2016).

Eye Image Capture

The user is provided with two options to upload their image for the physical cataract test to be conducted (i.e.) Using a smartphone, the user can either capture the image from the camera or load image from the smart phone's gallery. The options provided are

1. Photo from the gallery
2. Take the photo from the camera

The accuracy depends on the clear input image with a good resolution rate and the aspect ratio could be 4:3. These days, most of the smartphone cameras have impressive capture quality.

Pre-Processing Steps

The loaded image is pre-processed thereby image is smoothed and de-noised. Pre-processing steps done are grayscale, contract enhancement and Gaussian filter (Kumar S et al., 2019)

Pre-Processing Step 1: Grayscale Conversion

The input bitmap image is converted into a comprised grid of Red, Green, Blue, Alpha pixels.

Pre-Processing Step 2: Gaussian Filter

Gaussian filter is the result of blurring an image by a Gaussian function. It is used to reduce image noise. The grayscale image is provided as an input for this filtering process. Convolution matrix is used here. This matrix and the grayscale image are parsed and the final Gaussian filtered bitmap image is obtained.

Feature Extraction and Texture Parameters Calculation

Cataracts usually occur in the lens that is noticeable in the pupil where cloudiness is caused and hence pupil is extracted. In the proposed application, the users have to manually crop their pupil as instructed in the application. Texture feature parameters like intensity and mean for the pre-processed image are calculated to differentiate normal and cataract eye (Valenti, R. & Gevers, T. 2012). The mean intensity (I) of the normal eye will be fed as the thresholds for the comparison of mean value intensities. To localize the inner part of the pupil, binarization and morphological mechanism can also be applied which is helpful to remove the errors.

Range of Mean Intensity

Normal: $12< I < 125$.
Mild: $125< I < 134$.
Severe: $I<120$.

Figure 2. Workflow of the cataract test phase

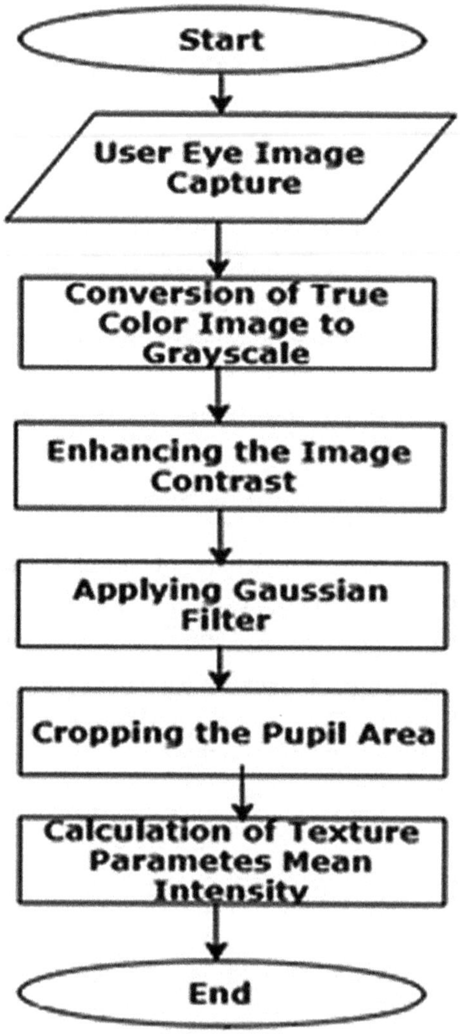

Usually, the input images are in jpeg or png or tiff formats. One another main issue here is the flash spotted images that will occur often while taking photographs using a smartphone camera, hence that should be given more focus to get the right results. The so-called red-eye dots or pixels on the image can be calculated and thereby identified using hue-saturation-value (HSV). With the help of extracting the brightness component it can be achieved (Ferman, A. M. 2008., Khan, 2017).

Vision Ability Test

In this phase, the user is asked to type the letter that appears on their screen as it is another usual practice in the eye care centers. This is done to ensure that the users are having a good vision. The users should wear their contact lenses or glasses if they normally wear them. They should hold their phone at arm's length and attend the test with the eye that is to be examined.

Test Results

This phase will summarize the test results of the above-discussed tests. The results of the individual tests can also be shown in both languages. The consolidated result considering all the three tests can be generated. All three tests are considered for the final result to ensure accuracy. The questions that are answered affirmatively by the user in the pre-assessment test will be displayed. The results of the cataract test will state if the person has a "normal/mild/severe" cataract. The vision ability test result will be the number of letters answered correctly by the user. A final report in a PDF format will be output by the application listing the results (Ferman, A. M. 2008) the users can see their result in the application itself i.e. in the test results page. The users can also download their reports in PDF format and send an mail.

Figure 3. Workflow of the application designed

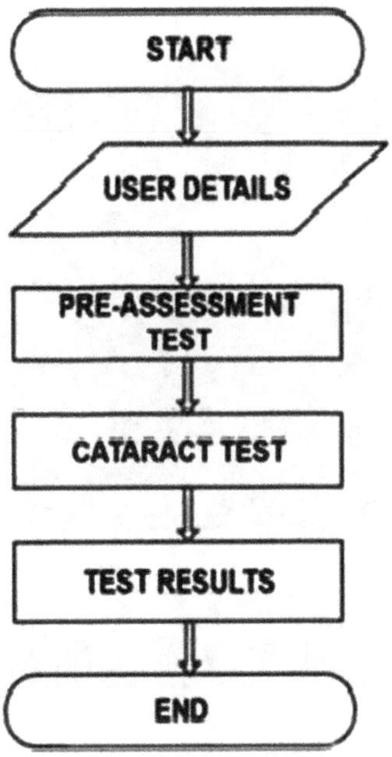

The PDF report will be downloaded in the local storage of the mobile phone and it can be available in the language that the user opted for.

Eye Advice

The possible factors that cause cataracts are stated as a part of the application. How the factors cause cataract is also described in this phase.

RESULTS AND DISCUSSION

The activities related to pre-diagnosis and further immediate treatment of cataract might be costly for the poor. The machine-based detection of cataract is more time consuming and costly, thereby crippling the efficiency of the practitioner. The creation of a simple, low-cost smart-phone based cataract detection mobile application helps detect cataract from anywhere at any time (Figure 4-12). The proposed app is trained with images of 40 pairs of human eyes. The captured images are in different categories like varying illumination details, left and right eye centers, scale, location, and head pose.

Figure 4. User input details

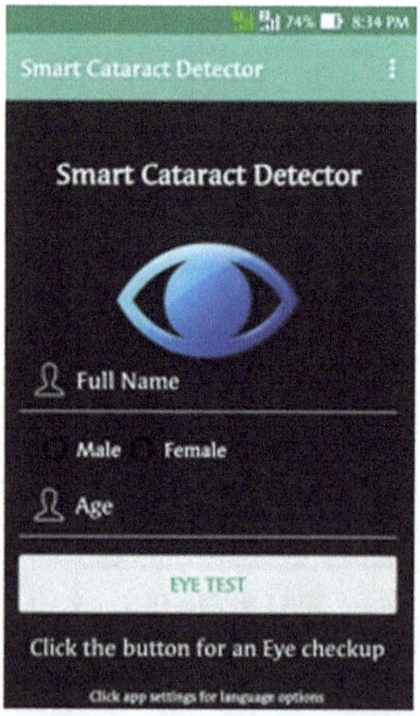

Figure 5. List of modules

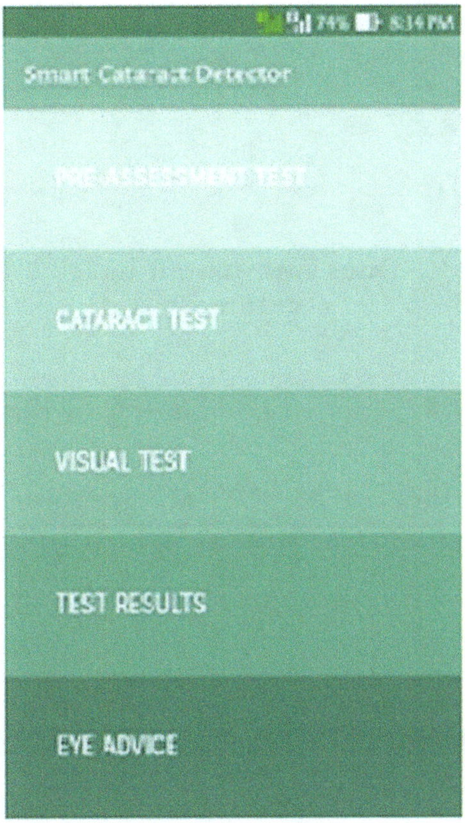

Figure 6. Pre-assessment test

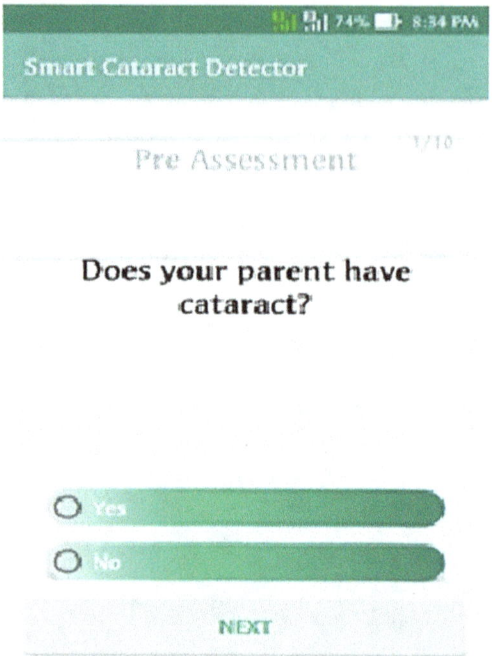

Figure 7. Cataract test

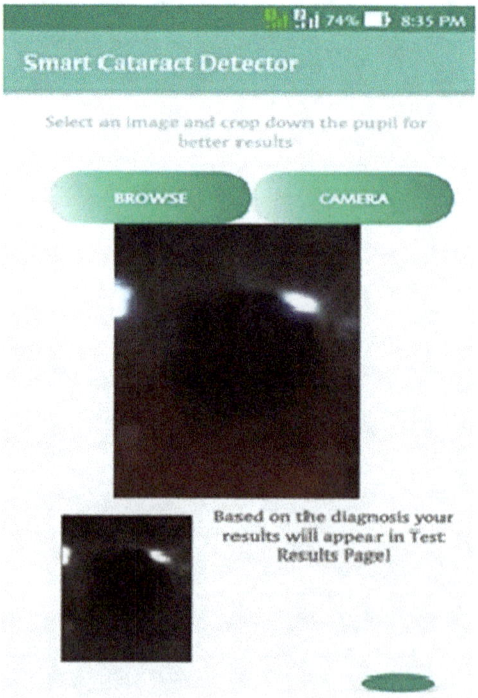

Figure 8. Vision test

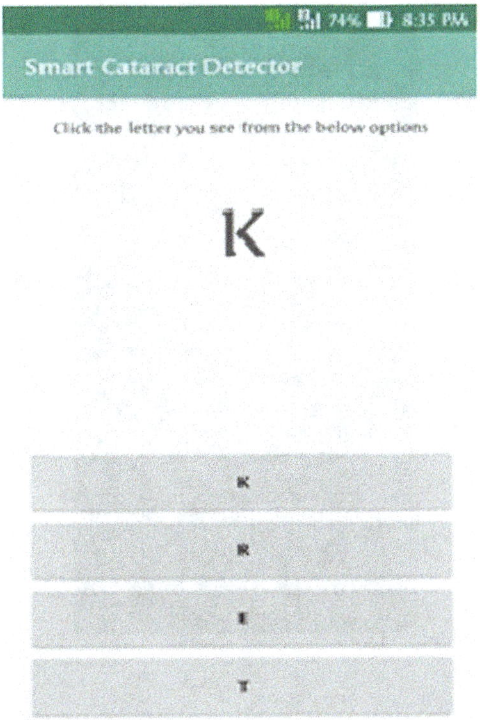

Figure 9. Test Result

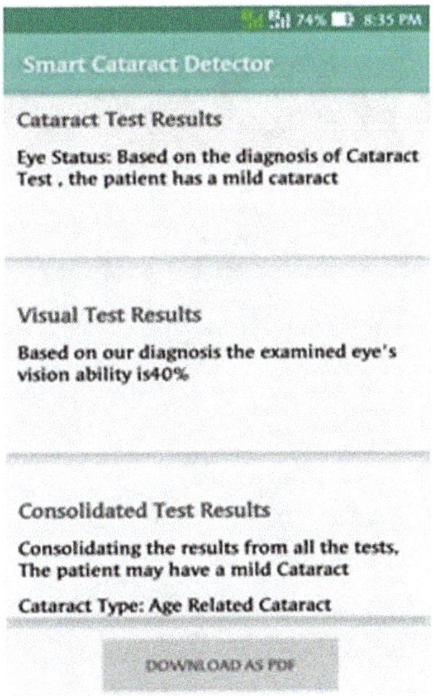

Figure 10. Eye advice

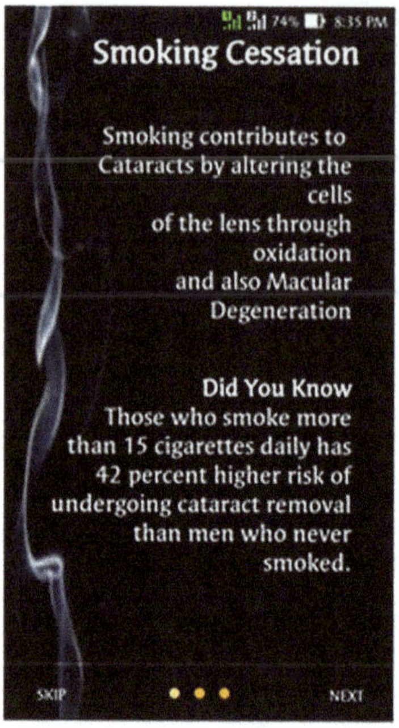

Figure 11. Report generated

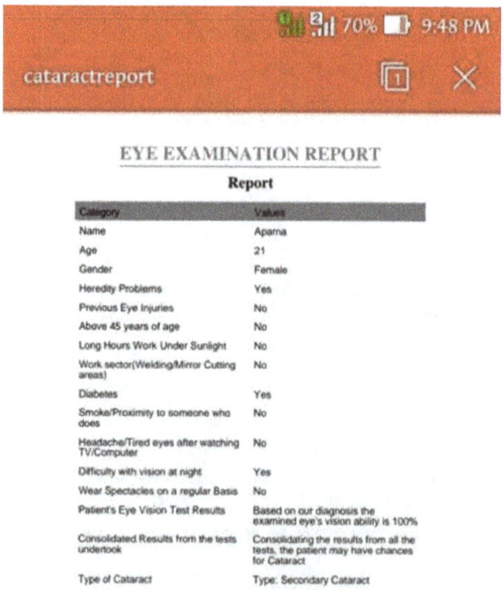

EYE EXAMINATION REPORT

Report

Category	Values
Name	Aparna
Age	21
Gender	Female
Heredity Problems	Yes
Previous Eye Injuries	No
Above 45 years of age	No
Long Hours Work Under Sunlight	No
Work sector(Welding/Mirror Cutting areas)	No
Diabetes	Yes
Smoke/Proximity to someone who does	No
Headache/Tired eyes after watching TV/Computer	No
Difficulty with vision at night	Yes
Wear Spectacles on a regular Basis	No
Patient's Eye Vision Test Results	Based on our diagnosis the examined eye's vision ability is 100%
Consolidated Results from the tests undertook	Consolidating the results from all the tests, the patient may have chances for Cataract
Type of Cataract	Type: Secondary Cataract

Figure 12. Language Settings

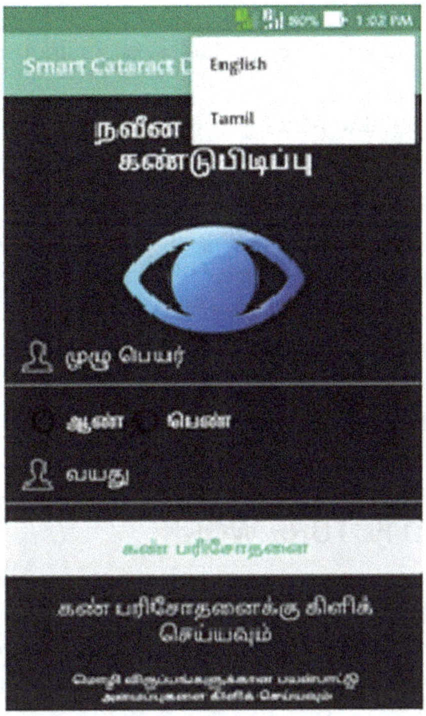

Accuracy

The captured images are tested on the proposed mobile application and the system reaches the expected accuracy during the validation time. The system provides an accuracy of about 64.30% to 87.50% based on the quality of the input image. Since the system does not use complex algorithms but uses geometric parameters, the computation speed is high and fast enough to find the presence of cataract in real-time. The system is able to scale any number of images using a threaded approach. The application also works well with varying image resolutions. But sometimes the true labels of the pupil are inaccurate which leads to less accuracy.

Error Possibilities

The possible errors discussed in this works might degrade the system. Some examples are,

1. Eye corner detection error

2. Eyebrow and eyelash detection error
3. Camera spotlight errors
4. Errors due to stray factors like spectacles, occlusions, and wrinkles.

This application is found to be a replacement for the existing methods used for cataract diagnosis which are quite sophisticated and involve the use of expensive machines. The mobile application developed offers mobility to the users as they can perform a diagnosis for cataract by sitting at home, office i.e. anytime anywhere access. Cataract is one of the major causes of blindness amongst the aging population; this app helps in the timely and convenient diagnosis. Cataract occurs due to the clouding of the lens and it could even lead to eye blindness. Cataract detection requires the most expensive machines and huge amount of time. It also requires good infrastructure and ophthalmologists.

CONCLUSION AND FUTURE WORK

Cataract is a very serious disease and it should be identified, monitored and treated at the right time. The cloudiness on the pupil causes loss of sight. This chapter presented a simple, low-cost smart-phone based cataract detection application. This application is found to be a replacement for the existing methods used for cataract diagnosis which are quite sophisticated and involve the use of expensive machines. The mobile application developed offers mobility to the users as they can perform a diagnosis for cataract by sitting at home, office i.e. anytime anywhere access.

The shortcomings of the software are that the image captured with a flash spot could have variations in the grayscale thus affecting the result. Efforts can be made to remove the flash spot from the image obtained from the camera. The future works include collecting the digital images of the eye that are provided as input to the application which would be used for analysis in a later period. Suggesting the users with near-by hospitals would help them to go for a check-up. Thus, the application designed is found to be user-friendly and it minimizes the time spent at the hospital to meet the doctor and also the cost needed to test the cataract detection at hospitals.

REFERENCES

Abraham, A. G., Duncan, D. D., Gange, S. J., & West, S. (2009). Computer-aided assessment of diagnostic images for epidemiological research. *BMC Medical Research Methodology*, *9*(1), 74. doi:10.1186/1471-2288-9-74 PMID:19906311

Acharya, U. R., Wong, L. Y., Ng, E. Y. K., & Suri, J. S. (2007). Automatic identification of anterior segment eye abnormality. *IRBM*, *28*(1), 35–41. doi:10.1016/j.rbmret.2007.02.002

Ahuja, K., Banerjee, R., Nagar, S., Dey, K., & Barbhuiya, F. (2016). Eye center localization and detection using radial mapping. *Proceedings 2016 IEEE International Conference on Image Processing (ICIP)*. DOI:10.1109/ICIP.2016.7532934

Ferman, A. M. (2008). Automatic detection of red-eye artifacts in digital color photos. *Proceedings 2008 15th IEEE International Conference on Image Processing*. DOI:10.1109/icip.2008.4711830

Khan, A. A., Akram, M. U., Tariq, A., Tahir, F., & Wazir, K. (2017). Automated Computer-Aided Detection of Cataract. Advances in Intelligent Systems and Computing, 340–349. Doi:10.1007/978-3-319-60834-1_34

Khan, A. A., Akram, M. U., Tariq, A., Tahir, F., & Wazir, K. (2017). Automated Computer-Aided Detection of Cataract. *Advances in Intelligent Systems and Computing,* 340–349. Doi:10.1007/978-3-319-60834-1_34

Kumar, S., Pathak, S., & Kumar, B. (2019). Automated Detection of Eye Related Diseases Using Digital Image Processing. In Handbook of Multimedia Information Security: Techniques and Applications, 513–544. Doi:10.1007/978-3-030-15887-3_25

Manikandakumar, M., & Ramanujam, E. (2018). Security and Privacy Challenges in Big Data Environment. *Advances in Information Security, Privacy, and Ethics*, 315–325. doi:10.4018/978-1-5225-4100-4.ch017

Pathak, S., & Kumar, B. (2016). A Robust Automated Cataract Detection Algorithm Using Diagnostic Opinion Based Parameter Thresholding for Telemedicine Application. *Electronics (Basel)*, *5*(4), 57. doi:10.3390/electronics5030057

Patwari, M. A. U., Arif, M. D., Chowdhury, M. N., Arefin, A., & Imam, M. I. (2011, May). Detection, categorization, and assessment of eye cataracts using digital image processing. *Proceedings The first international conference on interdisciplinary research and development* (pp. 22-1). Thailand. Academic Press.

Valenti, R., & Gevers, T. (2012). Accurate Eye Center Location through Invariant Isocentric Patterns. *IEEE Transactions on Pattern Analysis and Machine Intelligence*, *34*(9), 1785–1798. doi:10.1109/TPAMI.2011.251 PMID:22813958

Xu, Z., & Shi, P. (2006). A Robust and Accurate Method for Pupil Features Extra. Proceedings *18th International Conference on Pattern Recognition (ICPR'06)*. DOI:10.1109/icpr.2006.165

Chapter 12
A Survey and Analysis to Find Dental Implant Issues in India:
Dental Problems in India

Suchismita Satapathy
https://orcid.org/0000-0002-4805-1793
KIIT University, India

ABSTRACT

Presently, dental implantations are the ideal solution and best substitute option for missing teeth. Dental implants determined the replacements of root and non-working teeth after the loss of natural teeth. Strengthening dental materials helps to fix the loss teeth. For teeth with root disease and fault in bone density, dental implantation is very essential. While bridge work and dentures decline to reclaim the suitable chewing condition and turn the problem of missing teeth, dental implants trace the solution of missing teeth. For more progress in dental-concerned technology, an extensive growth in dental implants has been noticed during the last several years. So there is a large need of excellent, quality dental materials. The selection of the implant materials, their generation system, manufacturing method, age-long durability, bio compatibility with medical principle, and professional dental field of study are therefore essential.

DOI: 10.4018/978-1-7998-2581-4.ch012

INTRODUCTION

Dental implants are the frame or a component that attached with the jawbone to support crown, fixtures, abutment. These days, implantation is the perfect solution for the absence of tooth and being viewed as the best option for the replacement of the lost tooth. Regardless of the most recent advances in dental technology, implants are still subjected to decline. Tooth loss occurs due to root decay, infection, injury, fault in bone density, failure in the root canal, gum disease, congenital defects. Tooth loss can lead men and women to functional and aesthetic problems. The utilization of dental implants is offered to help for the substitution of missing teeth and determine the replacement of root and non-working teeth. The implant material should have ideal properties such as mechanical, physical, chemical and biological. The main parts of the dental implants are crown, abutment, implant body or fixtures. Crown is a cap-like structure that protects the covering of the implant and is placed into the jawbone. An abutment is the part of the implant that helps to support the frame selection of the implant materials and their manufacturing process are very essential. Materials like metal alloy, ceramics, polymer are mostly used for the fabrication of dental implants. Other materials like stainless steel, cobalt-based alloy found to be a little success in dental implants due to bad mechanical properties. Mechanical behavior of dental implants is very important to fix the lost tooth and lead to strengthening the material for long term implantation. So the latest research is to search and find the best material to perform effectively with the least cost.

The classification of the dental implants, which is introduced in the dentistry based on placement, includes endosteal type, subperiosteal type, and transosteal type. End osseous type implant further classified into blade form and ramus form. The endosseous type of implant is mainly attached to the jawbone and has the shape like a cylindrical or screw type. The endosseous type of implant has common usage in dentistry. Blade form is like a thin plate in the blade structure attached to the bone. Ramus form is like a horseshoe structure embedded into the mandible from one region of the retromolar pad to the other. The subperiosteal implant can easily be attached to the jawbone and likely to offer root for multiple teeth; it helps to guide the elementary bone supports and has limited usage due to loss of bone. Transosteal implant is also known as a staple bone implant; surrounds the alveolar bone through the entire thickness; penetrates the cortical bone, but not used much more in dentistry now. The implants can also be classified into various shapes based on their design like cylindrical, conical and threaded.

Many materials have been employed as an implant for a substitute of missing teeth. The properties of the implant material should possess bulk properties like modulus of elasticity, tensile, compressive and shear strength, hardness and toughness, ductility, yield strength, and fatigue strength. The choice of the implant material with modulus elasticity should be greater uniform stress distribution at the site of the implant and relative movement to minimize the bone-implant junction. The implant should possess high compressive and tensile strength. Owing to high tensile and compressive strength fractures can be prevented and developed the stability function he wears of the implant material can be decreased owing to the increase in the hardness, and fracture of the implant can be prevented due to the increase in toughness. Ductility is important for the implant when the implant material is subjected to shaping and essential for contouring. The yield strength and fatigue strength of the implant material should be high, so that brittle fractures can be prevented under repeated loading cycle. Based on the surface properties of the implant materials depends on surface roughness, surface tension, and surface energy. Surface roughness is influencing the reaction of the cells and tissues by expanding the surface zone of the implant that fused to the bone and promote the cell connection to the bone. Surface tension promotes the cleanliness of the implant region and stability. Absorption of the protein have been affected by the surface energy and improved the implant region adhesion. The biocompatibility properties of the dental implant that show great response in a biological environment in a specific function. The biocompatibility of the material can be determined by the degradation mechanism like corrosion and wear. The material which has good corrosion and wears resistance possess good biocompatibility of the implant Saini(2015)

Corrosion leads when the ions of the metals released in the adjacent environment from the metal surface. The corrosion can be classified into pitting corrosion, galvanic corrosion, electrochemical corrosion. In our oral environment, different types of electrochemical corrosions can take place due to the presence of aggressive anions in saliva such as chlorides. The release of dissolved metal ion bonding with the chlorides leads the pitting corrosion. It also leads to a roughening surface due to pit composition. Galvanic corrosion has occurred when a combination of two or more dissimilar metal is in physical contact with each other. When the metal associated with the fluid electrolyte and saturated solution can be formed due to dissolving ions and release the free electrons leads the electrochemical corrosion Saini (2015), Chaturvedi(2009)].

The future of the implant for better long-term stability depends on the good design of implant and biomechanical features. The various technique was used, in order to investigate the occurrence of forces, stress and strain deformation. FEA analysis is one of the popular techniques that used for dental implant for evaluating the prominent result of shear stress distribution, forces variation, load condition of the implant, and boundary condition; and it permits better modeling of the geometry of the implant framework. Our literature review was mainly based on the design of the implant and its parameter which affects the stress-strain concentration at the bone-implant interface, analysis technique of the implant for precise modeling, a mechanical complication of the implant and mechanical evaluation of different implant design to determine the success for the long term stability of the implant system.

LITERATURE REVIEW

Based on Biomedical Materials for Dental Implant

Commercially pure titanium is mainly used for dental implants. Titanium has a good record with excellent biocompatibility property that is used as an implant material and its surface property possesses stable oxide layers.

An α-phase i.e hexagonal closed packed during the process of heating at temperature 883°C, Ti, is converted into β-phase i.e body-centered cubic lattice. Ti surface act as a stable oxide layer and below temperature 882.5°C and also act as a dimorphic metal. Due to more passivity and resistance to chemical attack, Ti material is a perfect choice of the dental implant. Different types of Ti-based alloy is also used for dental implants. Ti-6AL-4V is a standout among the most critical appropriate alloy that extensively utilized for dental implants. Different types of elements such as Va, Zn, Fe, Ur, Al, Ar, Cu reacts with titanium. These types of elements are formed when pure titanium is heated with Al and Va. At specific conditions after hearing process, elements like Al and Va that mixed with titanium have been cooled and then Ti-6Al-4V alloy is formed. Heat-treated alloy helps to promote good strength. Generally, in Ti-6Al-4V, variety contains 6% Al and 4% Va that used for dental implants. Ceramics has it has good physical properties and high strength for which it has been used for surgical implant component but its use is limited in dental implant due to poor ductility and brittleness.

Prior to the generation of osseointegration, there had been numerous shapes of dental implants used to assist partial dentures with various fulfillment costs. The diverse substances used in implants are porcelain, and cobalt-chromium. However, the invention of titanium changed the path of implant history. Osseous integration has been defined by the Bran mark who radically influenced the implant ideas processed on bone marrow curative. Then titanium-like material and newly developed substance, which was biocompatible with the human body, had been used Rajput(2016).

Holmgren et al. (1998) have carried out FEA for determining the stress concentration at the implant-bone attachment, suggest that the bigger diameter the shape of the implant is not usually the satisfactory preference during the time of stress transmission to the adjacent bones, and also reveals that stepped cylindrical the design had better stress concentration at the adjacent to the jawbone and better implant shape for the stress concentration. Chun et al. (2002) have determined the various shape of dental implant carried out by finite element analysis and shows that thread like framework having greater stress concentration in the jawbone. Based on the thread property, consequences on the stress concentration of jawbone were valid to determine the most reliable dimensions of several dental implant parameters.

Vidyasagar et al. (2004) have suggested that the different bone aspects, various implant geometry, surface properties like roughness and design alteration could lead to a better result of the primary implant stability.

Jae-hoon lee et al. (2005) have suggested that the parameters of the implant design like length, diameter, slope could determine the better performance of an implant. He also determines that condition like stress and load, the behavior could be improved through the implant design parameters and also leads to determine the fracture resistance and implant strength.

Misch et al. (2008) have evaluated the study of bone density, which is required for the better performance of the implant, and also determine the stability of the implant.

Biaggi et al. (2008) have demonstrated the stress variation, shown that maximum stress occurs at the neck of the implant through numerical study, and also reveal that larger diameter of an implant at cortical bone shows low stress concentration, while larger length shows better stress concentration in cancellous bone. Misch et al. (2008) have revealed that conical design implant shows better stability than that of cylindrical.

Guan et al. (2009) demonstrates the finite element study to determine the analysis of bone and implant stability. Javed and Romanos (2010) have revealed the characteristics of various thread shapes, surface regions of an implant, parameters of various implant design, and comparisons of cylindrical and tapered implant clarifies that thread design implant shows different characteristics and it also reveals that thread structure implant with a tapered framework requires more surface region.

Faegh et al. (2010) have revealed the stress distribution was evaluated on the basis of external threads parameters like body dimension, length, diameter. It also reveals that at the implant-bone junction site it shows great alteration on external threads when subjected to the shear stress.

Abuhussein et al. (2010) have focused on the stability of the implant and analyze through various models of the implants and it shows that bone characteristics features, major surface region, the low angle at helix point, greater diameter, the broad thread would be a favorable condition for implant success was the as large pitch, smaller shaped implant, less threaded geometry, the restricted diameter of the implant resulted in the bad stability of the implant. Reddy and Thumati have (2014) have revealed that the choice of threaded design implant provides better results in clinical condition because of high uniform stress concentration was seen in a threaded implant than that of a smooth implant. Smooth implant shows progressive stress concentration at the tip of the implant.

George et al. (2015) have demonstrated the comparisons between the cylinder and tapered implant based on the placement and it reveals that the tapered had shown better stability than the cylindrical implant because tapered lead more torque insertion during the time of placement.

Rajput et al. (2016).have demonstrated the experiments about mechanical characteristics of the implants that deals with various condition. et al [2017] have demonstrated the different types of implant design that can lead the better stability for long term implantation. Mechanical characteristics, proper stress distribution at the implant junction can be determined through the various design of the implant.

Fangqiu Ji et al. (2018) have focused on the study of mechanical finite element analysis when the implant is integrated with the jawbone and it proposed that the level of density should be higher during integrating between abutment and implant to reduce the effect of stress shielding effect and enhance the stiffness property and strength of the implant.

BASED ON MECHANICAL COMPLICATION OF THE IMPLANT

Mechanical issues like Screw fracture, abutment breakdown, implant damage which leads the damage to the implant. **Berlundh et al** (2002) have suggested that implant the damage occurred due to overloading, the poor mechanical design of the implant and implant-bone adjustment site but it reveals that no implant damage was resulted during changing the single tooth process.Karl **et al**(2009) Suggest that Screw damage leads the rate of issues that varying from 9.3% and 18.5% with follow up 5 and 10 years.

RESEARCH METHODOLOGY

To find problems of dental patients a standard is designed by literature review and expert analysis and a cross-sectional questionnaire study was carried out in Dental Colleges to find several dental problems faced by patients and frequency of visit. One hundred and fifty patients participated in this study. The patients were asked to answer a questionnaire on dental problems faced within the last 5 years. Likert scale of 1to 5 is used to collect data .1= Totally disagree,2=disagree, 3=no opinion,4=agree,5=totally agree. To find barriers and customer satisfaction of Dental implants a questionnaire survey of 150 patients was conducted including experts opinion and literature survey. Experts are selected consisting of 5 experts of medical college,10 dental surgeons,6 academicians. A Likert scale of 1 to 5 is used. 1=Totally disagree,2=disagree,,3=no opinion,4=agree,5=totally agree. Then

Promethee-II is implemented to find the most important barriers that discard dental implants. Then dental implantation is measured by measuring customer satisfaction in successive implantation.

RESULT AND DISCUSSION

Table 1. Dental problems of patients visiting OPD.

Cause for Visit to OPD	Number of Patient (%)
Dental problem faced due to cavity	126 (86.88)
Pain due to toothache	111 (77.08)
Use of drugs and tabaco decays tooth and cause of hanging teeth	120 (83.33)
Chocolates & sweets creates tooth problem	14 (9.72)
Half broken teeth	09 (6.25)
Fall down and accidents	16 (11.11)
Mouth cancer	28 (20.05)
Diabetics	13 (9.02)
Bleeding Due to irregular brushing habit	138 (95.83)
Drinking habits	129 (89.58)
Age problem	07 (4.25)
Mouth smell	06(3.11)
Dental implants	141(96.05)
Regular check up	11 (8.62)
For shaping teeth	108 (90.83)
Root canal	121 (83.58)

Dental implants are artificial tooth roots that provide a permanent base for fixed, replacement teeth. Compared to dentures, bridges, and crowns, dental implants are popular and effective the long-term solution for people who suffer from missing teeth, failing teeth or chronic dental problems. Although patient suffering and doctors suggesting, dental implants are still not preferred by patients. Still patients afraid of implants due to fear, and try to avoid it. India is still not popular. Patients have many questions about cost, effectiveness, durability procedure, etc. Thus, this effort was taken to find barriers that hindering dental implants in India. Then Promethee-II is implemented to find the most important barriers that discard dental implants.

Drivers or the motivation for tooth implants. At present days dental implantation is the ideal solution and best substitute option for missing teeth. Dental implants determined the replacements of root and non-working teeth after the loss of natural teeth. strengthening dental materials helps to fix the lost teeth. The teeth, which are concerned by root disease, fault in bone density, dental implantation, is very essential, While bridgework and dentures decline to reclaim the suitable chewing condition and turn the problem of missing teeth. Dental implant traces the solution of missing teeth. For more progress in dental concerned technology, extensive growth in dental implants has been noticed during the last several years. Thus there is a large need for excellent quality dental materials.

1. Enablers: Personal Life
2. Enjoyment of Food
3. Physical Comfort
4. Self Confidence
5. Appearance
6. Professional Life
7. Food Choices
8. Oral Health
9. Pain relief

Table 2 shows assigned input weight.

Table 2. Assigned input eight

Enablers	Averaged Values	Normalized Values
A	3.88	0.615385
B	4	0.846154
C	3.84	0.538462
D	3.72	0.307692
E	3.56	0
F	4.08	1
G	3.72	0.307692
H	4	0.846154
I	4	0.846154

Table 3 shows preference functions table.

Table 3. Preference functions table

Barrier Pairs	Normalized Values
AB	0
AC	0.076923
AD	0.307693
AE	0.615385
AF	0
AG	0.307693
AH	0
AI	0
BA	0.230769
BC	0.307692
BD	0.538462
BE	0.846154
BF	0
BG	0.538462
BH	0
BI	0
CA	0
CB	0
CD	0.23077
CE	0.538462
CF	0
CG	0.23077
CH	0
CI	0
DA	0
DB	0
DC	0
DE	0.307692
DF	0
DG	0
DH	0
DI	0
EA	0
EB	0
EC	0
ED	0
EF	0
EG	0
EH	0
EI	0
FA	0.384615
FB	0.153846
FC	0.461538
FD	0.692308
FE	1

continued on following page

Table 3 continued

Barrier Pairs	Normalized Values
FG	0.692308
FH	0.153846
FI	0.153846
GA	0
GB	0
GC	0
GD	0
GE	0.307692
GF	0
GH	0
GI	0
HA	0.230769
HB	0
HC	0.307692
HD	0.538462
HE	0.846154
HF	0
HG	0.538462
HI	0
IA	0.230769
IB	0
IC	0.307692
ID	0.538462
IE	0.846154
IF	0
IG	0.538462
IH	0

Table 4. Aggregated preference functions matrix

	A	B	C	D	E	F	G	H	I
A	0	0	0.077	0.308	0.615	0	0.308	0	0
B	0.231	0	0.308	0.538	0.846	0	0.538	0	0
C	0	0	0	0.231	0.538	0	0.231	0	0
D	0	0	0	0	0.308	0	0	0	0
E	0	0	0	0	0	0	0	0	0
F	0.385	0.154	0.462	0.692	1	0	0.692	0.154	0.154
G	0	0	0	0	0.308	0	0	0	0
H	0.231	0	0.308	0.538	0.846	0	0.538	0	0
I	0.231	0	0.308	0.538	0.846	0	0.538	0	0

Table 4 shows aggregated preference functions matrix.
Table 5 shows ranking table.

Table 5. Ranking table

Enablers	Φnablersg tabl	Ranks		
A	1.307694	1.076922	0.230772	5
B	2.461539	0.153846	2.307693	4
C	1.000002	1.461537	-0.461535	6
D	0.307692	2.846157	-2.538465	8
E	0	5.307693	-5.307693	9
F	3.692307	0	3.692307	1
G	0.307692	2.846157	-2.538465	7
H	2.461539	0.153846	2.307693	2
I	2.461539	0.153846	2.307693	3

Promethee-II

The PROMETHEE II method allows one to establish a complete ranking between possible movements based on outranking relations.

Procedure of Promethee-II:

Normalization of Decision matrix using the following equation (Min-Max Normalizasiton):

$$R_{ij} = [X_{ij}\text{-min}(X_{ij})]/[\max(X_{ij})\text{-min}(X_{ij})] \ (i=1, 2..n;j=1,2..m)$$

where X_{ij} is the performance measure of ith factor with respect to j^{th} criterion.

Computation of evaluative differences of ith factor with respect to other factors.

This step involved the calculation of differences in criteria values between different factors pairwise.

Calculation of preference function Pj (i, i′) using the following equation:

Preference Functions Values:

$$P(i, i') = 0 \text{ If } R_i \leq R_{i'}$$

$P(i, i') = (R_i - R_{i'})$ If $R_i > R_{i'}$

$R_1 - R_2 = 0$

Table 6 shows input weights assigned for barriers.

Table 6. Input weights assigned for Barriers

	Barriers	Averaged Value
A	Mental preparedness for replace of teeth	3.1
B	Technical design for proper implantation	3.472
C	Fear of surgery & pain	3.312
D	Success in implantations and lasting	3.068
E	Strength of material used in implantation and its durability	3.088
F	Lack of knowledge and education.	3.028
G	Not got clear information from dentist	3.112
H	Suitable Material selection for implantation	3.484
I	High cost	3.532
J	Not clear about procedure	3.068

Table 7 shows normalized value of barriers.

Table 7. Normalized value

	Barriers	Normalized Value
A	Mental preparedness for replace of teeth	0.879
B	Technical design for proper implantation	0.83
C	Fear of surgery& pain	0.973
D	Success in implantations and lasting	0.868
E	Strength of material used in implantation and its durability	0.874
F	Lack of knowledge and education.	.857
G	Not got clear information from dentist	0.88
H	Suitable Material selection for implantation	0.986
I	High cost	1
J	Not clear about procedure	0.868

Table 8 shows preference function value of barriers.

Table 8. Preference function value of barriers

Barrier Pairs	Values
AB	0
AC	0.219526
AD	0
AE	0
AF	0
AG	0.150263
AH	0
AI	0
AJ	0
BA	0.507
BC	0.789
BD	0.0552
BE	0
BF	0.5670
BG	0.6584
BH	0
BI	0.5126
BJ	0.0152
CA	0
CB	0
CD	0
CE	0
CF	0
CG	0
CH	0
CI	0
CJ	0
DA	0.5323
DB	0
DC	0.7736
DE	0

continued on following page

Table 8 continued

Barrier Pairs	Values
DF	0.5026
DG	0.6231
DH	0
DI	0.447
DJ	0
EA	0.7089
EB	0.4211
EC	0
ED	0.2362
EF	0.7678
EG	0.8809
EH	0.0152
EI	0.7036
EJ	0.0261
FA	0
FB	0
FC	0.2231
FD	0
FE	0
FG	0.10049
FH	0
FI	0
FJ	0
GA	0
GB	0
GC	0.1019
GD	0
GE	0
GF	0
GH	0
GI	0
GJ	0
HA	0.6773
HB	0.1057

continued on following page

Table 8 continued

Barrier Pairs	Values
HC	0.9334
HD	0.2210
HE	0
HF	0.7731
HG	0.7984
HI	0.6684
HJ	0.2561
IA	0.1052
IB	0
IC	0.3326
ID	0
IE	0
IF	0.2057
IG	0.11057
IH	0
IJ	0
JA	0.5552
JB	0
JC	0.7073
JD	0
JE	0
JF	0.4952
JG	0.561
JH	0
JI	0.4337

Table 9 shows aggregated preference functions matrix.
Table 10 shows ranking of barriers of dental implants.

Table 9. Aggregated preference functions matrix

	A	B	C	D	E	F	G	H	I	J
A	0	0	0.211	0	0	0	0.105	0	0	0
B	0.579	0	0.789	0.053	0	0.579	0.684	0	0.526	0.053
C	0	0	0	0	0	0	0	0	0	0
D	0.526	0	0.737	0	0	0.526	0.632	0	0.474	0
E	0.789	0.211	1	0.263	0	0.789	0.895	0.053	0.737	0.263
F	0	0	0.211	0	0	0	0.105	0	0	0
G	0	0	0.105	0	0	0	0	0	0	0
H	0.737	0.158	0.947	0.211	0	0.737	0.842	0	0.684	0.211
I	0.053	0	0.263	0	0	0.053	0.158	0	0	0
J	0.526	0	0.737	0	0	0.526	0.632	0	0.474	0

Table 10. Ranking table

Barriers	Φ+	Φ-	Φ(Total)	Ranks
A	0.315789	3.210528	-2.894739	7
B	3.263161	0.36842	2.894741	3(3rd)
C	0	4.999999	-4.999999	10
D	2.894737	0.526316	2.368421	4
E	5.000001	0	5.000001	1(1st)
F	0.315789	3.210528	-2.894739	8
G	0.105263	4.052632	-3.947369	9
H	4.526313	0.052632	4.473681	2(2nd)
I	0.526317	2.894736	-2.368419	6
J	2.894737	0.526316	2.368421	5

After ranking, it is found that strength of the material used in implantation and its durability is the most important barrier ranked first, technical design for proper implantation ranked second and suitable material selection for implantation is ranked third. It shows that these are the cause of patients not preferring dental implantation. So to avoid these barriers suitably technology, materials, and design aspects must be considered which can make artificial implants not only look natural but it also can function long-term like natural teeth. The selection of the implant materials, their generation system, manufacturing method, age-long durability, biocompatibility with medical principles and professional dental field of studies are therefore essential. Today, precision investment casting and manufacturing processes of dental implants produce many defects and faults since imperfect castings and their mechanical properties cannot satisfy the standard. The implant made by this process cannot exactly measure the elastic modulus. Materials, for example, metal alloys and ceramics are broadly utilized for the manufacture of dental implants. Ceramic production either makes up the whole implants or can be connected as a covering the metallic core. A perfect implant should have higher strength character, biocompatibility, fatigue nature and fracture toughness characteristics and capable to withstand the reactive environment that exposed within the human body. Several types of metallic material are used for the implant, among them, the stainless steel has been limited due to its bad fatigue strength and galvanic corrosion.

CONCLUSION

The improvement of the dental implant has been a trending topic in the field of implant research at present days. With the help of various analysis techniques and research, the performance of the implant may develop clinically with better success results. Several mechanical evaluations of the implant design, biomechanical features, biomaterials properties, bone-implant interface condition, mechanical the complication and design requirements have been focused in this context but it is still necessary to further research on mechanical consideration, testing, and analysis of implant design and material properties for better clinical performance and long term stability of the implant.

REFERENCES

Abuhussein, H., Pagni, G., Rebaudi, A., & Wang, H. L. (2010). The effect of thread pattern upon implant osseointegration. *Clinical Oral Implants Research, 21*(2), 129–136. doi:10.1111/j.1600-0501.2009.01800.x PMID:19709058

Baggi, L., Cappelloni, I., Di Girolamo, M., Maceri, F., & Vairo, G. (2008). The influence of implant diameter and length on stress distribution of osseointegrated implants related to crestal bone geometry: A three-dimensional finite element analysis. *The Journal of Prosthetic Dentistry, 100*(6), 422–431. doi:10.1016/S0022-3913(08)60259-0 PMID:19033026

Berglundh, T., Persson, L., & Klinge, B. (2002). A systematic review of the incidence of biological and technical complications in implant dentistry reported in prospective longitudinal studies of at least 5 years. *Journal of Clinical Periodontology*, *29*, 197–212.

Bicudo, P., Reis, J., Deus, A. M., Reis, L., & Vaz, M. F. (2016). Mechanical behaviour of dental implants. *Procedia Structural Integrity*, *1*, 26–33. doi:10.1016/j.prostr.2016.02.005

Chaturvedi, T. P. (2009). An overview of the corrosion aspect of dental implants (titanium and its alloys). *Indian Journal of Dental Research*, *20*(1), 91. doi:10.4103/0970-9290.49068 PMID:19336868

Chun, H. J., Cheong, S. Y., Han, J. H., Heo, S. J., Chung, J. P., Rhyu, I. C., ... Kim, M. H. (2002). Evaluation of design parameters of osseointegrated dental implants using finite element analysis. *Journal of Oral Rehabilitation*, *29*(6), 565–574. doi:10.1046/j.1365-2842.2002.00891.x PMID:12071926

de Andrade, C. L., Carvalho, M. A., Bordin, D., da Silva, W. J., Del Bel Cury, A. A., & Sotto-Maior, B. S. (2017). Biomechanical Behavior of the Dental Implant Macrodesign. *International Journal of Oral & Maxillofacial Implants*, *32*(2).

Faegh, S., & Müftü, S. (2010). Load transfer along the bone–dental implant interface. *Journal of Biomechanics*, *43*(9), 1761–1770. doi:10.1016/j.jbiomech.2010.02.017 PMID:20202639

George, A., Khalil, A., & Hassan, N. (2015). Comparison between cylinder and tapered implants in delayed immediate placement. *Alexandria Dental Journal*, *40*(2), 221–228. doi:10.21608/adjalexu.2015.59156

Gil, F. J., Herrero-Climent, M., Lázaro, P., & Rios, J. V. (2014). Implant–abutment connections: Influence of the design on the microgap and their fatigue and fracture behavior of dental implants. *Journal of Materials Science. Materials in Medicine*, *25*(7), 1825–1830. doi:10.100710856-014-5211-7 PMID:24719176

Guan, H., van Staden, R., Loo, Y. C., Johnson, N., Ivanovski, S., & Meredith, N. (2009). Influence of bone and dental implant parameters on stress distri-bution in the mandible: A finite element study. *Int J Oral Maxillofac Implants*, *24*, 866–876. PMID:19865627

Hanif, A., Qureshi, S., Sheikh, Z., & Rashid, H. (2017). Complications in implant dentistry. *European Journal of Dentistry*, *11*(1), 135–140. doi:10.4103/ejd.ejd_340_16 PMID:28435381

Holmgren, E. P., Seckinger, R. J., Kilgren, L. M., & Mante, F. (1998). Evaluating parameters of osseointegrated dental implants using finite element analysis—A two-dimensional comparative study examining the effects of implant diameter, implant shape, and load direction. *The Journal of Oral Implantology*, *24*(2), 80–88. doi:10.1563/1548-1336(1998)024<0080:EPOODI>2.3.CO;2 PMID:9835834

Javed, F., & Romanos, G. E. (2010). The role of primary stability for successful immediate loading of dental implants. A literature review. *Journal of Dentistry*, *38*(8), 612–620. doi:10.1016/j.jdent.2010.05.013 PMID:20546821

Ji, F., Zhang, C., & Chen, X. (2018, March). Structure Optimization of Porous Dental Implant Based on 3D Printing. *Proceedings IOP Conference Series: Materials Science and Engineering*, 324, 1, p. 012060. IOP Publishing.

Karl, M., & Kelly, J. R. (2009). Influence of loading frequency on implant failure under cyclic fatigue conditions. *Dental Materials*, *25*(11), 1426–1432. doi:10.1016/j.dental.2009.06.015 PMID:19643468

Kim, J. W., Baek, S. H., Kim, T. W., & Chang, Y. I. (2008). Comparison of stability between cylindrical and conical type mini-implants: Mechanical and histologic properties. *The Angle Orthodontist*, *78*(4), 692–698. doi:10.2319/0003-3219(2008)078[0692:COSBCA]2.0.CO;2 PMID:18302470

Lee, J. H., Frias, V., Lee, K. W., & Wright, R. F. (2005). Effect of implant size and shape on implant success rates: A literature review. *The Journal of Prosthetic Dentistry*, *94*(4), 377–381. doi:10.1016/j.prosdent.2005.04.018 PMID:16198176

Misch, C. (2008). *Density of bone: effects on surgical approach and healing. Contemporary Implant Dentistry*. Mosby.

Pjetursson, B. E., Thoma, D., Jung, R., Zwahlen, M., & Zembic, A. (2012). A systematic review of the survival and complication rates of implants upported fixed dental prostheses (FDP s) after a mean observation period of at least 5 years. *Clinical Oral Implants Research*, *23*, 22–38. doi:10.1111/j.1600-0501.2012.02546.x PMID:23062125

Rajput, R., Chouhan, Z., Sindhu, M., Sundararajan, S., & Chouhan, R. R. S. (2016). A Brief Chronological Review of Dental Implant History. *International Dental Journal of Students Research, 4*.

Reddy, K. R., & Thumati, P. (2014). Influence of implant with different dimensions and designs in ideal stress distribution in bone for application in compromised situations: Analysis by three-dimensional finite element method. *Journal of Dental Implants*, *4*(2), 109. doi:10.4103/0974-6781.140848

Saini, M., Singh, Y., Arora, P., Arora, V., & Jain, K. (2015). Implant biomaterials: A comprehensive review. *World Journal of Clinical Cases: WJCC*, *3*(1), 52. doi:10.12998/wjcc.v3.i1.52 PMID:25610850

Vidyasagar, L., & Apse, P. (2004). Dental implant design and biological effects on bone-implant interface. *Stomatologija*, *6*(2), 51–54.

Compilation of References

Abbas, F., Feng, D., Habib, S., Rahman, U., Rasool, A., & Yan, Z. (2018). Short term residential load forecasting: An Improved optimal nonlinear auto regressive (NARX) method with exponential weight decay function. *Electronics (Basel)*, *7*(12), 432. doi:10.3390/electronics7120432

Abiyev, R. H., & Ma'aitah, M. K. S. (2018). Deep Convolutional Neural Networks for Chest Diseases Detection. *Journal of Healthcare Engineering*, 1–11. doi:10.1155/2018/4168538 PMID:30154989

About Chronic Diseases | CDC. (n.d.). Retrieved August 31, 2019, from https://www.cdc.gov/chronicdisease/about/index.htm

Abraham, A. G., Duncan, D. D., Gange, S. J., & West, S. (2009). Computer-aided assessment of diagnostic images for epidemiological research. *BMC Medical Research Methodology*, *9*(1), 74. doi:10.1186/1471-2288-9-74 PMID:19906311

Abuhussein, H., Pagni, G., Rebaudi, A., & Wang, H. L. (2010). The effect of thread pattern upon implant osseointegration. *Clinical Oral Implants Research*, *21*(2), 129–136. doi:10.1111/j.1600-0501.2009.01800.x PMID:19709058

Acharya, U. R., Wong, L. Y., Ng, E. Y. K., & Suri, J. S. (2007). Automatic identification of anterior segment eye abnormality. *IRBM*, *28*(1), 35–41. doi:10.1016/j.rbmret.2007.02.002

Adeloye, A. J., & De Munari, A. (2006). Artificial neural network based generalized storage–yield–reliability models using the Levenberg–Marquardt algorithm. *Journal of Hydrology (Amsterdam)*, *326*(1-4), 215–230. doi:10.1016/j.jhydrol.2005.10.033

Afkham, L., Abdi, F., & Komijan, A. (2012). Evaluation of service quality by using fuzzy MCDM: A case study in Iranian health-care centers. *Management Science Letters*, *2*(1), 291–300. doi:10.5267/j.msl.2011.08.009

Aghazadeh, S. M., Mohammadi, M., & Naderi, B. (2017). Multi objective organ transplant supply chain with effective location and time consideration. *Journal of Industrial and Systems Engineering*, *10*(4), 158–176.

Ahmadvand, S., & Pishvaee, M. S. (2018). An efficient method for kidney allocation problem: A credibility-based fuzzy common weights data envelopment analysis approach. *Health Care Management Science, 21*(4), 587–603. doi:10.100710729-017-9414-6 PMID:28795254

Ahuja, K., Banerjee, R., Nagar, S., Dey, K., & Barbhuiya, F. (2016). Eye center localization and detection using radial mapping. *Proceedings 2016 IEEE International Conference on Image Processing (ICIP)*. DOI:10.1109/ICIP.2016.7532934

Akay, E. Ç. (2018). A New Horizon in Econometrics: Big Data and Machine Learning. *Social Sciences Research Journal, 7*(2), 41–53.

Akdag, H., Kalaycı, T., Karagöz, S., Zülfikar, H., & Giz, D. (2014). The evaluation of hospital service quality by fuzzy MCDM. *Applied Soft Computing, 23*, 239–248. doi:10.1016/j.asoc.2014.06.033

Aktas, A., Cebi, S., & Temiz, I. (2015). A new evaluation model for service quality of health care systems based on AHP and information axiom. *Journal of Intelligent & Fuzzy Systems, 28*(3), 1009–1021. doi:10.3233/IFS-141385

Akyuz, E., & Celik, E. (2015). A fuzzy DEMATEL method to evaluate critical operational hazards during gas freeing process in crude oil tankers. *Journal of Loss Prevention in the Process Industries, 38*, 243–253. doi:10.1016/j.jlp.2015.10.006

Al Shayea, Q., El Refae, G., & Yaseen, S. (2013). Artificial neural networks for medical diagnosis using biomedical dataset. *International Journal of Behavioural & Healthcare Research, 4*(1), 45–63. doi:10.1504/IJBHR.2013.054519

Alashwal, H., El Halaby, M., Crouse, J. J., Abdalla, A., & Moustafa, A. A. (2019). The application of unsupervised clustering methods to Alzheimer's disease. *Frontiers in Computational Neuroscience, 13*(May), 1–9. doi:10.3389/fncom.2019.00031 PMID:31178711

Ali, S. S., Basu, A., & Ware, N. (2018). Quality measurement of Indian commercial hospitals– using a SERVQUAL framework. *Benchmarking: an international journal, 25*(3), 815-837.

Ali, M., & Raza, S. A. (2017). Service quality perception and customer satisfaction in Islamic banks of Pakistan: The modified SERVQUAL model. *Total Quality Management & Business Excellence, 28*(5-6), 559–577. doi:10.1080/14783363.2015.1100517

Almubarak, H. (2018). *Deep Learning and Localized Features Fusion for Medical Image Classification*. Retrieved from http://search.proquest.com/docview/2068551083/

Al-Neyadi, H. S., Abdallah, S., & Malik, M. (2018). Measuring patient's satisfaction of healthcare services in the UAE hospitals: Using SERVQUAL. *International Journal of Healthcare Management, 11*(2), 96–105. doi:10.1080/20479700.2016.1266804

Al-Shayea, Q., & Bahia, I. (2010). Urinary system diseases diagnosis using artificial neural networks. *IJCSNS, 10*(7). Retrieved from https://resolver.1science.com/proquest/?id=f586b4f2b6fce265b0bd04f39031ff86e6e16dfd

Altuntas, S., Dereli, T., & Yilmaz, M. K. (2012). Multi-criteria decision-making methods based weighted SERVQUAL scales to measure perceived service quality in hospitals: A case study from Turkey. *Total Quality Management & Business Excellence, 23*(11-12), 1379–1395. doi:10.1080/14783363.2012.661136

Antonoglou, D., Kastanioti, C., & Niakas, D. (2017). ABC and VED Analysis of Medical Materials of a General Military Hospital in Greece. *Journal of Health Management, 19*(1), 170–179. doi:10.1177/0972063416682643

Anyanwu, K. (2011). Overview and Applications of Artificial Intelligence, (June).

Armstrong, J. S. (n.d.). Long-range forecasting: from crystal ball to computer / J. Scott Armstrong. In *Long-range forecasting : from crystal ball to computer* (2nd ed.). New York: Wiley.

Arora, M., & Gigras, Y. (2018). Importance of Supply Chain Management in Healthcare of Third World Countries. *International Journal of Supply and Operations Management, 5*(1), 101–106.

Arora, R., & Suman, S. (2012). Comparative analysis of classification algorithms on different datasets using WEKA. *International Journal of Computers and Applications, 54*(13).

Artificial intelligence | Definition, Examples, and Applications | Britannica.com. (n.d.). Retrieved August 31, 2019 from https://www.britannica.com/technology/artificial-intelligence/Reasoning

Aygn, O., Gokdemir, O., Bulut, L., Yaprak, S., & Gldal, D. (2016). Evaluation of Primary Health Care Services Which Is Provided To Refugees Within a Public Health Center. *Turkish Journal of Family Medicine & Primary Care, 10*(1), 6. doi:10.5455/tjfmpc.199143

Baba, N. (1989). A new approach for finding the global minimum of error function for neural networks. *Neural Networks, 2*(5), 367–373. doi:10.1016/0893-6080(89)90021-X

Baggi, L., Cappelloni, I., Di Girolamo, M., Maceri, F., & Vairo, G. (2008). The influence of implant diameter and length on stress distribution of osseointegrated implants related to crestal bone geometry: A three-dimensional finite element analysis. *The Journal of Prosthetic Dentistry, 100*(6), 422–431. doi:10.1016/S0022-3913(08)60259-0 PMID:19033026

Bala, V., & Goyal, S. (1998). Learning from Neighbours. *The Review of Economic Studies, 65*(3), 595–621. doi:10.1111/1467-937X.00059

Balin, A., Demirel, H., Celik, E., & Alarcin, F. (2018). A fuzzy DEMATEL model proposal for the cause and effect of the fault occurrıng ın the auxılıary systems of the shıps' maın engıne. *International Journal of Maritime Engineering, 160*(A2), A141–A153. doi:10.3940/rina.ijme.2018.a2.465

Ballinger, B., Hsieh, J., Singh, A., Sohoni, N., Wang, J., & Tison, G. H., … Pletcher, M. J. (2018). Deepheart: Semi-supervised sequence learning for cardiovascular risk prediction. *32nd AAAI Conference on Artificial Intelligence, AAAI 2018*, 2079–2086. AAAI press.

Ban, A. I., & Coroianu, L. (2012). Nearest interval, triangular and trapezoidal approximation of a fuzzy number preserving ambiguity. *International Journal of Approximate Reasoning*, *53*(5), 805–836. doi:10.1016/j.ijar.2012.02.001

Bang, Y. K., & Lee, C. H. (2011). Fuzzy time series prediction using hierarchical clustering algorithms. *Expert Systems with Applications*, *38*(4), 4312–4325. doi:10.1016/j.eswa.2010.09.100

Banihabib, M. E., Ahmadian, A., & Valipour, M. (2018). Hybrid MARMA-NARX model for flow forecasting based on the large-scale climate signals, sea-surface temperatures, and rainfall. *Hydrology Research*, *49*(6), 1788–1803. doi:10.2166/nh.2018.145

Barbato, M., Barclay, G., Potter, J., Yeo, W., & Chung, J. (2017). Correlation Between Observational Scales of Sedation and Comfort and Bispectral Index Scores. *Journal of Pain and Symptom Management*, *54*(2), 186–193. doi:10.1016/j.jpainsymman.2016.12.335 PMID:28063863

Başhan, V., & Demirel, H. (2019). Application of fuzzy DEMATEL technique to assess most common critical operational faults of marine boilers. *Politeknik Dergisi*, *22*(3), 545–555.

Baştürk, A., Badem, H., Caliskan, A., & Yüksel, M. E. (2019). Application of Deep Neural Networks for Disease Diagnosis Through Medical Data Sets. In V. E. Balas, S. S. Roy, D. Sharma, & P. Samui (Eds.), *Handbook of Deep Learning Applications* (pp. 259–292)., doi:10.1007/978-3-030-11479-4_12

Batista, G. E., Prati, R. C., & Monard, M. C. (2004). A study of the behavior of several methods for balancing machine learning training data. ACM SIGKDD explorations newsletter, 6(1), 20-29.

Bays, H. E., Chapman, R. H., & Grandy, S.SHIELD Investigators' Group. (2007). The relationship of body mass index to diabetes mellitus, hypertension, and dyslipidaemia: Comparison of data from two national surveys. *International Journal of Clinical Practice*, *61*(5), 737–747. doi:10.1111/j.1742-1241.2007.01336.x PMID:17493087

Baytas, I. M., Xiao, C., Zhang, X., Wang, F., Jain, A. K., & Zhou, J. (2017). Patient subtyping via time-aware LSTM networks. *Proceedings of the ACM SIGKDD International Conference on Knowledge Discovery and Data Mining, Part F129685*, 65–74. 10.1145/3097983.3097997

Beale, R. (1990). Neural computing: an introduction / R. Beale and T. Jackson. In Neural computing: an introduction. Bristol, UK: Hilger.

Begik, M., Hamurcu, M., & Eren, T. (2017). Stok kontrolde ABC analizi ve analitik ağ süreci yönteminin ısı cihazları firmasında uygulanması. *Kırıkkale Üniversitesi Sosyal Bilimler Dergisi*, *7*(1), 197–216.

Behdioğlu, S., Acar, E., & Burhan, H. A. (2019). Evaluating service quality by fuzzy SERVQUAL: A case study in a physiotherapy and rehabilitation hospital. *Total Quality Management & Business Excellence*, *30*(3-4), 301–319. doi:10.1080/14783363.2017.1302796

Behzadian, M., Otaghsara, S. K., Yazdani, M., & Ignatius, J. (2012). A state-of the-art survey of TOPSIS applications. *Expert Systems with Applications*, *39*(17), 13051–13069. doi:10.1016/j.eswa.2012.05.056

Beliën, J., De Boeck, L., Colpaert, J., Devesse, S., & Van den Bossche, F. (2013). Optimizing the facility location design of organ transplant centers. *Decision Support Systems*, *54*(4), 1568–1579. doi:10.1016/j.dss.2012.05.059

Bennett, K. P., & Demiriz, A. (1998). Semi-Supervised Support Vector Machines. In M. S. Kearns, S. A. Solla, & D. A. Cohn (Eds.), Vol. 11). Advances in Neural Information Processing Systems Cambridge, MA: MIT Press; Retrieved from http://books.nips.cc/papers/files/nips11/0368.pdf

Berglind, J. (2019). Temporal convolutional networks for forecasting of patient volumes in a digital healthcare setting. Degree project in computer science and engineering, Second cycle, Stockholm, Sweden.

Berglundh, T., Persson, L., & Klinge, B. (2002). A systematic review of the incidence of biological and technical complications in implant dentistry reported in prospective longitudinal studies of at least 5 years. *Journal of Clinical Periodontology*, *29*, 197–212.

Bergs, J., Heerinckx, P., & Verelst, S. (2014). Knowing what to expect, forecasting monthly emergency department visits: A time-series analysis. *International Emergency Nursing*, *22*(2), 112–115. doi:10.1016/j.ienj.2013.08.001 PMID:24055373

Bhattacharya, A., Sarkar, B., & Mukherjee, S. K. (2007). Distance-based consensus method for ABC analysis. *International Journal of Production Research*, *45*(15), 3405–3420. doi:10.1080/00207540600847145

Bicudo, P., Reis, J., Deus, A. M., Reis, L., & Vaz, M. F. (2016). Mechanical behaviour of dental implants. *Procedia Structural Integrity*, *1*, 26–33. doi:10.1016/j.prostr.2016.02.005

Bilge, U. (2007). Tıpta Yapay Zeka ve Uzman Sistemler. In *IV* (pp. 113–118). Antalya: Ulusal Tıp Bilişimi Kongresi.

Bishop, C. (2006). *Pattern Recognition and Machine Learning*. Retrieved from https://www.springer.com/gp/book/9780387310732

Boser, B. E., Guyon, I. M., & Vapnik, V. N. (1992). A Training Algorithm for Optimal Margin Classifiers. *Proceedings of the Fifth Annual Workshop on Computational Learning Theory*, 144–152. 10.1145/130385.130401

Bouhentala, M., Mouna G., & Kheireddine, C. (2018). Interval-valued membership function estimation for fuzzy modeling, *Fuzzy Sets and Systems*, Available online July 4, 2018.

Bruni, M. E., Conforti, D., Sicilia, N., & Trotta, S. (2006). A new organ transplantation location–allocation policy: A case study of Italy. *Health Care Management Science*, *9*(2), 125–142. doi:10.100710729-006-7661-z PMID:16895308

Caetano, S. J., Sonpavde, G., & Pond, G. R. (2018). C-statistic: A brief explanation of its construction, interpretation and limitations. *European Journal of Cancer, 90*, 130, 132.

Cakir, O., & Canbolat, M. S. (2008). A web-based decision support system for multi-criteria inventory classification using fuzzy AHP methodology. *Expert Systems with Applications*, *35*(3), 1367–1378. doi:10.1016/j.eswa.2007.08.041

Caliskan, A. (2017). *Derin sinir ağının sınıflandırma başarımının artırılması için yeni bir eğitim stratejisi geliştirilmesi ve biyomedikal veri setleri üzerinde test edilmesi*. Erciyes Üniversitesi Fen Bilimleri Enstitüsü Biyomedikal Mühendisliği Anabilim Dalı, Doktora Tezi.

Caliskan, A., Badem, H., Basturk, A., & Yuksel, M. E. (2017). Diagnosıs of the Parkınson dısease by usıng deep neural network classıfıer. *Istanbul University - Journal of Electrical and Electronics Engineering (Oradea)*, *17*(2), 3311–3318.

Caliskan, A., & Yuksel, M. E. (2017). Classification of coronary artery disease data sets by using a deep neural network. *The EuroBiotech Journal*, *1*(4), 271–277. doi:10.24190/ISSN2564-615X/2017/04.03

Caliskan, A., Yuksel, M. E., Badem, H., & Basturk, A. (2017). A Deep Neural Network Classifier for Decoding Human Brain Activity Based on Magnetoencephalography. *Elektronika ir Elektrotechnika*, *23*(2), 63–67. doi:10.5755/j01.eie.23.2.18002

Carpenter, G. A., & Markuzon, N. (1998). ARTMAP-IC and medical diagnosis: Instance counting and inconsistent cases. *Neural Networks*, *11*(2), 323–336. doi:10.1016/S0893-6080(97)00067-1 PMID:12662841

Caruso, V., & Daniele, P. (2018). A network model for minimizing the total organ transplant costs. *European Journal of Operational Research*, *266*(2), 652–662. doi:10.1016/j.ejor.2017.09.040

Celik, E., & Akyuz, E. (2016). Application of interval type-2 fuzzy sets DEMATEL methods in maritime transportation: the case of ship collision. *International Journal of Maritime Engineering*, *158*(A 4), A359-A371.

Çetin, O., Temurtaş, F., & Gülgönül, Ş. (2015). An application of multilayer neural network on hepatitis disease diagnosis using approximations of sigmoid activation function. *Dicle Medical Journal / Dicle Tip Dergisi*, *42*(2). doi:10.5798/diclemedj.0921.2015.02.0550

Chakravarty, A. (2011). Evaluation of service quality of hospital outpatient department services. *Medical Journal, Armed Forces India*, *67*(3), 221–224. doi:10.1016/S0377-1237(11)60045-2 PMID:27365810

Chanas, S. (2001). On the interval approximation of a fuzzy number. *Fuzzy Sets and Systems*, *122*(2), 353–356. doi:10.1016/S0165-0114(00)00080-4

Chang, D. Y. (1996). Applications of the extent analysis method on fuzzy AHP. *European Journal of Operational Research*, *95*(3), 649–655. doi:10.1016/0377-2217(95)00300-2

Chang, F. J., Chen, P. A., Liu, C. W., Liao, V. H. C., & Liao, C. M. (2013). Regional estimation of groundwater arsenic concentrations through systematical dynamic-neural modeling. *Journal of Hydrology (Amsterdam)*, *499*, 265–274. doi:10.1016/j.jhydrol.2013.07.008

Chang, T. H. (2014). Fuzzy VIKOR method: A case study of the hospital service evaluation in Taiwan. *Information Sciences*, *271*, 196–212. doi:10.1016/j.ins.2014.02.118

Chang, X., & Lilly, J. H. (2004). Evolutionary design of a fuzzy classifier from data. *IEEE Transactions on Systems, Man, and Cybernetics. Part B, Cybernetics*, *34*(4), 1894–1906. doi:10.1109/TSMCB.2004.831160 PMID:15462454

Chaturvedi, T. P. (2009). An overview of the corrosion aspect of dental implants (titanium and its alloys). *Indian Journal of Dental Research*, *20*(1), 91. doi:10.4103/0970-9290.49068 PMID:19336868

Chen, C. H., Hong, T.-P., & Tseng, V. S. (2009). An improved approach to find membership functions and multiple minimum supports in fuzzy data mining. *Expert Systems with Applications*, *36*(6). doi:10.1016/j.eswa.2009.01.067

Cheng, C. H., Cheng, G. V., & Wang, J. W. (2008). Multi-attribute fuzzy time series method based on fuzzy clustering. *Expert Systems with Applications*, *3*(2), 1235–1242. doi:10.1016/j.eswa.2006.12.013

Cheng, Y., Wang, F., Zhang, P., & Hu, J. (2016). Risk prediction with electronic health records: A deep learning approach. *Proceedings 16th SIAM International Conference on Data Mining 2016, SDM 2016*, 432–440. 10.1137/1.9781611974348.49

Chen, J., Huang, H., Tian, S., & Qu, Y. (2009). Feature selection for text classification with Naïve Bayes. *Expert Systems with Applications*, *36*(3 PART 1), 5432–5435. doi:10.1016/j.eswa.2008.06.054

Chen, S. H., Jakeman, A. J., & Norton, J. P. (2008). Artificial Intelligence techniques: An introduction to their use for modelling environmental systems. *Mathematics and Computers in Simulation*, *78*(2–3), 379–400. doi:10.1016/j.matcom.2008.01.028

Che, Z., & Liu, Y. (2017). Deep learning solutions to computational phenotyping in health care. *IEEE International Conference on Data Mining Workshops, ICDMW, 2017-November*, 1100–1109. 10.1109/ICDMW.2017.156

Che, Z., Purushotham, S., Cho, K., Sontag, D., & Liu, Y. (2018). Recurrent Neural Networks for Multivariate Time Series with Missing Values. *Scientific Reports*, *8*(1), 6085. doi:10.103841598-018-24271-9 PMID:29666385

Choi, B. I., & Rhee, F. C. H. (2009). Interval Type-2 fuzzy membership function generation methods for pattern recognition. *Information Sciences*, *179*(13), 2102–2122. doi:10.1016/j.ins.2008.04.009

Choi, E., Bahadori, M. T., Schuetz, A., Stewart, W. F., & Sun, J. (2016). Doctor AI: Predicting Clinical Events via Recurrent Neural Networks. *JMLR Workshop and Conference Proceedings*, *56*, 301–318. Retrieved from http://www.ncbi.nlm.nih.gov/pubmed/28286600 PMID:28286600

Choi, E., Schuetz, A., Stewart, W. F., & Sun, J. (2017). Using recurrent neural network models for early detection of heart failure onset. *Journal of the American Medical Informatics Association*, *24*(2), 361–370. doi:10.1093/jamia/ocw112 PMID:27521897

Chou, H. C., Cheng, C. H., & Chang, J. R. (2007). Extracting drug utilization knowledge using self-organizing map and rough set theory. *Expert Systems with Applications*, *33*(2), 499–508. doi:10.1016/j.eswa.2006.05.020

Chun, H. J., Cheong, S. Y., Han, J. H., Heo, S. J., Chung, J. P., Rhyu, I. C., ... Kim, M. H. (2002). Evaluation of design parameters of osseointegrated dental implants using finite element analysis. *Journal of Oral Rehabilitation*, *29*(6), 565–574. doi:10.1046/j.1365-2842.2002.00891.x PMID:12071926

Çıtak, Ş. (2013). *Bir Elektronik Firmasında Çok Ölçütlü Stok Sınıflandırma*. Yüksek Lisans Tezi, Gazi Üniversitesi, Fen Bilimleri Enstitüsü.

Cohen, M. A., & Ernst, R. (1988). Multi-Item Classification and Generic Inventory Stock Contr. *Production and Inventory Management Journal*, *29*(3), 6.

Cordeau, J.-F., Furini, F., & Ljubić, I. (2019). Benders decomposition for very large-scale partial set covering and maximal covering location problems. *European Journal of Operational Research*, *275*(3), 882–896. doi:10.1016/j.ejor.2018.12.021

Cortes, Corinna, and V. V. (1995). Photonic neural networks and learning machines. *IEEE Expert*, *7*(5), 63–72. doi:10.1109/64.163674

Crowther, P. S., & Cox, R. J. (2005, September). A method for optimal division of data sets for use in neural networks. *Proceedings International Conference on Knowledge-Based and Intelligent Information and Engineering Systems* (pp. 1-7). Berlin, Germany: Springer. 10.1007/11554028_1

Cruz-Roa, A., Basavanhally, A., González, F., Gilmore, H., Feldman, M., & Ganesan, S. … Madabhushi, A. (2014). Automatic detection of invasive ductal carcinoma in whole slide images with convolutional neural networks. In M. N. Gurcan, & A. Madabhushi (Eds.), Medical Imaging 2014: Digital Pathology (Vol. 9041, pp. 1–15). doi:10.1117/12.2043872

Dalli, A. (2003). *Adaptation of the F-measure to cluster-based lexicon quality evaluation*. doi:10.3115/1641396.1641404

Daskin, M. S. (2008). What you should know about location modeling. *Naval Research Logistics*, *55*(4), 283–294. doi:10.1002/nav.20284

de Andrade, C. L., Carvalho, M. A., Bordin, D., da Silva, W. J., Del Bel Cury, A. A., & Sotto-Maior, B. S. (2017). Biomechanical Behavior of the Dental Implant Macrodesign. *International Journal of Oral & Maxillofacial Implants*, *32*(2).

Deepa, M., & Revathy, P. (2012). Validation of Document Clustering based on Purity and Entropy measures. *International Journal of Advanced Research in Computer and Communication Engineering*, *1*(3), 147–152.

Demirer, Ö., & Bülbül, H. (2014). Kamu ve özel hastanelerde hizmet kalitesi, hasta tatmini ve tercihi arasındaki ilişki: Karşılaştırmalı bir analiz. *Amme Idaresi Dergisi*, *47*(2), 95–119.

Demir, H., & Gümüşoğlu, Ş. (2003). *Üretim Yönetimi*. İstanbul, Turkey: Beta Basım Yayım Dağıtım.

Demírhan, A., Alper Kilic, Y., Güler, İ., Üniversitesi Teknoloji Fakültesi, G., & Mühendisliği Bölümü, B. (2010). *Tıpta Yapay Zeka Uygulamaları* Artificial Intelligence Applications in Medicine. Yoğun Bakım Dergisi*, *9*.

Demir, P., Gul, M., & Guneri, A. F. (2018). Evaluating occupational health and safety service quality by SERVQUAL: A field survey study. *Total Quality Management & Business Excellence*, 1–18. doi:10.1080/14783363.2018.1433029

Deo, S. S., Gore, S. D., Deobagkar, D. N., & Deobagkar, D. D. (2006). Study of inheritance of diabetes mellitus in Western Indian population by pedigree analysis. *JAPI*, *54*, 441–443. PMID:16909690

Devi, R. D. H., Bai, A., & Nagarajan, N. (2019). A Novel Hybrid Approach for Diagnosing Diabetes Mellitus using Farthest First and Support Vector Machine Algorithms. Obesity Medicine, 100152.

Di Piazza, A., Di Piazza, M. C., & Vitale, G. (2016). Solar and wind forecasting by NARX neural networks. *Renewable Energy and Environmental Sustainability*, *1*, 39. doi:10.1051/rees/2016047

Ding, S., Zhu, Z., & Zhang, X. (2017). An overview on semi-supervised support vector machine. *Neural Computing & Applications*, *28*(5), 969–978. doi:10.100700521-015-2113-7

Draszawka, K., & Szymański, J. (2011). External validation measures for nested clustering of text documents. *Studies in Computational Intelligence*, *369*, 207, 225.

Du, K.-L. (2014). Neural Networks and Statistical Learning [electronic resource] / In K.-L. Du, & M. N. S. Swamy (Eds.), Neural Networks and Statistical Learning (1st ed. 20). London, UK: Springer London.

Duan, P., Wang, T., Cui, M., Sang, H., & Sun, Q. (2019). Multi-person pose estimation based on a deep convolutional neural network. *Journal of Visual Communication and Image Representation*, *62*, 245, 252.

Dwivedi, S., & Kothiyal, P. (2012). Inventory management: A tool of identifying items that need greater attention for control. *The Pharma Innovation*, *1*(7, Part A), 125.

Elkady, S. K., & Abdelsalam, H. M. (2016). A modified multi-objective particle swarm optimisation algorithm for healthcare facility planning. *International Journal of Business and Systems Research*, *10*(1), 1–22. doi:10.1504/IJBSR.2016.073685

Elkady, S. K., & Abdelsalam, H. M. (2016a). A modified particle swarm optimization algorithm for solving capacitated maximal covering location problem in healthcare systems. *Intelligent Systems Reference Library*, *96*, 117–133. doi:10.1007/978-3-319-21212-8_5

Ertuğrul, İ. (2013). Stok Kontrolde ABC Yöntemi ve AHP Analizlerinin İplik İşletmesine Uygulanması. *Uluslararası Alanya İşletme Fakültesi Dergisi*, *5*(1), 41–52.

Esteva, A., Kuprel, B., Novoa, R. A., Ko, J., Swetter, S. M., Blau, H. M., & Thrun, S. (2017). Dermatologist-level classification of skin cancer with deep neural networks. *Nature*, *542*(7639), 115–118. doi:10.1038/nature21056 PMID:28117445

Faegh, S., & Müftü, S. (2010). Load transfer along the bone–dental implant interface. *Journal of Biomechanics*, *43*(9), 1761–1770. doi:10.1016/j.jbiomech.2010.02.017 PMID:20202639

Fan, R.-E., Chang, K.-W., Hsieh, C.-J., Wang, X.-R., & Lin, C.-J. (2008). LIBLINEAR: A Library for Large Linear Classification. *Journal of Machine Learning Research*, *9*(Aug), 1871–1874.

Faraway, J. J. (2016). Extending the linear model with R : generalized linear, mixed effects and nonparametric regression models / Julian J. Faraway, University of Bath, UK. In *Extending the linear model with R : generalized linear, mixed effects and nonparametric regression models (2nd ed.)*. Boca Raton, FL: CRC Press. doi:10.1201/b21296

Fawcett, T. (2006). An introduction to ROC analysis. *Pattern Recognition Letters*, *27*(8), 861, 874.

Fekihal, M. A., & Yousif, J. H. (2012). Self-Organizing Map Approach for Identifying Mental Disorders. *International Journal of Computer Applications*, *45*(7), 25, 30. Retrieved from https://resolver.1science.com/proquest/?id=9d8b94ada26ae94ece6c6ec6524c845f5e289ee5

Feng, Y., Min, X., Chen, N., Chen, H., Xie, X., Wang, H., & Chen, T. (2017). Patient outcome prediction via convolutional neural networks based on multi-granularity medical concept embedding. *Proceedings - 2017 IEEE International Conference on Bioinformatics and Biomedicine, BIBM 2017, 2017-January*, 770–777. 10.1109/BIBM.2017.8217753

Ferman, A. M. (2008). Automatic detection of red-eye artifacts in digital color photos. *Proceedings 2008 15th IEEE International Conference on Image Processing*. DOI:10.1109/icip.2008.4711830

Fitriana, I., Satria, R. G. D., & Setiawan, D. C. B. (2018). Medicine Inventory Management by ABC-VED Analysis in the Pharmacy Store of Veterinary Hospital, Yogyakarta, Indonesia. *Asian Journal of Animal and Veterinary Advances*, *13*, 85–90. doi:10.3923/ajava.2018.85.90

Flores, B. E., & Clay Whybark, D. J. I. J. O. O. (1986). Multiple criteria ABC analysis. *International Journal of Operations & Production Management*, *6*(3), 38–46. doi:10.1108/eb054765

Fo, A. R. A. V., & Mota, I. S. (2012). Optimization models in the location of healthcare facilities: A real case in Brazil. *Journal of Applied Operational Research*, *4*(1), 37–50.

Foresee, F. D., & Hagan, M. T. 1997: Gauss-Newton approximation to Bayesian learning. *Proceedings IEEE International Conference on Neural Networks, 3,* 1930-1935. 10.1109/ICNN.1997.614194

Fukunaga, K., & Hayes, R. R. (1989). The Reduced Parzen Classifier. *IEEE Transactions on Pattern Analysis and Machine Intelligence*, *11*(4), 423–425. doi:10.1109/34.19040

Fu, Y., Lai, K. K., Miao, Y., & Leung, J. W. (2016). A distance-based decision-making method to improve multiple criteria ABC inventory classification. *International Transactions in Operational Research*, *23*(5), 969–978. doi:10.1111/itor.12193

George, A., Khalil, A., & Hassan, N. (2015). Comparison between cylinder and tapered implants in delayed immediate placement. *Alexandria Dental Journal*, *40*(2), 221–228. doi:10.21608/adjalexu.2015.59156

Ghane, M., & Tavakkoli-Moghaddam, R. (2018). A stochastic optimization approach to a location-allocation problem of organ transplant centers. *Journal of Optimization in Industrial Engineering*, *11*(1), 103–111.

Ghanvatkar, S., & Rajan, V. (2019). Deep recurrent neural networks for mortality prediction in intensive care using clinical time series at multiple resolutions. *Proceedings of ICIS*. Munich, Germany. Academic Press.

Ghazavi, S. N., & Liao, T. W. (2008). Medical data mining by fuzzy modeling with selected features. *Artificial Intelligence in Medicine*, *43*(3), 195–206. doi:10.1016/j.artmed.2008.04.004 PMID:18534831

Gil, D., Johnsson, M., Garcia Chamizo, J. M., Paya, A. S., & Fernandez, D. R. (2009). Application of artificial neural networks in the diagnosis of urological dysfunctions. *Expert Systems with Applications*, *36*(3), 5754–5760. doi:10.1016/j.eswa.2008.06.065

Gil, F. J., Herrero-Climent, M., Lázaro, P., & Rios, J. V. (2014). Implant–abutment connections: Influence of the design on the microgap and their fatigue and fracture behavior of dental implants. *Journal of Materials Science. Materials in Medicine*, *25*(7), 1825–1830. doi:10.100710856-014-5211-7 PMID:24719176

GODT. (2019). Global Observatory on Donation and Transplantation. Retrieved from http://www.transplant-observatory.org/data-charts-and-tables/chart/, Access date: 22.10.2019.

Goldstein, B. A., Navar, A. M., & Carter, R. E. (2016). Moving beyond regression techniques in cardiovascular risk prediction: Applying machine learning to address analytic challenges. *European Heart Journal*, *38*(23). doi:10.1093/eurheartj/ehw302 PMID:27436868

Golmohammadi, D. (2016). Predicting hospital admissions to reduce emergency department boarding. *International Journal of Production Economics*, *182*, 535–544. doi:10.1016/j.ijpe.2016.09.020

Gonçalves, L. B., Vellasco, M. M. B. R., Pacheco, M. A. C., & de Souza, F. J. (2006). Inverted hierarchical neuro-fuzzy BSP system: A novel neuro-fuzzy model for pattern classification and rule extraction in databases. *IEEE Transactions on Systems, Man and Cybernetics. Part C, Applications and Reviews*, *36*(2), 236–248. doi:10.1109/TSMCC.2004.843220

Goodfellow, I., Bengio, Y., & Courville, A. (2016). Deep learning. MIT press. Retrieved from MIT Press website: https://books.google.com.mx/books?hl=en&lr=&id=omivDQAAQBAJ&oi=fnd&pg=PR5&dq=deep+learning+ian+goodfellow&ots=MMT-hrrBQQ&sig=Ue-yavSqPS_vg2AQFhGKKaBY-5U&redir_esc=y#v=onepage&q=deep learning ian goodfellow&f=false

Graves, A. (2012). Supervised sequence labelling. In Supervised sequence labelling with recurrent neural networks (pp. 5-13). Berlin, Germany: Springer.

Greenfield, S., & Chiclana, F. (2018). Type-Reduced Set structure and the truncated type-2 fuzzy set. *Fuzzy Sets and Systems*, *352*, 119–141. doi:10.1016/j.fss.2018.02.012

Gridach, M. (2017). Character-level neural network for biomedical named entity recognition. *Journal of Biomedical Informatics, 70*, 85, 91.

Guan, H., van Staden, R., Loo, Y. C., Johnson, N., Ivanovski, S., & Meredith, N. (2009). Influence of bone and dental implant parameters on stress distri-bution in the mandible: A finite element study. *Int J Oral Maxillofac Implants*, *24*, 866–876. PMID:19865627

Gul, M., & Guneri, A. F. (2012). *A computer sımulatıon model to reduce patıent length of stay and to ımprove resource utılızatıon rate ın an emergency department servıce system.* 12.

Gul, M., & Celik, E. (2018). An exhaustive review and analysis on applications of statistical forecasting in hospital emergency departments. *Health Systems (Basingstoke, England)*, 1–22. doi:10.1080/20476965.2018.1547348

Gul, M., Celik, E., Aydin, N., Gumus, A. T., & Guneri, A. F. (2016). A state-of-the-art literature review of VIKOR and its fuzzy extensions on applications. *Applied Soft Computing*, *46*, 60–89. doi:10.1016/j.asoc.2016.04.040

Gül, M., & Güneri, A. F. (2015a). Forecastıng patıent length of stay ın an emergency department by artıfıcıal neural networks. *Journal of Aeronautics and Space Technologies*, *8*(2), 43–48.

Gül, M., & Güneri, A. F. (2015b). A comprehensive review of emergency department simulation applications for normal and disaster conditions. *Computers & Industrial Engineering*, *83*, 327–344. doi:10.1016/j.cie.2015.02.018

Gul, M., & Guneri, A. F. (2016). Planning the future of emergency departments: Forecasting ED patient arrivals by using regression and neural network models. *International Journal of Industrial Engineering*, *23*(2), 137–154.

Gul, M., Guneri, A. F., & Derin, B. (2014). Evaluation of service quality criteria for a private medical center by using SERVQUAL and DEMATEL methods. *Sigma*, *32*, 240–253.

Gülmez, H. (2013). Factors that Affecting Quality of Life of Employees. *Turkish Journal of Family Medicine & Primary Care*, *7*(4), 1. doi:10.5455/tjfmpc.38192

Gupta, S., & Sunil, K. (2000). *Hospital stores management: An integrated approach* (pp. 14–1). India: Jaypee. doi:10.5005/jp/books/10360

Guvenir, H. A., & Erel, E. (1998). Multicriteria inventory classification using a genetic algorithm. *European Journal of Operational Research, 105*(1), 29–37. doi:10.1016/S0377-2217(97)00039-8

Guzman, S. M., Paz, J. O., & Tagert, M. L. M. (2017). The use of NARX neural networks to forecast daily groundwater levels. *Water Resources Management, 31*(5), 1591–1603. doi:10.100711269-017-1598-5

Hadavandi, E., Shavandi, H., Ghanbari, A., & Abbasian-Naghneh, S. (2012). Developing a hybrid artificial intelligence model for outpatient visits forecasting in hospitals. *Applied Soft Computing, 12*(2), 700–711. doi:10.1016/j.asoc.2011.09.018

Hadi-Vencheh, A. (2010). An improvement to multiple criteria ABC inventory classification. *European Journal of Operational Research, 201*(3), 962–965. doi:10.1016/j.ejor.2009.04.013

Handayani, P. W., Hidayanto, A. N., Sandhyaduhita, P. I., & Ayuningtyas, D. (2015). Strategic hospital services quality analysis in Indonesia. *Expert Systems with Applications, 42*(6), 3067–3078. doi:10.1016/j.eswa.2014.11.065

Hanif, A., Qureshi, S., Sheikh, Z., & Rashid, H. (2017). Complications in implant dentistry. *European Journal of Dentistry, 11*(1), 135–140. doi:10.4103/ejd.ejd_340_16 PMID:28435381

Han, J., Kamber, M., & Pei, J. (2011). *Data mining: concepts and techniques. The Morgan Kaufmann series of data management systems* (pp. 230–240). Elsevier.

Han, J., Pei, J., & Kamber, M. (2011). *Data mining: concepts and techniques*. Elsevier.

Haszlinna Mustaffa, N., & Potter, A. (2009). Healthcare supply chain management in Malaysia: A case study. *Supply Chain Management, 14*(3), 234–243. doi:10.1108/13598540910954575

Hatefi, S. M., Torabi, S. A., & Bagheri, P. (2014). Multi-criteria ABC inventory classification with mixed quantitative and qualitative criteria. *International Journal of Production Research, 52*(3), 776–786. doi:10.1080/00207543.2013.838328

Heckerman, D., Geiger, D., & Chickering, D. M. (1995). Learning Bayesian Networks: The Combination of Knowledge and Statistical Data. *Machine Learning, 20*(3), 197–243. doi:10.1007/BF00994016

Hertzum, M. (2017). Forecasting Hourly Patient Visits in the Emergency Department to Counteract Crowding. *The Ergonomics Open Journal, 10*(1).

Hertzum. M. (2017). Forecasting Hourly Patient Visits in the Emergency Department to Counteract Crowding. *The Ergonomics Open Journal, 10*(1).

He, W., Williard, N., Chen, C., & Pecht, M. (2014). State of charge estimation for Li-ion batteries using neural network modeling and unscented Kalman filter-based error cancellation. *International Journal of Electrical Power & Energy Systems, 62*, 783–791. doi:10.1016/j.ijepes.2014.04.059

Holm, L. B., & Dahl, F. A. (2011). Using soft systems methodology as a precursor for an emergency department simulation model. *OR insight, 24*(3), 168-189.

Holmgren, E. P., Seckinger, R. J., Kilgren, L. M., & Mante, F. (1998). Evaluating parameters of osseointegrated dental implants using finite element analysis—A two-dimensional comparative study examining the effects of implant diameter, implant shape, and load direction. *The Journal of Oral Implantology*, *24*(2), 80–88. doi:10.1563/1548-1336(1998)024<0080:EPOODI>2.3.CO;2 PMID:9835834

Hoot, N. R., & Aronsky, D. (2008). Systematic review of emergency department crowding: Causes, effects, and solutions. *Annals of Emergency Medicine*, *52*(2), 126–136. doi:10.1016/j.annemergmed.2008.03.014 PMID:18433933

Howard, A. G., Zhu, M., Chen, B., Kalenichenko, D., Wang, W., Weyand, T., … Adam, H. (2017). *MobileNets: Efficient Convolutional Neural Networks for Mobile Vision Applications.*

Hubicka, K., Marcjasz, G., & Weron, R. (2018). A note on averaging day-ahead electricity price forecasts across calibration windows. *IEEE Transactions on Sustainable Energy*, *10*(1), 321–323. doi:10.1109/TSTE.2018.2869557

Hu, Y. H., Tai, C. T., Chen, S. C. C., Lee, H. W., & Sung, S. F. (2017). Predicting return visits to the emergency department for pediatric patients: Applying supervised learning techniques to the Taiwan National Health Insurance Research Database. *Computer Methods and Programs in Biomedicine*, *144*, 105–112. doi:10.1016/j.cmpb.2017.03.022 PMID:28494994

Infoclimat, France. Retrieved from (http://www.infoclimat.fr) [Access in 30.05.2019]

IRODaT. (2018). International Registry in Organ Donation and Transplantation. Retrieved from http://www.irodat.org/img/database/pdf/IRODaT%20Newsletter%202017.pdf, Access date: 22.10.2019.

Isa, N. A. M., & Mamat, W. M. F. W. (2011). Clustered-hybrid multilayer perceptron network for pattern recognition application. *Applied Soft Computing*, *11*(1), 1457–1466. doi:10.1016/j.asoc.2010.04.017

Jain, A. K., Mao, J., & Mohiuddin, K. M. (1996). Artificial neural networks: A tutorial. *Computer*, *29*(3), 31–44. doi:10.1109/2.485891

Jauregi Unanue, I., Zare Borzeshi, E., & Piccardi, M. (2017). Recurrent neural networks with specialized word embeddings for health-domain named-entity recognition. *Journal of Biomedical Informatics*, *76*, 102–109. doi:10.1016/j.jbi.2017.11.007 PMID:29146561

Javed, F., & Romanos, G. E. (2010). The role of primary stability for successful immediate loading of dental implants. A literature review. *Journal of Dentistry*, *38*(8), 612–620. doi:10.1016/j.jdent.2010.05.013 PMID:20546821

Jha, R. K., Sahay, B. S., Chattopadhyay, M., & Gajpal, Y. (2018). A visual approach to enhance coordination among diagnostic units using self-organizing map. *Decision (Washington, D.C.)*, *45*(1), 27–41. doi:10.100740622-017-0170-8

Ji, S., Xu, W., Yang, M., & Yu, K. (2013). 3D Convolutional Neural Networks for Human Action Recognition. *IEEE Transactions on Pattern Analysis and Machine Intelligence*, *35*(1), 221, 231.

Ji, F., Zhang, C., & Chen, X. (2018, March). Structure Optimization of Porous Dental Implant Based on 3D Printing. *Proceedings IOP Conference Series: Materials Science and Engineering*, 324, 1, p. 012060. IOP Publishing.

Jihad, A. S., & Tahiri, M. (2018). Forecasting the heating and cooling load of residential buildings by using a learning algorithm "gradient descent", Morocco. *Case Studies in Thermal Engineering*, *12*, 85–93. doi:10.1016/j.csite.2018.03.006

Jilani, T., Housley, G., Figueredo, G., Tang, P. S., Hatton, J., & Shaw, D. (2019). Short- and Long-Term Predictions of Hospital Emergency Department Attendances. *International Journal of Medical Informatics*, *129*, 167–174. doi:10.1016/j.ijmedinf.2019.05.011 PMID:31445251

Johnson, D. R., & Creech, J. C. (1983). Ordinal measures in multiple indicator models: A simulation study of categorization error. *American Sociological Review*, *48*(3), 398–407. doi:10.2307/2095231

Jones, S. S., Evans, R. S., Allen, T. L., Thomas, A., Haug, P. J., Welch, S. J., & Snow, G. L. (2009). A multivariate time series approach to modeling and forecasting demand in the emergency department. *Journal of Biomedical Informatics*, *42*(1), 123–139. doi:10.1016/j.jbi.2008.05.003 PMID:18571990

Kabir, G., & Sumi, R. S. (2014). Power substation location selection using fuzzy analytic hierarchy process and PROMETHEE: A case study from Bangladesh. *Energy*, *72*, 717–730. doi:10.1016/j.energy.2014.05.098

Kahramanli, H., & Allahverdi, N. (2008). Design of a hybrid system for the diabetes and heart diseases. *Expert Systems with Applications*, *35*(1-2), 82–89. doi:10.1016/j.eswa.2007.06.004

Kamnitsas, K., Ledig, C., Newcombe, V. F. J., Simpson, J. P., Kane, A. D., Menon, D. K., ... Glocker, B. (2017). Efficient multi-scale 3D CNN with fully connected CRF for accurate brain lesion segmentation. *Medical Image Analysis*, *36*, 61–78. doi:10.1016/j.media.2016.10.004 PMID:27865153

Kannadasan, K., Edla, D. R., & Kuppili, V. (2018). *Type 2 diabetes data classification using stacked autoencoders in deep neural networks*. Clinical Epidemiology and Global Health.

Kannan, R., & Vasanthi, V. (2019). Machine Learning Algorithms with ROC Curve for Predicting and Diagnosing the Heart Disease. In Springer Briefs in Applied Sciences and Technology (pp. 63–72). doi:10.1007/978-981-13-0059-2_8

Kar, S., & Majumder, D. (2017). A mathematical theory of shape and neuro-fuzzy methodology-based diagnostic analysis: a comparative study on early detection and treatment planning of brain cancer. *International Journal of Clinical Oncology, 22*(4), 667, 681.

Karan, O., Bayraktar, C., Gümüşkaya, H., & Karlık, B. (2012). Diagnosing diabetes using neural networks on small mobile devices. *Expert Systems With Applications, 39*(1), 54, 60.

Karl, M., & Kelly, J. R. (2009). Influence of loading frequency on implant failure under cyclic fatigue conditions. *Dental Materials*, *25*(11), 1426–1432. doi:10.1016/j.dental.2009.06.015 PMID:19643468

Kaufmann, M., Meier, A., & Stoffel, K. (2015). IFC-Filter: Membership function generation for inductive fuzzy classification. *Expert Systems with Applications*, *42*(21), 8369–8379. doi:10.1016/j.eswa.2015.06.034

Kayapınar, S., & Erginel, N. (2017). Designing the airport service with fuzzy QFD based on SERVQUAL integrated with a fuzzy multi-objective decision model. *Total Quality Management & Business Excellence*, 1–20.

Khaldi, R., El Afia, A., & Chiheb, R. (2019). Forecasting of weekly patient visits to emergency department: Real case study. *Procedia Computer Science*, *148*, 532–541. doi:10.1016/j.procs.2019.01.026

Khan, A. A., Akram, M. U., Tariq, A., Tahir, F., & Wazir, K. (2017). Automated Computer-Aided Detection of Cataract. Advances in Intelligent Systems and Computing, 340–349. Doi:10.1007/978-3-319-60834-1_34

Kilic, A., Aygün S., Keskin, G. A., & Baynal, K. (2014). Çok kriterli ABC analizi problemine farklı birbakış açısı: bulanık analitik hiyerarşi prosesi-ideal çözüme yakınlığa göre tercih sıralama tekniği. *Pamukkale üniversitesi mühensilik bilimleri dergisi*, 20(5), 179-188.

Kim, Y. (2014). *Convolutional Neural Networks for Sentence Classification*. Retrieved from https://arxiv.org/abs/1408.5882

Kim, J. W., Baek, S. H., Kim, T. W., & Chang, Y. I. (2008). Comparison of stability between cylindrical and conical type mini-implants: Mechanical and histologic properties. *The Angle Orthodontist*, *78*(4), 692–698. doi:10.2319/0003-3219(2008)078[0692:COSBCA]2.0.CO;2 PMID:18302470

Kingma, D. P., & Ba, J. (2014). Adam: A method for stochastic optimization. *Proceedings International Conference on Learning Representations* (pp. 1-15). Academic Press.

Kobu, B. (2017). *Üretim yönetimi*. İstanbul, Turkey: Beta Basım.

Koc, S. (2014). Forensic Medicine Related Physician Liability and Malpractice. *Toraks Cerrahisi Bulteni*, *5*(1), 14–22. doi:10.5152/tcb.2014.002

Koizumi, N., Ganesan, R., Gentili, M., Chen, C. H., Waters, N., & Das Gupta, D. (2013). Redesigning organ allocation boundaries for liver transplantation in the United States. *Proceedings of the International Conference On Health Care Systems Engineering* (pp. 15–27).

Kong, N., Schaefer, A. J., Hunsaker, B., & Roberts, M. S. (2010). Maximizing the efficiency of the US liver allocation system through region design. *Management Science*, *56*(12), 2111–2122. doi:10.1287/mnsc.1100.1249

Kubler, S., Robert, J., Derigent, W., Voisin, A., & Le Traon, Y. (2016). A state-of the-art survey & testbed of fuzzy AHP (FAHP) applications. *Expert Systems with Applications*, *65*, 398–422. doi:10.1016/j.eswa.2016.08.064

Kumar, S., Pathak, S., & Kumar, B. (2019). Automated Detection of Eye Related Diseases Using Digital Image Processing. In Handbook of Multimedia Information Security: Techniques and Applications, 513–544. Doi:10.1007/978-3-030-15887-3_25

Kumar, S., & Chakravarty, A. (2015). ABC–VED analysis of expendable medical stores at a tertiary care hospital. *Medical Journal, Armed Forces India, 71*(1), 24–27. doi:10.1016/j.mjafi.2014.07.002 PMID:25609859

Kwon, I. W. G., Kim, S. H., & Martin, D. G. (2016). Healthcare supply chain management; strategic areas for quality and financial improvement. *Technological Forecasting and Social Change, 113*, 422–428. doi:10.1016/j.techfore.2016.07.014

Ladhari, T., Babai, M. Z., & Lajili, I. (2016). Multi-criteria inventory classification: New consensual procedures. *IMA Journal of Management Mathematics, 27*(2), 335–351. doi:10.1093/imaman/dpv003

Lakhani, P., & Sundaram, B. (2017). Deep learning at chest radiography: Automated classification of pulmonary tuberculosis by using convolutional neural networks. *Radiology, 284*(2), 574–582. doi:10.1148/radiol.2017162326 PMID:28436741

Lawrence, S., Giles, C. L., Tsoi, A. C., & Back, A. D. (1997). Face recognition: A convolutional neural-network approach. *IEEE Transactions on Neural Networks, 8*(1), 98, 113. doi:10.1109/72.554195 PMID:18255614

LeCun, Y., Bengio, Y., & Hinton, G. (2015). Deep Learning. *Nature, 521*(7553), 436–444. doi:10.1038/nature14539 PMID:26017442

Lee, H., Delene, L. M., Bunda, M. A., & Kim, C. (2000). Methods of measuring health-care service quality. *Journal of Business Research, 48*(3), 233–246. doi:10.1016/S0148-2963(98)00089-7

Lee, J. H., Frias, V., Lee, K. W., & Wright, R. F. (2005). Effect of implant size and shape on implant success rates: A literature review. *The Journal of Prosthetic Dentistry, 94*(4), 377–381. doi:10.1016/j.prosdent.2005.04.018 PMID:16198176

Leontaritis, I., & Billings, S. (1985a). Input–output parametric models for non-linear systems—Part I:deterministicnon-linearsystems. *International Journal of Control, 41*(2), 303–328. doi:10.1080/0020718508961129

Levandowsky, M., & Winter, D. (1971). Distance between sets [5]. *Nature, 234*(5323), 34,35.

Lewis, C. D. (1982). *Industrial and business forecasting methods: A practical guide to exponential smoothing and curve fitting*. Butterworth-Heinemann.

Li, J.-S., Tian, Y., Liu, Y.-F., Shu, T., & Liang, M.-H. (2013). Applying a BP Neural Network Model to Predict the Length of Hospital Stay. In G. Huang, X. Liu, J. He, F. Klawonn, & G. Yao (Eds.), Health Information Science (pp. 18–29). Berlin, Germany: Springer. doi:10.1007/978-3-642-37899-7_2

Liao, T. W. (2017). A Procedure for the generation of type-2 membership functions from data. *Applied Soft Computing*, *52*, 925–936. doi:10.1016/j.asoc.2016.09.034

Liaw, A., & Wiener, M. (2002). *Classification and Regression by RandomForest*. Retrieved from https://www.researchgate.net/publication/228451484

Li, D. C., Liu, C. W., & Hu, S. C. (2011). A fuzzy-based data transformation for feature extraction to increase classification performance with small medical data sets. *Artificial Intelligence in Medicine*, *52*(1), 45–52. doi:10.1016/j.artmed.2011.02.001 PMID:21493051

Likas, A., Vlassis, N., & Verbeek, J. (2003). The global k-means clustering algorithm. *Pattern Recognition*, *36*(2), 451–461. doi:10.1016/S0031-3203(02)00060-2

Lin, Q. L., Liu, L., Liu, H. C., & Wang, D. J. (2013). Integrating hierarchical balanced scorecard with fuzzy linguistic for evaluating operating room performance in hospitals. *Expert Systems with Applications*, *40*(6), 1917–1924. doi:10.1016/j.eswa.2012.10.007

Lin, T. N., Giles, C. L., Horne, B. G., & Kung, S. Y. (1997). A delay damage model selection algorithm for NARX neural networks. *IEEE Transactions on Signal Processing*, *45*(11), 2719–2730. doi:10.1109/78.650098

Liou, T. S., & Wang, M. J. J. (1992). Ranking fuzzy numbers with integral value. *Fuzzy Sets and Systems*, *50*(3), 247–255. doi:10.1016/0165-0114(92)90223-Q

Lipton, Z. C., Berkowitz, J., & Elkan, C. (2015). *A Critical Review of Recurrent Neural Networks for Sequence Learning*. Academic Press.

Lipton, Z. C., Kale, D. C., & Wetzel, R. (2016). *Modeling Missing Data in Clinical Time Series with RNNs*. Academic Press.

Lipton, Z. C., Kale, D. C., Elkan, C., & Wetzel, R. (2017). Learning to Diagnose with LSTM Recurrent *Neural Networks*. Academic Press.

Lipu, M. H., Hussain, A., Saad, M. H. M., Ayob, A., & Hannan, M. A. (2018, April). Improved recurrent NARX neural network model for state of charge estimation of lithium-ion battery using pso algorithm. *Proceedings 2018 IEEE Symposium on Computer Applications & Industrial Electronics (ISCAIE)* (pp. 354-359). IEEE. 10.1109/ISCAIE.2018.8405498

Liu, C., Sun, H., Du, N., Tan, S., Fei, H., & Fan, W. … Zhang, C. (2017). Augmented LSTM framework to construct medical self-diagnosis android. *Proceedings - IEEE International Conference on Data Mining, ICDM*, 251–260. 10.1109/ICDM.2016.157

Liu, A., Guo, X., Liu, T., Zhang, Y., Tsai, S. B., Zhu, Q., & Hsu, C. F. (2019). A GRA-Based Method for Evaluating Medical Service Quality. *IEEE Access: Practical Innovations, Open Solutions*, *7*, 34252–34264. doi:10.1109/ACCESS.2019.2903684

Liu, C. L., Sako, H., & Fujisawa, H. (2004). Discriminative learning quadratic discriminant function for handwriting recognition. *IEEE Transactions on Neural Networks*, *15*(2), 430–444. doi:10.1109/TNN.2004.824263 PMID:15384535

Liu, S., Tang, B., Chen, Q., & Wang, X. (2016). Drug-Drug Interaction Extraction via Convolutional Neural Networks. *Computational and Mathematical Methods in Medicine, 2016*, 1–8. doi:10.1155/2016/6918381 PMID:26941831

Liu, Y. H., Qiu, D. J., Jia, L., Tan, J. T., Kang, J. M., Xie, T., & Xu, H. M. (2019). Depth of anesthesia measured by bispectral index and postoperative mortality: A meta-analysis of observational studies. *Journal of Clinical Anesthesia*, *56*, 119–125. doi:10.1016/j.jclinane.2019.01.046 PMID:30771713

Lloyd, G. R., Wongravee, K., Silwood, C. J. L., Grootveld, M., & Brereton, R. G. (2009). Self Organising Maps for variable selection: Application to human saliva analysed by nuclear magnetic resonance spectroscopy to investigate the effect of an oral healthcare product. *Chemometrics and Intelligent Laboratory Systems*, *98*(2), 149–161. doi:10.1016/j.chemolab.2009.06.002

Lolli, F., Ishizaka, A., & Gamberini, R. (2014). New AHP-based approaches for multi-criteria inventory classification. *International Journal of Production Economics*, *156*, 62–74. doi:10.1016/j.ijpe.2014.05.015

Luo, H., Yang, Y., Tong, B., Wu, F., & Fan, B. (2018). Traffic Sign Recognition Using a Multi-Task Convolutional Neural Network. *IEEE Transactions on Intelligent Transportation Systems, 19*(4), 1100,1111.

Lupo, T. (2013). A fuzzy ServQual based method for reliable measurements of education quality in Italian higher education area. *Expert Systems with Applications*, *40*(17), 7096–7110. doi:10.1016/j.eswa.2013.06.045

Lupo, T. (2016). A fuzzy framework to evaluate service quality in the healthcare industry: An empirical case of public hospital service evaluation in Sicily. *Applied Soft Computing*, *40*, 468–478. doi:10.1016/j.asoc.2015.12.010

Luukka, P. (2011). Feature selection using fuzzy entropy measures with similarity classifier. *Expert Systems with Applications*, *38*(4), 4600–4607. doi:10.1016/j.eswa.2010.09.133

Luukka, P., & Leppälampi, T. (2006). Similarity classifier with generalized mean applied to medical data. *Computers in Biology and Medicine*, *36*(9), 1026–1040. doi:10.1016/j.compbiomed.2005.05.008 PMID:16159657

MacKay, D. J. (1992). A practical Bayesian framework for backpropagation networks. *Neural Computation*, *4*(3), 448–472. doi:10.1162/neco.1992.4.3.448

Maclin, R., & Opitz, D. (1997). *An Empirical Evaluation of Bagging and Boosting Advice Refinement in Knowledge-Based SVMs View project An Empirical Evaluation of Bagging and Boosting*. AAAI Press. Retrieved from https://www.researchgate.net/publication/2262068

Ma, F., Chitta, R., Zhou, J., You, Q., Sun, T., & Gao, J. (2017). Dipole: Diagnosis prediction in healthcare via attention-based bidirectional recurrent neural networks. *Proceedings of the ACM SIGKDD International Conference on Knowledge Discovery and Data Mining, Part F129685*, 1903–1911. 10.1145/3097983.3098088

Manikandakumar, M., & Ramanujam, E. (2018). Security and Privacy Challenges in Big Data Environment. *Advances in Information Security, Privacy, and Ethics*, 315–325. doi:10.4018/978-1-5225-4100-4.ch017

Maragatham, G., & Devi, S. (2019). LSTM Model for Prediction of Heart Failure in Big Data. *Journal of Medical Systems, 43*(5), 1, 13.

Marcjasz, G., Uniejewski, B., & Weron, R. (2018). On the importance of the long-term seasonal component in day-ahead electricity price forecasting with NARX neural networks. *International Journal of Forecasting*.

McCullagh, P. (1980). Regression models for ordinal data. *Journal of the Royal Statistical Society. Series B. Methodological*, *42*(2), 109–127. doi:10.1111/j.2517-6161.1980.tb01109.x

McKeigue, P. M., Shah, B., & Marmot, M. G. (1991). Relation of central obesity and insulin resistance with high diabetes prevalence and cardiovascular risk in South Asians. *Lancet*, *337*(8738), 382–386. doi:10.1016/0140-6736(91)91164-P PMID:1671422

Medasani, S., Kim, J., & Krishnapuram, R. (1998). An overview of membership function generation techniques for pattern recognition. *International Journal of Approximate Reasoning*, *19*(3-4), 391–417. doi:10.1016/S0888-613X(98)10017-8

Menke, N. B., Caputo, N., Fraser, R., Haber, J., Shields, C., & Menke, M. N. (2014). A retrospective analysis of the utility of an artificial neural network to predict ED volume. *The American Journal of Emergency Medicine*, *32*(6), 614–617. doi:10.1016/j.ajem.2014.03.011 PMID:24736127

Mete, S., Cil, Z. A., & Özceylan, E. (2018). Location and coverage analysis of bike-sharing stations in university campus. *Business Systems Research*, *9*(2), 80–95. doi:10.2478/bsrj-2018-0021

Miljkovic, D. (2017). Brief review of self-organizing maps. *Proceedings 2017 40th International Convention on Information and Communication Technology, Electronics and Microelectronics (MIPRO)*, 1061–1066. 10.23919/MIPRO.2017.7973581

Millstein, M. A., Yang, L., & Li, H. (2014). Optimizing ABC inventory grouping decisions. *International Journal of Production Economics*, *148*, 71–80. doi:10.1016/j.ijpe.2013.11.007

Milner, P. C. (1997). Ten-year follow-up of ARIMA forecasts of attendances at accident and emergency departments in the Trent region. *Statistics in Medicine*, *16*(18), 2117–2125. doi:10.1002/(SICI)1097-0258(19970930)16:18<2117::AID-SIM649>3.0.CO;2-E PMID:9308136

Ministry of Health in Republic of Turkey. (2017). Health Statistics Yearbook 2016. Republic of Turkey Ministry of Health General Directorate of Health Research, Ankara, Turkey.

Minsky, M. L., & Papert, S. (1969). *Perceptrons: an introduction to computational geometry*. USA: MIT Press.

Misch, C. (2008). *Density of bone: effects on surgical approach and healing. Contemporary Implant Dentistry*. Mosby.

Moa, H., Wang, F.-Y., Zhou, M., Li, R., & Xiao, Z. (2014). Footprint of uncertainty for type-2 fuzzy sets. *Information Sciences*, *272*, 96–110. doi:10.1016/j.ins.2014.02.092

Montgomery, D. C., Peck, E. A., & Vining, G. G. (2012). *Introduction to linear regression analysis* (Vol. 821). John Wiley & Sons.

Muhammad, H., Fuchs, T. J., De Cuir, N., De Moraes, C. G., Blumberg, D. M., Liebmann, J. M., ... Hood, D. C. (2017). Hybrid Deep Learning on Single Wide-field Optical Coherence tomography Scans Accurately Classifies Glaucoma Suspects. *Journal of Glaucoma*, *26*(12), 1086–1094. doi:10.1097/IJG.0000000000000765 PMID:29045329

Muhuri, P. K., & Shukla, A. K. (2017). Semi-elliptic membership function: Representation, generation, operations, deffuzification, ranking and its application to the real-time task scheduling problem. *Engineering Applications of Artificial Intelligence*, *60*, 71–82. doi:10.1016/j.engappai.2016.12.020

Murata, M., Ariji, Y., Ohashi, Y., Kawai, T., Fukuda, M., Funakoshi, T., ... Ariji, E. (2019). Deep-learning classification using convolutional neural network for evaluation of maxillary sinusitis on panoramic radiography. *Oral Radiology*, *35*(3), 301–307. doi:10.100711282-018-0363-7 PMID:30539342

Murtagh, F. (1991). Multilayer perceptrons for classification and regression. *Neurocomputing*, *2*(5–6), 183–197. doi:10.1016/0925-2312(91)90023-5

Nag, K., & Helal, M. (2018, December). Multicriteria Inventory Classification of Diabetes Drugs Using a Comparison of AHP and Fuzzy AHP Models. *Proceedings 2018 IEEE International Conference on Industrial Engineering and Engineering Management (IEEM)* (pp. 1456-1460). IEEE. 10.1109/IEEM.2018.8607678

Nasibov, E. N., & Ulutagay, G. (2010). Comparative clustering analysis of bispectral index series of brain activity. *Expert Systems with Applications*, *37*(3), 2495–2504. doi:10.1016/j.eswa.2009.07.071

Nasibov, E., & Peker, S. (2011). Exponential Membership Function Based on Frequency. *Asian Journal of Mathematics and Statistics*, *4*(1), 8–20. doi:10.3923/ajms.2011.8.20

Nawel, Z., Nabiha, A., Nilanjan, D., & Mokhtar, S. (2016). Adaptive semi supervised support vector machine semi supervised learning with features cooperation for breast cancer classification. *Journal of Medical Imaging and Health Informatics*, *6*(1), 53–62. doi:10.1166/jmihi.2016.1591

Ngan, S.-C. (2018). Revisiting fuzzy set operations: A rational approach for designing set operators for type-2 fuzzy sets and type-2 like fuzzy sets. *Expert Systems with Applications*, *107*, 255–284. doi:10.1016/j.eswa.2018.03.061

Nguyen, P., Tran, T., Wickramasinghe, N., & Venkatesh, S. (2017). Deepr: A Convolutional Net for Medical Records. *IEEE Journal of Biomedical and Health Informatics*, *21*(1), 22–30. doi:10.1109/JBHI.2016.2633963 PMID:27913366

Ng, W. L. (2007). A simple classifier for multiple criteria ABC analysis. *European Journal of Operational Research, 177*(1), 344–353. doi:10.1016/j.ejor.2005.11.018

Nigah, R., Devnani, M., & Gupta, A. K. (2010). ABC and VED analysis of the pharmacy store of a tertiary care teaching, research and referral healthcare institute of India. *Journal of Young Pharmacists, 2*(2), 201-205.

Norman, G. (2010). Likert scales, levels of measurement and the "laws" of statistics. *Advances in Health Sciences Education: Theory and Practice, 15*(5), 625–632. doi:10.100710459-010-9222-y PMID:20146096

Ordu, M., Demir, E., & Tofallis, C. (2019). A comprehensive modelling framework to forecast the demand for all hospital services. *The International Journal of Health Planning and Management, 34*(2), 1257–1271. doi:10.1002/hpm.2771 PMID:30901132

Organ. (2019). *Turkey organ transplant statistics*. Retrieved from https://organ.saglik.gov.tr

Osisanwo, F. Y., Akinsola, J. E. T., Awodele, O., Hinmikaiye, J. O., Olakanmi, O., & Akinjobi, J. (2017). Supervised machine learning algorithms: classification and comparison. *International Journal of Computer Trends and Technology, 48*(3), 128-138.

Ozcan, A., & Oguducu, S. G. (2018). Link prediction in evolving heterogeneous networks using the NARX neural networks. *Knowledge and Information Systems, 55*(2), 333–360. doi:10.100710115-017-1073-x

Ozdemir, A., & Zveri, O. (2004). Çok Kriterli Envanter Sınıflandırmasında Analitik Hiyerarşi Süreci Analizinin Uygulanması. *Dokuz Eylül Üniversitesi İktisadi ve İdari Bilimler Fakültesi Dergisi, 19*(2), 137-154.

Ozguven, N. (2011). Vakif üniversitesi tercihinin analitik hiyerarşi süreci ile belirlenmesi. *Dumlupınar Üniversitesi Sosyal Bilimler Dergisi*, (30), 279-290.

Ozudogru, A. G., & Gorener, A. (2016). Method Selection for Demand Forecasting: Application in a Private Hospital. *International Journal of Decision Sciences & Applications-IJDSA, 1*(1), 22–34.

Parasuraman, A., Zeithaml, V. A., & Berry, L. L. (1988). Servqual: A multiple-item scale for measuring consumer perc. *Journal of Retailing, 64*(1), 12.

Park, S. U., Park, J. H., Al-Masni, M. A., Al-Antari, M. A., Uddin, M. ., & Kim, T.-S. (2016). A Depth Camera-based Human Activity Recognition via Deep Learning Recurrent Neural Network for Health and Social Care Services. *Procedia Computer Science, 100*, 78, 84.

Park, J., Bae, H., & Bae, J. (2014). Cross-evaluation-based weighted linear optimization for multi-criteria ABC inventory classification. *Computers & Industrial Engineering, 76*, 40–48. doi:10.1016/j.cie.2014.07.020

Partovi, F. Y., & Anandarajan, M. (2002). Classifying inventory using an artificial neural network approach. *Computers & Industrial Engineering, 41*(4), 389–404. doi:10.1016/S0360-8352(01)00064-X

Partovi, F. Y., & Burton, J. (1993). Using the analytic hierarchy process for ABC analysis. *International Journal of Operations & Production Management*, *13*(9), 29–44. doi:10.1108/01443579310043619

Patel, V. L., Shortliffe, E. H., Stefanelli, M., Szolovits, P., Berthold, M. R., Bellazzi, R., & Abu-Hanna, A. (2009). The coming of age of artificial intelligence in medicine. *Artificial Intelligence in Medicine*, *46*(1), 5–17. doi:10.1016/j.artmed.2008.07.017 PMID:18790621

Pathak, S., & Kumar, B. (2016). A Robust Automated Cataract Detection Algorithm Using Diagnostic Opinion Based Parameter Thresholding for Telemedicine Application. *Electronics (Basel)*, *5*(4), 57. doi:10.3390/electronics5030057

Patole, V., Kulkarni, D., & Pachghare, V. K. (2010). Self-Organizing Maps to Build Intrusion Detection System. *International Journal of Computer Applications, 1*(8), 1, 4. Retrieved from https://resolver.1science.com/proquest/?id=3ffd17e15fc7228301415445ba5972a3a06ab95a

Patwari, M. A. U., Arif, M. D., Chowdhury, M. N., Arefin, A., & Imam, M. I. (2011, May). Detection, categorization, and assessment of eye cataracts using digital image processing. *Proceedings The first international conference on interdisciplinary research and development* (pp. 22-1). Thailand. Academic Press.

Peek, N., Combi, C., Marin, R., & Bellazzi, R. (2015). Thirty years of artificial intelligence in medicine (AIME) conferences: A review of research themes. *Artificial Intelligence in Medicine*, *65*(1), 61–73. doi:10.1016/j.artmed.2015.07.003 PMID:26265491

Pekkaya, M., Pulat İmamoğlu, Ö., & Koca, H. (2019). Evaluation of healthcare service quality via Servqual scale: An application on a hospital. *International Journal of Healthcare Management*, *12*(4), 340–347. doi:10.1080/20479700.2017.1389474

Petrovic, S. (2006). A Comparison Between the Silhouette Index and the Davies-Bouldin Index in Labelling IDS Clusters. *11th Nordic Workshop on Secure IT-Systems*, 53–64. Retrieved from https://xp-dev.com/svn/b_frydrych.../silhuetteIndexRegulaStopu.pdf

Pham, T., Tran, T., Phung, D., & Venkatesh, S. (2016). DeepCare: A deep dynamic memory model for predictive medicine. Lecture Notes in Computer Science (Including Subseries Lecture Notes in Artificial Intelligence and Lecture Notes in Bioinformatics), 9652, 30, 41. Springer Verlag.

Pham, H. T., & Yang, B. S. (2010). A hybrid of nonlinear autoregressive model with exogenous input and autoregressive moving average model for long-term machine state forecasting. *Expert Systems with Applications*, *37*(4), 3310–3317. doi:10.1016/j.eswa.2009.10.020

Pisoni, E., Farina, M., Carnevale, C., & Piroddi, L. (2009). Forecasting peak air pollution levels using NARX models. *Engineering Applications of Artificial Intelligence*, *22*(4-5), 593–602. doi:10.1016/j.engappai.2009.04.002

Pjetursson, B. E., Thoma, D., Jung, R., Zwahlen, M., & Zembic, A. (2012). A systematic review of the survival and complication rates of implants upported fixed dental prostheses (FDP s) after a mean observation period of at least 5 years. *Clinical Oral Implants Research*, *23*, 22–38. doi:10.1111/j.1600-0501.2012.02546.x PMID:23062125

Polat, K., Güneş, S., & Arslan, A. (2008). A cascade learning system for classification of diabetes disease: Generalized discriminant analysis and least square support vector machine. *Expert Systems with Applications*, *34*(1), 482–487. doi:10.1016/j.eswa.2006.09.012

Pouraliakbari, M., Mohammadi, M., & Mirzazadeh, A. (2018). Analysis of maximal covering location-allocation model for congested healthcare systems in user choice environment. *International Journal of Industrial and Systems Engineering*, *28*(2), 240–274. doi:10.1504/IJISE.2018.089139

Pourkia, J., Rahimi, S., & Baghaei, K. T. (2019). Hospital Data Interpretation: A Self-Organizing Map Approach. In R. B. Kearfott, I. Batyrshin, M. Reformat, M. Ceberio, & V. Kreinovich (Eds.), *Fuzzy Techniques: Theory and Applications* (pp. 493–504). Cham, Switzerland: Springer International Publishing. doi:10.1007/978-3-030-21920-8_44

Primary health care. (n.d.). Retrieved August 31, 2019, from https://www.who.int/news-room/fact-sheets/detail/primary-health-care

Quinlan, J. R. (1986). Induction of decision trees. *Machine Learning*, *1*(1), 81–106. doi:10.1007/BF00116251

Rabbani, M., & Talebi, E. (2019). A comprehensive mathematical model for designing an organ transplant supply chain network under uncertainty. *International Journal of Engineering*, *32*(6), 835–841.

Radha, M., Fonseca, P., Moreau, A., Ross, M., Cerny, A., Anderer, P., ... Aarts, R. M. (2019). Sleep stage classification from heart-rate variability using long short-term memory neural networks. *Scientific Reports*, *9*(1), 1–11. doi:10.103841598-019-49703-y PMID:31578345

Rahimi, Z., Shafri, H. Z. M., & Norman, M. (2018). A GNSS-based weather forecasting approach using Nonlinear Auto Regressive Approach with Exogenous Input (NARX). *Journal of Atmospheric and Solar-Terrestrial Physics*, *178*, 74–84. doi:10.1016/j.jastp.2018.06.011

Rais, A., & Vianaa, A. (2011). Operations research in healthcare: A survey. *International Transactions in Operational Research*, *18*(1), 1–31. doi:10.1111/j.1475-3995.2010.00767.x

Rajmohan, M., Theophilus, C., Sumalatha, M. R., & Saravanakumar, S. (2017). Facility location of organ procurement organizations in Indian health care supply chain management. *South African Journal of Industrial Engineering*, *28*(1), 90–102. doi:10.7166/28-1-1508

Rajput, R., Chouhan, Z., Sindhu, M., Sundararajan, S., & Chouhan, R. R. S. (2016). A Brief Chronological Review of Dental Implant History. *International Dental Journal of Students Research, 4.*

Rakel, R. E., & Rakel, D. (n.d.). *Textbook of family medicine.*

Rakshita, P., Saha, S., Konar, A., & Saha, S. (2016). A type-2 fuzzy classifier for gesture induced pathological disorder recognition. *Fuzzy Sets and Systems*, *305*, 95–130. doi:10.1016/j.fss.2016.05.001

Ramanathan, R. (2006). ABC Inventory Classification With Multiple- Criteria Using Weighted Linear Optimization. *Computers & Operations Research*, *33*(3), 695–700. doi:10.1016/j.cor.2004.07.014

Ramesh, A. N., Kambhampati, C., Monson, J., & Drew, P. J. (2004). Artificial intelligence in medicine. *Annals of the Royal College of Surgeons of England*, *86*(5), 334–338. doi:10.1308/147870804290 PMID:15333167

Raziei, Z., Torabi, S. A., Tabrizian, S., & Zahiri, B. (2018). A Hybrid GDM-SERVQUAL-QFD Approach for Service Quality Assessment in Hospitals. *Engineering Management Journal*, *30*(3), 179–190. doi:10.1080/10429247.2018.1443670

Reddy, K. R., & Thumati, P. (2014). Influence of implant with different dimensions and designs in ideal stress distribution in bone for application in compromised situations: Analysis by three-dimensional finite element method. *Journal of Dental Implants*, *4*(2), 109. doi:10.4103/0974-6781.140848

Reitermanov, Z. (2010). Data splitting. *WDS'10 Proceedings of Contributed Papers, Part I*, 31–36.

Rendón, E., Abundez, I., Arizmendi, A., & Quiroz, E. (2011). Internal versus external cluster validation indexes. *International Journal of Computers and Communications*, *5*(1), 27, 34. Retrieved from https://resolver.1science.com/proquest/?id=bf2a5cfbebe590efcee9d581287c290126a44cc7

Rezaei, M., & Franti, P. (2016). Set Matching Measures for External Cluster Validity. *IEEE Transactions on Knowledge and Data Engineering*, *28*(8), 2173,2186.

Rogrilie, M., & Shi, A. W. P. (2007). Optimizing the effectiveness of organ allocation. *Academic Journal*, *28*(2), 1–17.

Røislien, J., van den Berg, P. L., Lindner, T., Zakariassen, E., Aardal, K., & van Essen, J. T. (2017). Exploring optimal air ambulance base locations in Norway using advanced mathematical modeling. *Injury Prevention*, *23*(1), 10–15. doi:10.1136/injuryprev-2016-041973 PMID:27325670

Rosenberg, A., & Hirschberg, J. (2007). V-Measure: A Conditional Entropy-Based External Cluster Evaluation Measure. *Proceedings of the 2007 Joint Conference on Empirical Methods in Natural Language Processing and Computational Natural Language Learning*, 410-420. Prague, Czech Republic: Association for Computational Linguistics.

Roy, J., Adhikary, K., Kar, S., & Pamucar, D. (2018). A rough strength relational DEMATEL model for analysing the key success factors of hospital service quality. *Decision Making: Applications in Management and Engineering*, *1*(1), 121–142.

Rumelhart, D. E., Hinton, G. E., & Williams, R. J. (1986): Learning internal representations by error propagation. In Parallel distributed processing: Explorations in the microstructure of cognition, 1, 318-362, Bradford Books.

Rutkowski, L., Jaworski, M., Pietruczuk, L., & Duda, P. (2014). The CART decision tree for mining data streams. *Information Sciences*, *266*, 1–15. doi:10.1016/j.ins.2013.12.060

Saeedi, P., Petersohn, I., Salpea, P., Malanda, B., Karuranga, S., Unwin, N., ... Shaw, J. E. (2019). WITHDRAWN: Global and regional diabetes prevalence estimates for 2019 and projections for 2030 and 2045: results from the International Diabetes Federation Diabetes Atlas. *Diabetes Research and Clinical Practice*. doi:10.1016/j.diabres.2019.107843 PMID:31518657

Safavian, S. R., & Landgrebe, D. A. (1990). *A Survey of Decision Tree Classifier Methodology*. Retrieved from https://books.google.com.tr/books?id=Y0G2SgAACAAJ

Sahoo, S., & Jha, M. K. (2013). Groundwater-level prediction using multiple linear regression and artificial neural network techniques: A comparative assessment. *Hydrogeology Journal*, *21*(8), 1865–1887. doi:10.100710040-013-1029-5

Saini, I., Singh, D., & Khosla, A. (2013). QRS detection using K-Nearest Neighbor algorithm (KNN) and evaluation on standard ECG databases. *Journal of Advanced Research*, *4*(4), 331–344. doi:10.1016/j.jare.2012.05.007 PMID:25685438

Saini, M., Singh, Y., Arora, P., Arora, V., & Jain, K. (2015). Implant biomaterials: A comprehensive review. *World Journal of Clinical Cases: WJCC*, *3*(1), 52. doi:10.12998/wjcc.v3.i1.52 PMID:25610850

Samant, P., & Agarwal, R. (2018). Machine learning techniques for medical diagnosis of diabetes using iris images. *Computer Methods and Programs in Biomedicine*, *157*, 121–128. doi:10.1016/j.cmpb.2018.01.004 PMID:29477420

Samuel, C., Gonapa, K., Chaudhary, P. K., & Mishra, A. (2010). Supply chain dynamics in healthcare services. *International Journal of Health Care Quality Assurance*, *23*(7), 631–642. doi:10.1108/09526861011071562 PMID:21125959

Sariyer, G. (2018b). Acil Servislerde Talebin Zaman Serileri Modelleri ile Tahmin Edilmesi. *Uluslararası Mühendislik Araştırma ve Geliştirme Dergisi*, *10*(1), 66–77.

Sariyer, G. (2018a). Sizing capacity levels in emergency medical services dispatch centers: Using the newsvendor approach. *The American Journal of Emergency Medicine*, *36*(5), 804–815. doi:10.1016/j.ajem.2017.10.027 PMID:29055616

Sarıyer, G., Ataman, M. G., & Kızıloğlu, İ. (2018). Factors affecting length of stay in the emergency department: A research from an operational viewpoınt. *International Journal of Healthcare Management*, 1–10.

Sariyer, G., Taşar, C. Ö., & Cepe, G. E. (2019). Use of data mining techniques to classify length of stay of emergency department patients. *Bio-Algorithms and Med-Systems*, *15*(1). doi:10.1515/bams-2018-0044

Sarkar, R., Julai, S., Hossain, S., Chong, W. T., & Rahman, M. (2019). A Comparative Study of Activation Functions of NAR and NARX Neural Network for Long-Term Wind Speed Forecasting in Malaysia. *Mathematical Problems in Engineering*.

Savaşer, S., Kınay, Ö. B., Kara, B. Y., & Cay, P. (2019). Organ transplantation logistics: A case for Turkey. *OR-Spektrum*, *41*(2), 327–356. doi:10.100700291-018-0538-y

Seera, M., & Lim, C. P. (2014). A hybrid intelligent system for medical data classification. *Expert Systems with Applications*, *41*(5), 2239–2249. doi:10.1016/j.eswa.2013.09.022

Şen, C. G., & Çınar, G. (2010). Evaluation and pre-allocation of operators with multiple skills: A combined fuzzy AHP and max-min approach. *Expert Systems with Applications*, *37*(3), 2043–2053. doi:10.1016/j.eswa.2009.06.075

Shahmoradi, S., & Shouraki, S. B. (2018). Evaluation of a novel fuzzy sequential pattern recognition tool (fuzzy elastic matching machine) and its applications in speech and handwriting recognition. *Applied Soft Computing*, *62*, 315–327. doi:10.1016/j.asoc.2017.10.036

Shariff, S. S. R., Moin, N. H., & Omar, M. (2012). Location allocation modeling for healthcare facility planning in Malaysia. *Computers & Industrial Engineering*, *62*(4), 1000–1010. doi:10.1016/j.cie.2011.12.026

Shariff, S. S. R., Omar, M., Moin, N. H., & Smith, D. K. (2010). Locational analysis of public health facilities: A case study of Telok Panglima Garang, Selangor, Malaysia. *Malaysian Journal of Science*, *29*(2), 98–118. doi:10.22452/mjs.vol29no2.2

Shen, L., Chen, H., Yu, Z., Kang, W., Zhang, B., Li, H., ... Liu, D. (2016). Evolving support vector machines using fruit fly optimization for medical data classification. *Knowledge-Based Systems*, *96*, 61–75. doi:10.1016/j.knosys.2016.01.002

Shieh, J. I., Wu, H. H., & Huang, K. K. (2010). A DEMATEL method in identifying key success factors of hospital service quality. *Knowledge-Based Systems*, *23*(3), 277–282. doi:10.1016/j.knosys.2010.01.013

Shukla, A., Tiwari, R., Kaur, P., & Janghel, R. R. (2009). Diagnosis of thyroid Disorders using Artificial Neural Networks. *Proceedings 2009 IEEE International Advance Computing Conference, IACC 2009*, 1016, 1020. 10.1109/IADCC.2009.4809154

Shukla, A. K., & Muhuri, P. K. (2019). Big-data clustering with interval type-2 fuzzy uncertainty modeling in gene expression datasets. *Engineering Applications of Artificial Intelligence*, *77*, 268–282. doi:10.1016/j.engappai.2018.09.002

Singaravel, S., Suykens, J., & Geyer, P. (2018). Deep-learning neural-network architectures and methods: Using component-based models in building-design energy prediction. *Advanced Engineering Informatics, 38*, 81, 90.

Singh, A., & Prasher, A. (2019). Measuring healthcare service quality from patients' perspective: Using Fuzzy AHP application. *Total Quality Management & Business Excellence*, *30*(3-4), 284–300. doi:10.1080/14783363.2017.1302794

Sisodia, D., & Sisodia, D. S. (2018). Prediction of diabetes using classification algorithms. *Procedia Computer Science*, *132*, 1578–1585. doi:10.1016/j.procs.2018.05.122

Solanki, A., & Pandey, S. (2019). Music instrument recognition using deep convolutional neural networks, *International Journal of Information Technology*, 1-10.

Solano, G., & Ghany, M. (2012). *Visualization of Multivariate Health Data using Self-Organizing Maps*. Porto, Portugal: Mathematical Models and Methods in Modern Science.

Sousa, M. J., Moutinho, A., & Almeida, M. (2019). Classification of potential fire outbreaks: A fuzzy modeling approach based on thermal images. *Expert Systems with Applications*, *129*, 216–232. doi:10.1016/j.eswa.2019.03.030

Soylu, B., & Akyol, B. (2014). Multi-criteria inventory classification with reference items. *Computers & Industrial Engineering*, *69*, 12–20. doi:10.1016/j.cie.2013.12.011

Srinivasa, K. G., Venugopal, K. R., & Patnaik, L. M. (2007). A self-adaptive migration model genetic algorithm for data mining applications. *Information Sciences*, *177*(20), 4295–4313. doi:10.1016/j.ins.2007.05.008

Stahl, J. E., Kong, N., Shechter, S. M., Schaefer, A. J., & Roberts, M. S. (2005). A methodological framework for optimally reorganizing liver transplant regions. *Medical Decision Making*, *25*(1), 35–46. doi:10.1177/0272989X04273137 PMID:15673580

Sullivan, G., & Artino, A. R. Jr. (2013). Analyzing and Interpreting Data From Likert-Type Scales. *Journal of Graduate Medical Education*, *5*(4), 541–542. doi:10.4300/JGME-5-4-18 PMID:24454995

Suo, Q., Ma, F., Canino, G., Gao, J., Zhang, A., Veltri, P., & Agostino, G. (2017). A Multi-Task Framework for Monitoring Health Conditions via Attention-based Recurrent Neural Networks. *AMIA ... Annual Symposium Proceedings. AMIA Symposium*, *2017*, 1665–1674.

Suykens, J. A. K., & Vandewalle, J. (1999). Least Squares Support Vector Machine Classifiers. *Neural Processing Letters*, *9*(3), 293–300. doi:10.1023/A:1018628609742

Swapna, G., Vinayakumar, R., & Soman, K. P. (2018). Diabetes detection using deep learning algorithms. *ICT Express*, *4*(4), 243–246. doi:10.1016/j.icte.2018.10.005

Tajbakhsh, N., Shin, J. Y., Gurudu, S. R., Hurst, R. T., Kendall, C. B., Gotway, M. B., & Liang, J. (2016). Convolutional Neural Networks for Medical Image Analysis: Full Training or Fine Tuning? *IEEE Transactions on Medical Imaging*, *35*(5), 1299–1312. doi:10.1109/TMI.2016.2535302 PMID:26978662

Tanrıverdi, Y. (2010). *Tedarik Zinciri Ve Stok Yönetimi Üzerine Bir Uygulama*. Yüksek Lisans Tezi, Pamukkale Üniversitesi, Sosyal Bilimler Enstitüsü.

Taşar, C. Ö., & Sariyer, G. (April, 2018). The use of data mining and neural networks for forecasting patient volume in an emergency department (abstract). 4th International Researchers, Statisticians, and Young Statisticians Congress. Izmir, Turkey

Taşkin, H., Kahraman, Ü. A., & Kubat, C. (2015). Evaluation of the hospital service in Turkey using fuzzy decision-making approach. *Journal of Intelligent Manufacturing*, 1–12.

Taylor, J. W. (2008). A comparison of univariate time series methods for forecasting intraday arrivals at a call center. *Management Science*, *54*(2), 253–265. doi:10.1287/mnsc.1070.0786

Teng, C. I., Ing, C. K., Chang, H. Y., & Chung, K. P. (2007). Development of service quality scale for surgical hospitalization. *Journal of the Formosan Medical Association*, *106*(6), 475–484. doi:10.1016/S0929-6646(09)60297-7 PMID:17588841

Ticknor, J. L. (2013). A Bayesian regularized artificial neural network for stock market forecasting. *Expert Systems with Applications*, *40*(14), 5501–5506. doi:10.1016/j.eswa.2013.04.013

Tirunagari, S., Poh, N., Hu, G., & Windridge, D. (2015). *Identifying Similar Patients Using Self-Organising Maps: A Case Study on Type-1 Diabetes Self-care Survey Responses*. Retrieved from http://arxiv.org/abs/1503.06316

Tomioka, R., Aihara, K., & Müller, K.-R. (2007). Logistic Regression for Single Trial EEG Classification. In B. Schölkopf, J. C. Platt, & T. Hoffman (Eds.), Advances in Neural Information Processing Systems, Retrieved from http://papers.nips.cc/paper/3134-logistic-regression-for-single-trial-eeg-classification.pdf

Topol, E. J. (2019). High-performance medicine: The convergence of human and artificial intelligence. *Nature Medicine*, *25*(1), 44–56. doi:10.103841591-018-0300-7 PMID:30617339

Toregas, C., Swain, R., ReVelle, C., & Bergman, L. (1971). The location of emergency service facilities. *Operations Research*, *19*(6), 1259–1551. doi:10.1287/opre.19.6.1363

Torres-Blanc, C., Hernández-Varela, P., & Cubillo, S. (2018). Self-contradiction for type-2 fuzzy sets whose membership degrees are normal and convex functions. *Fuzzy Sets and Systems*, *352*, 73–91. doi:10.1016/j.fss.2017.12.015

Tsai, C. Y., & Yeh, S. W. (2008). A multiple objective particle swarm optimization approach for inventory classification. *International Journal of Production Economics*, *114*(2), 656–666. doi:10.1016/j.ijpe.2008.02.017

Tuckova, J., Bartu, M., Zetocha, P., & Grill, P. (2011). Self-organizing maps as data classifiers in medical applications. *NCTA 2011 - Proceedings of the International Conference on Neural Computation Theory and Applications*. 10.5220/0003722604220429

Turabieh, H., Abu Salem, A., & Abu-El-Rub, N. (2018). Dynamic L-RNN recovery of missing data in IoMT applications. *Future Generation Computer Systems*, *89*, 575–583. doi:10.1016/j.future.2018.07.006

Tuzkaya, G., Sennaroglu, B., Kalender, Z. T., & Mutlu, M. (2019). Hospital service quality evaluation with IVIF-PROMETHEE and a case study. *Socio-Economic Planning Sciences*, *68*, 100705. doi:10.1016/j.seps.2019.04.002

Uthayakumar, R., & Priyan, S. (2013). Pharmaceutical supply chain and inventory management strategies: Optimization for a pharmaceutical company and a hospital. *Operations Research for Health Care*, *2*(3), 52–64. doi:10.1016/j.orhc.2013.08.001

Vahidnia, M. H., Alesheikh, A. A., & Alimohammadi, A. (2009). Hospital site selection using fuzzy AHP and its derivatives. *Journal of Environmental Management, 90*(10), 3048–3056. doi:10.1016/j.jenvman.2009.04.010 PMID:19477577

Valenti, R., & Gevers, T. (2012). Accurate Eye Center Location through Invariant Isocentric Patterns. *IEEE Transactions on Pattern Analysis and Machine Intelligence, 34*(9), 1785–1798. doi:10.1109/TPAMI.2011.251 PMID:22813958

Valipour, M. T., Nedjati, A., & Kazemi, R. (2013). Solving health care facility location problems with new heuristic algorithm method. *International Journal of Modeling and Optimization, 3*(1), 12–14. doi:10.7763/IJMO.2013.V3.225

van der Westhuizen, J., & Lasenby, J. (2017). *Techniques for visualizing LSTMs applied to electrocardiograms*. Retrieved from http://arxiv.org/abs/1705.08153

Vidyasagar, L., & Apse, P. (2004). Dental implant design and biological effects on bone-implant interface. *Stomatologija, 6*(2), 51–54.

Wang, Y., Chen, W., Zhang, J., Dong, T., Shan, G., & Chi, X. (2011). Efficient volume exploration using the gaussian mixture model. *IEEE Transactions on Visualization and Computer Graphics, 17*(11), 1560–1573. doi:10.1109/TVCG.2011.97 PMID:21670489

What is artificial intelligence? (n.d.). Retrieved September 1, 2019, from https://www.brookings.edu/research/what-is-artificial-intelligence/

What, Is. Machine Learning? | How It Works, Techniques & Applications - MATLAB & Simulink. (n.d.). Retrieved September 2, 2019, from https://www.mathworks.com/discovery/machine-learning.html

WHO. (2018). *Projections of mortality and causes of death, 2016 to 2060*. WHO.

WHO. | Integrated chronic disease prevention and control. (2010). *WHO*. Retrieved from https://www.who.int/chp/about/integrated_cd/en/

World Health Organization. (1978). Declaration of Alma-Ata: International Conference on Primary Health Care, Alma-Ata, USSR, September 6-12, 1978. Retrieved February, 14, 2006.

Wrenn, J., Jones, I., Lanaghan, K., Congdon, C. B., & Aronsky, D. (2005). Estimating patient's length of stay in the Emergency Department with an artificial neural network. *AMIA ... Annual Symposium Proceedings. AMIA Symposium, 2005*, 1155–1155.

Wunsch, A., Liesch, T., & Broda, S. (2018). Forecasting groundwater levels using nonlinear autoregressive networks with exogenous input (NARX). *Journal of Hydrology (Amsterdam), 567*, 743–758. doi:10.1016/j.jhydrol.2018.01.045

Xu, M., Wong, T. C., & Chin, K. S. (2013). Modeling daily patient arrivals at Emergency Department and quantifying the relative importance of contributing variables using artificial neural network. *Decision Support Systems, 54*(3), 1488–1498. doi:10.1016/j.dss.2012.12.019

Xu, Q., Tsui, K. L., Jiang, W., & Guo, H. (2016). A hybrid approach for forecasting patient visits in emergency department. *Quality and Reliability Engineering International*, *32*(8), 2751–2759. doi:10.1002/qre.2095

Xu, Z., & Shi, P. (2006). A Robust and Accurate Method for Pupil Features Extra. Proceedings *18th International Conference on Pattern Recognition (ICPR'06)*. DOI:10.1109/icpr.2006.165

Yamashita, R., Nishio, M., Do, R., & Togashi, K. (2018). Convolutional neural networks: an overview and application in radiology. *Insights into Imaging*, *9*(4), 611, 629.

Yang, C. C., & Bose, N. K. (2006). Generating fuzzy membership function with self-organizing feature map. *Pattern Recognition Letters*, *27*(5), 356–365. doi:10.1016/j.patrec.2005.08.026

Yasaka, K., Akai, H., Abe, O., & Kiryu, S. (2018). Deep learning with convolutional neural network for differentiation of liver masses at dynamic contrast-enhanced CT: A preliminary study. *Radiology*, *286*(3), 887–896. doi:10.1148/radiol.2017170706 PMID:29059036

Yeh, C.-C., & Yang, M.-S. (2017). Evaluation measures for cluster ensembles based on a fuzzy generalized Rand index. *Applied Soft Computing*, *57*, 225, 234.

Yeh, J. Y., & Lin, W. S. (2007). Using simulation technique and genetic algorithm to improve the quality care of a hospital emergency department. *Expert Systems with Applications*, *32*(4), 1073–1083. doi:10.1016/j.eswa.2006.02.017

Yeşilyurt, Ö., Sulak, H., & Bayhan, M. (2014). Sağlık Sektöründe Stok Kontrol Faaliyetlerinin ABC ve VED Analizleriyle Değerlendirilmesi: Isparta Devlet Hastanesi Örneği. *Süleyman Demirel Üniversitesi İktisadi ve İdari Bilimler Fakültesi Dergisi*, *20*(1), 365–376.

Yucesan, M., & Gul, M. (2020). Hospital service quality evaluation: an integrated model based on Pythagorean fuzzy AHP and fuzzy TOPSIS. *Soft Computing*,1-19, 24, 3237-3255. doi:10.1007/s00500-019-04084-2.

Yucesan, M., Gul, M., & Erkan, E. (2017). Application of artificial neural networks using Bayesian training rule in sales forecasting for furniture industry. *Drvna industrija: Znanstveni časopis za pitanja drvne tehnologije*, *68*(3), 219-228.

Yucesan, M., Gul, M., & Celik, E. (2018). A multi-method patient arrival forecasting outline for hospital emergency departments. *International Journal of Healthcare Management*, 1–13. doi: 10.1080/20479700.2018.1531608

Yucesan, M., Gul, M., Mete, S., & Celik, E. (2019). A forecasting model for patient arrivals of an emergency department in healthcare management systems. In *Intelligent Systems for Healthcare Management and Delivery* (pp. 266–284). IGI Global. doi:10.4018/978-1-5225-7071-4.ch012

Zahiri, B., Tavakkoli-Moghaddam, R., Mohammadi, M., & Julab, P. (2014a). Multi-objective design of an organ transplant network under uncertainty. *Transportation Research Part E, Logistics and Transportation Review*, *72*, 101–124. doi:10.1016/j.tre.2014.09.007

Zahiri, B., Tavakkoli-Moghaddam, R., & Pishvaee, M. S. (2014b). A robust possibilistic programming approach to multi–period location–allocation of organ transplant centers under uncertainty. *Computers & Industrial Engineering*, *74*, 139–148. doi:10.1016/j.cie.2014.05.008

Zaiwalla, Z. (2018). To EEG or not EEG. *Paediatrics & Child Health*, *28*(6), 289–292. doi:10.1016/j.paed.2018.04.013

Zhang, T., & Iyengar, V. S. (2002). Recommender Systems Using Linear Classifiers. *Journal of Machine Learning Research*, *2*(3), 313–334. doi:10.1162/153244302760200641

Zhang, Y., & An, M. (2017). Deep Learning- and Transfer Learning-Based Super Resolution Reconstruction from Single Medical Image. *Journal of Healthcare Engineering*, *2017*, 20. doi:10.1155/2017/5859727 PMID:29065625

Zheng, H., Wang, H., & Black, N. (2008). Human activity detection in smart home environment with self-adaptive neural networks. *Proceedings of 2008 IEEE International Conference on Networking, Sensing and Control, ICNSC*, 1505–1510. 10.1109/ICNSC.2008.4525459

Zhou, P., & Fan, L. (2007). A note on multi-criteria ABC inventory classification using weighted linear optimization. *European Journal of Operational Research*, *182*(3), 1488–1491. doi:10.1016/j.ejor.2006.08.052

Zhu, Z., Liang, D., Zhang, S., Huang, X., Li, B., & Hu, S. (2016). Traffic-Sign Detection and Classification in the Wild. *Proceedings of the IEEE Computer Society Conference on Computer Vision and Pattern Recognition*, *2016*, 2110, 2118. IEEE Computer Society. 10.1109/CVPR.2016.232

Zhu, C., Byrd, R. H., Lu, P., & Nocedal, J. (1997). Algorithm 778: L-BFGS-B: Fortran subroutines for large-scale bound-constrained optimization. *ACM Transactions on Mathematical Software*, *23*(4), 550–560. doi:10.1145/279232.279236

Zou, L., Yu, S., Meng, T., Zhang, Z., Liang, X., & Xie, Y. (2019). A Technical Review of Convolutional Neural Network-Based Mammographic Breast Cancer Diagnosis. *Computational and Mathematical Methods in Medicine*, *2019*, 1–16. doi:10.1155/2019/6509357 PMID:31019547

Zumbo, B. D., & Zimmerman, D. W. (1993). Is the selection of statistical methods governed by level of measurement? *Canadian Psychology*, *34*(4), 390–400. doi:10.1037/h0078865

About the Contributors

Muhammet Gul is PhD and has been working as an Associate Professor at the Department of Industrial Engineering, Munzur University, Tunceli, Turkey. He received his MSc in Industrial Engineering from Yildiz Technical University. His research interests are in simulation modeling, healthcare system management, occupational safety and risk assessment, multi-criteria decision-making and fuzzy sets. His papers appeared in International high-cited journals such as Computers & Industrial Engineering, Knowledge-Based Systems, Applied Soft Computing, Journal of Safety Research, Journal of Cleaner Production and Journal of the Operational Research Society. Now, he is the editor in chief of two book projects that will be released in 2020: Computational Intelligence and Soft Computing Applications in Healthcare Management Science (IGI-Global) and Fine–Kinney-based multi-criteria risk assessment: Approaches, Case studies and Python applications (Springer). He will also conduct a new thematic issue in 2021 for a Bentham Science journal Current Chinese Computer Science (CCCS) called as Operations Research/ Management Science in Healthcare: New Methodologies and Applications.

Erkan Celik received BSc and MSc degree in Industrial Engineering from Selcuk University, Konya, Turkey in 2008 and 2011, respectively. He also received PhD in Industrial Engineering from Yildiz Technical University, İstanbul, Turkey in 2015. He is now Associate Professor in Industrial Engineering from Munzur University, Tunceli, Turkey. He has published many papers in highly cited journals as Transportation Research Part E, Transportation Research Part A, Computers & Industrial Engineering, International Journal of Production Research, European Journal of Industrial Engineering and etc. His research interests are in decision analysis, humanitarian logistic, fuzzy sets. Now, he is the editor in chief of two book projects that will be released in 2020: Computational Intelligence and Soft Computing Applications in Healthcare Management Science (IGI-Global) and Fine–Kinney-based multi-criteria risk assessment: Approaches, Case studies and Python applications (Springer).

Suleyman Mete, Ph.D., is an Assistant Professor employed at Industrial Engineering Department, Faculty of Engineering, Gaziantep University in Turkey. He received his Ph.D. from Gaziantep University Industrial Engineering in 2017. His research interests include optimization, assembly line balancing, disassembly line balancing, mathematical modelling, heuristics and supply chain network design. Now, he is the editor in chief of two book projects that will be released in 2020: Computational Intelligence and Soft Computing Applications in Healthcare Management Science (IGI-Global) and Fine–Kinney-based multi-criteria risk assessment: Approaches, Case studies and Python applications (Springer).

Faruk Serin, Ph.D., is an Assistant Professor employed at Computer Engineering Department, Faculty of Engineering, Munzur University in Turkey. He received his Ph.D. from Inonu University Computer Engineering in 2017. His research interests include optimization, graph theory, medical image processing, software development and intelligent transportation. Now, he is the editor in chief of two book projects that will be released in 2020: Computational Intelligence and Soft Computing Applications in Healthcare Management Science (IGI-Global) and Fine–Kinney-based multi-criteria risk assessment: Approaches, Case studies and Python applications (Springer).

*****

Abdullah Caliskan is PhD and has currently been working as Assistant Professor at the Department of Biomedical Engineering, Iskenderun Technical University, Hatay, Turkey. He received B.Sc. degree in June-2011 from the Department of Electrical-Electronic Engineering at Gaziantep University. He received his PhD degrees in Biomedical Engineering from Erciyes University in November, 2017. His research interests include image processing, deep learning and signal processing in biomedical application.

Zeynel Abidin Çil is PhD and has been working as Assistant Professor at the Department of Industrial Engineering, Izmir Democracy University, Izmir, Turkey. He received his MSc degree in Department of Manufacturing Engineering and Management from The University of Nottingham, UK, in 2012 and received PhD degree Department of Industrial Engineering from Gaziantep University in 2017. His research interests include integer programming, robotics, manufacturing systems, heuristics and image processing.

Sundus Dag is an Assistant Professor in the department of Business Administration, at Istanbul University, Istanbul, Turkey. She got her MSc and PhD from Istanbul University, Turkey. Her research focus is on operations planning and management and supply chain management. Dr. Dag teaches production systems, advanced quality techniques and six sigma, design of quality systems courses at the undergraduate and graduate level.

Camila P. E. De Souza is PhD and is an Assistant Professor at the Department of Statistics and Actuarial Sciences at Western University, Canada. She was previously a postdoctoral fellow at the Shah Lab for Computational Cancer Biology at the BC Cancer Agency Research Centre. She completed her PhD in Statistics at the University of British Columbia (UBC). She is originally from Brazil where she received her Master's and Bachelor's Degrees in Statistics at the University of Campinas. Her main research areas of interest include method development and analysis of genomic data, single-cell sequencing, functional data analysis, latent variable modeling, nonparametric regression, semi-parametric models, machine learning and big data analytics.

Hakan Gulmez was born in 1980 in İzmir. He completed his primary, secondary and high school education in Karşıyaka. He graduated from Ege University Faculty of Medicine in 2004. After graduation, he worked as a physician and manager in primary health care until 2009. In 2009, he started his specialty education in Baskent University Faculty of Medicine, Department of Family Medicine. In 2012, he received the title of Family Medicine Specialist. He was appointed to Konya Hadim State Hospital as an expert doctor within the scope of compulsory service. Between 2012-2017 he worked as a family physician in family health center and other primary and secondary health care institutions. In 2017, he was appointed to Düzce University Faculty of Medicine, Department of Family Medicine as an assistant professor. In 2018, he was appointed as a faculty member to İzmir Democracy University Medical Faculty. He is still working as an assistant professor and vice dean at the Faculty of Medicine of İzmir Democracy University. He is married and has two children. Gülmez has many articles published in national and international scientific journals and papers presented in national and international congresses.

Nihan Kabadayı is an Assistant Professor in the department of Business Administration, at Istanbul University, Istanbul, Turkey. She got her MSc and PhD from Istanbul University, Turkey. Her research focus is on operations planning and management and supply chain management. Dr. Kabadayı teaches production management, supply chain management, modern production systems, warehouse management, quality improvement techniques, international logistics management courses at the undergraduate and graduate level.

Rasha Kashef is PhD and is an Assistant Professor at the Department of Electrical, Computer and Biomedical Engineering at Ryerson University, Toronto, Ontario, Canada. She received her Ph.D. from the University of Waterloo, Department of Electrical and Computer Engineering in 2008. She is a professional engineer in Ontario. She worked as Assistant Professor at the school of computing at the AAST institute in 2009-2011. She also worked as a Research Associate at Microsoft Corp. In 2010 she succeeded with her Machine learning research, and she received the "Early Researcher Award." Her research interests span the use of machine learning in big data analysis in different applications including healthcare, revenue management, and software engineering. She worked as a post-doctoral fellow at the department of applied mathematics at the University of Waterloo from 2011 until 2013. She also joined the department of management science at the University of Waterloo from 2013-2016. she had been hired as an assistant professor at the IVEY business School in Management science group with a focus on Data Analytics from 2016-2019. Her main research areas include data science, machine learning, big data, IOT, smart systems, operation research, management science, healthcare, autonomous systems, distributed computing.

M Manikandakumar is PhD and received the Master degree in Computer Science and Engineering and pursuing research degree at Anna University, Chennai. He is currently an Assistant Professor with the department of Information Technology, Thiagarajar College of Engineering, Madurai, India. His research interest includes Security, Internet of Things, Machine Learning and Big Data.

Efendi N. Nasibov received the B.Sc. and M.Sc. degrees in Applied Mathematics Department from Baku State University, Azerbaijan in 1983, and the Ph.D. degree in Mathematical Cybernetics (Moscow) and Dr.Sc. in Computer Science degree from Institute of Cybernetics of Academy of Science of Azerbaijan in 1987 and 2003, respectively. He is currently a full Professor of Department of Computer Science, Dokuz Eylul University, Izmir, Turkey. His research interests are in the application of Fuzzy Modeling and Data Mining techniques in Decision Making problems.

Eren Ozceylan is an Associate Professor of Industrial Engineering Department at the University of Gaziantep. He received a B.S. degree in Industrial Engineering and a Ph.D. degree in Computer Engineering from Selçuk University in 2007 and 2013, respectively. Dr. Özceylan has postdoctoral research experience at the University of Northeastern in 2019. His research interests are in mathematical modeling and GIS-based multi-criteria decision making of a variety of problems in production & distribution planning, including network design, location-allocation, and disassembly line balancing. His work appeared in journals such as Transportation Research Parts, Journal of the Operational Research Society, International Journal of Production Research and Computers and Industrial Engineering.

Barış Özkan is an Assistant Professor of Industrial Engineering Department at the University of Ondokuz Mayıs. He received a B.S. degree in Industrial Engineering from Selçuk University in 2010 and a Ph.D. degree from Eskişehir Osmangazi University in 2018, respectively. His research interests are in geographic information systems, multiple criteria decision making and fuzzy decision making.

Ebru Pekel Özmen is a PhD candidate. She is now a PhD student at Istanbul University-Cerrahpasa. She receives her MSc in Smart Systems Engineering from Ondokuz Mayıs University. His research interests are metaheuristic methods and machine learning.

Engin Pekel is PhD and has been working as Assistant Professor at the Department of Industrial Engineering, Hitit University, Çorum, Turkey. He receives a PhD in Industrial Engineering in 2018 from Yildiz Technical University. His research interests are artificial neural networks, metaheuristic methods, simulation, mathematical modeling and optimization. His papers appeared in international high-cited journals such as Applied Artificial Intelligence, Fuel Processing Technology, International Journal of Coal Preparation and Utilization, Applied Soft Computing, Theoretical and Applied Climatology, International Journal of Oil, Gas and Coal Technology, Promet – Traffic & Transportation, Sigma journal and International Journal of Simulation and Process Modelling.

Sinem Peker received the B.Sc. degree in Statistics Department from Ege University, Turkey in 2001, the M.Sc. degree from Graduate School of Natural and Applied Science from Ege University in 2004 and the Ph.D. degree in Econometrics from Graduate School of Social Sciences, Dokuz Eylül University, Turkey in 2010. She is currently a full Assistant Prof. (PhD) in the Department of Mathematics at Yaşar University, Izmir, Turkey. Her research interests are the Fuzzy Sets Theory, and Multivariate Statistical Techniques.

Felipe F. Rodrigues is PhD and is a Professor of Operations Management and Data Analytics at the School of Management, Economics and Mathematics at King's University College, Canada.

Görkem Sarıyer is an Assistant Professor in the department of Business Administration, at Yasar University, in Izmir, Turkey. She got her Ph.D., from Koç University in the Department of Industrial Engineering and Operations Management, in İstanbul, Turkey. Her research focus is on operations planning and management, quantitative decision making, statistical analysis and data mining. Dr. Sarıyer holds Assistant Professor position at her university and teaches business analytics, forecasting, research methodology, management science and production and operations management courses at the undergraduate and graduate level. Her e-mail address is gorkem.ataman@yasar.edu.tr.

Suchismita Satapathy is PhD and has currently been working at the School of Mechanical Engineering, KIIT University, India. She is currently working as an Associate Professor and has published many journal papers.

Zahra Shirazi is a PhD candidate. She is now a PhD student at in the Department of Statistics and Actuarial Sciences at Western University, Canada. Her research interests are deep learning and artificial neural networks.

Ceren Öcal Taşar is PhD and received her PhD degree from the Department of Computer Engineering at Yaşar University, Izmir, Turkey. He received his MSc degree from Ege University, Izmir, Turkey. His research interests include image processing, deep learning and software engineering.

Melih Yucesan is PhD and has been working as Assistant Professor at the Department of Mechanical Engineering, Munzur University, Tunceli, Turkey. He received his MSc in Mechanical Engineering from Karadeniz Technical University. His research interests are in production planning, sales forecasting, multi-criteria decision-making and fuzzy sets. His papers appeared in international journals such as Energy Policy, Soft Computing, Mathematics, Drvna industrija, Granular Computing, International Journal of Healthcare Management, Beni-Suef University Journal of Basic and Applied Sciences and Intelligent Systems for Healthcare Management and Delivery.

Index

www.ingramcontent.com/pod-product-compliance
Lightning Source LLC
LaVergne TN
LVHW080901300926
849162LV00003B/501

* 9 7 8 1 7 9 9 8 2 5 8 1 4 *